Second Edition

# Medicinal Chemistry III

Course Code **BP 601T**

*for* **Sixth Semester Bachelor in Pharmacy**

As per the latest syllabus prescribed by Pharmacy Council of India

**K Ilango** MPharm PhD FIC
Professor and Principal
Tagore College of Pharmacy
Chennai – 600 127

**P Valentina** MPharm PhD
Professor and Principal
PERI College of Pharmacy
Chennai – 600 048

CBSPD

**CBS Publishers & Distributors** Pvt Ltd

New Delhi • Bengaluru • Chennai • Kochi • Kolkata • Lucknow • Mumbai
Gujarat • Hyderabad • Jharkhand • Nagpur • Patna • Pune • Uttarakhand

Disclaimer

Science and technology are constantly changing fields. New research and experience broaden the scope of information and knowledge. The authors have tried their best in giving information available to them while preparing the material for this book. Although all efforts has been made to ensure optimum accuracy of the material, yet it is quite possible some errors might have been left uncorrected. The publisher, the printer and the authors will not be held responsible for any inadvertent errors or inaccuracies.

Second Edition

# Medicinal Chemistry III

Course Code **BP 601T**

*for* **Sixth Semester Bachelor in Pharmacy**

As per the latest syllabus prescribed by Pharmacy Council of India

ISBN: 978-93-49057-05-0



**Second Edition: 2025**
Reprint: **2026**
First Edition: 2019



Published by Satish Kumar Jain and produced by Varun Jain for
CBS Publishers and Distributors Pvt Ltd
4819/XI Prahlad Street, 24 Ansari Road, Daryaganj, New Delhi 110 002, India.
Ph: 011-23289259, 23266838 Website: www.cbspd.com
e-mail: delhi@cbspd.com

*Corporate Office:* 204 FIE, Industrial Area, Patparganj, Delhi 110 092, India
Ph: 011-49344934 Fax: 011-49344935 e-mail: publishing@cbspd.com; publicity@cbspd.com

***Branches***

- **Bengaluru:** Seema House 2975, 17th Cross, K.R. Road, Banasankari 2nd Stage, Bengaluru 560 070, Karnataka, India
  Ph: +91-80-26771678/79 Fax: +91-80-26771680 e-mail: bangalore@cbspd.com
- **Chennai:** 18/8B, Subbarayan Street, Shenoy Nagar, Chennai 600 030, Tamil Nadu, India
  Ph: +91-44-42032115, 26681266 e-mail: chennai@cbspd.com
- **Kochi:** 42/1325, 1326, Power House Road, Opposite KSEB, Power House, Ernakulam 682 018, Kochi, Kerala, India
  Ph: +91-484-4059061–65 Fax: +91-484-4059065 e-mail: kochi@cbspd.com
- **Kolkata:** 147 Hind Ceramics Compound, 1st Floor, Nilgunj Road, Belghoria, Kolkata 700 056, West Bengal, India
  Ph: +91-33-25633055/56 e-mail: kolkata@cbspd.com
- **Lucknow:** Basement, Khushnuma Complex, 7-Meerabai Marg (Behind Jawahar Bhawan), Lucknow 226 001, Uttar Pradesh, India
  Ph: +91-522-4000032 e-mail:tiwari.lucknow@cbspd.com
- **Mumbai:** PWD Shed, Gala No. 25/26, Ramchandra Bhatt Marg, Next to JJ Hospital, Gate No. 2, Opp Union Bank of India, Noorbaug, Mumbai 400009, Maharashtra, India
  Ph: +91-22-66661880, 66661889 e-mail: mumbai@cbspd.com

***Representatives***

| | | | | | |
|---|---|---|---|---|---|
| • **Gujarat** | 0-9879558667 | • **Hyderabad** | 0-9885175004 | • **Jharkhand** | 0-9811541605 |
| • **Nagpur** | 0-8692091830 | • **Patna** | 0-9334159340 | • **Pune** | 0-9664372571 |
| • **Uttarakhand** | 0-9716462459 | | | | |

*Printed at:* SRK Graphics, Delhi, India

Second Edition

# Medicinal Chemistry III

Course Code **BP 601T**

*for* **Sixth Semester Bachelor in Pharmacy**

As per the latest syllabus prescribed by Pharmacy Council of India

# Preface

This introduction highlights the significance of Medicinal Chemistry in the context of drug discovery and development (DDD), emphasizing its multidisciplinary nature, which involves collaboration among biologists, toxicologists, pharmacologists, medicinal chemists, microbiologists, and bio-pharmacists. It underscores the authors' experience, with over 25 years of teaching and interaction with graduate students across various universities. This book is intended to provide a handy but comprehensive textbook for the undergraduate students preparing for medicinal chemistry. The book is written in an easy and straightforward style according to the revised syllabus of Pharmacy Council of India.

The book, *Medicinal Chemistry III,* is designed to be a comprehensive resource tailored to undergraduate students studying medicinal chemistry, adhering to the revised syllabus. Following the success of previous works, the authors are motivated to present this volume, which focuses on 12 chapters covering essential topics like Antibiotics, Prodrugs, Antimalarials, Antitubercular agents, and several others related to anti-infective agents and drug design.

Each chapter offers an introduction, classification, structure activity relationship (SAR), and detailed information on individual drugs, making it easier for students to understand. The authors acknowledge the support of their institution, family, friends, and the broader academic community, and they invite feedback for further improvement of the book.

**K Ilango**
**P Valentina**

# Contents


| | |
|---|---|
| *Preface* | *v* |
| *Syllabus* | *xi* |
| **1. Antibiotics** | **1–63** |
| 1. Introduction | 1 |
| 2. Classification of Antibiotics | 2 |
| 2.1 β-*Lactam* Antibiotics | 5 |
| 2.1.1 Penicillins | 6 |
| 2.1.2 Cephalosporins | 26 |
| 2.1.3 β-*Lactamase* Inhibitors | 40 |
| 2.1.4 Monobactams | 42 |
| 2.2 Aminoglycoside antibiotics | 45 |
| 2.3 Tetracyclines | 49 |
| 2.4 Macrolide Antibiotics | 57 |
| 2.5 Lincomycin | 61 |
| 2.6 Miscellaneous | 62 |
| **2. Prodrugs** | **64–88** |
| 1. Introduction | 64 |
| 2. Prodrug Strategy in Drug Design | 65 |
| 3. Ideal Requirements of Prodrug | 67 |
| 4. Types of Prodrug | 67 |
| 4.1 Carrier Linked Prodrug | 67 |
| 4.2 Bio-precursor Prodrug | 73 |
| 5. Applications of Prodrugs | 74 |
| 5.1 Pharmaceutical Applications | 74 |
| 5.2 Pharmacological Applications | 78 |
| **3. Antimalarials** | **89–105** |
| 1. Introduction | 89 |
| 2. Classification | 92 |
| 2.1 Cinchona Alkaloids | 92 |
| 2.2 4-Amino Quinolines | 94 |
| 2.3 8 -Amino Quinolines | 97 |
| 2.4 9-Amino Acridines | 100 |

2.5 Biguanides 101
2.6 Dihydrotriazine 101
2.7 Pyrimidine Analogues 102
2.8 Sesquiterpene Lactones 103
2.9 Hydroxy Naphthoquinone 105
2.10 Quinoline 105

**4. Antitubercular Agents** **106–113**
1. Introduction 106
2. Classification 107
2.1 First-line Oral Drugs 107
2.2 Second-line Oral Drugs 109
2.3 Antibiotics 111

**5. Urinary Tract Anti-Infective Agents** **114–125**
1. Introduction 114
2. Classification 115
2.1 Quinolones 115
2.2 Nitrofurans 123
2.3 Methenamine and its Salts 125

**6. Antiviral Agents** **126–143**
1. Introduction 126
2. Classification 129
2.1 Purine Nucleoside and Nucleotide 130
2.2 Pyrimidine Nucleoside and Nucleotide 132
2.3 Adamantane Amines 134
2.4 Miscellaneous Agents 135
3. Anti-HIV Agents 136
3.1 Introduction 136
3.2 Classification 136
3.2.1 Reverse Transcriptase Inhibitors 137
3.2.2 Non-nucleoside Reverse Transcriptase Inhibitors 141
3.2.3 HIV Protease Inhibitors 142

**7. Antifungal Agents** **144–159**
1. Introduction 144
2. Classification 148
2.1 Antifungal Antibiotics 149
2.2 Allylamine and Related Compounds 153
2.3 Azole Antifungal Agents 154

**8. Antiprotozoal Agents** **160–166**
1. Introduction 160
2. Classification 161
2.1 Nitroimidazoles 161
2.2 Phenol and Benzoate Esters 164
2.3 8-Hydroxy Quinolines 164
2.4 Dibenzimidamide 165
2.5 Hydroxy Naphthoquinone 165
2.6 Fluoro amino acid 166

**9. Anthelmintic** **167–175**
1. Introduction 167
2. Classification 167
2.1 Piperazines Derivatives 168
2.2 Benzimidazoles 169
2.3 Heterocyclics 173
2.4 Amide 174
2.5 Natural Products 174

**10. Sulfonamides and Sulfones** **176–194**
1. Introduction 176
1.1 Nomenclature of Sulfonamides 177
1.2 General Properties 177
1.3 Crystalluria and pKa 177
1.4 Mechanism of Action 179
1.5 Structure Activity Relationship 180
1.6 Therapeutic Uses 181
1.7 General Method of Synthesis 182
2. Classification 184
2.1 Sulfonamides for General Infections 186
2.2 Sulfonamides for Urinary Tract Infection 188
2.3 Sulfonamides for Intestinal Infections 189
2.4 Sulfonamides for Local Infections 189
2.5 Sulfonamide for Dermatitis 191
2.6 Sulfonamide Combinations 192

**11. Drug Design** **195–224**
1. Introduction 195
1.1 Various Approaches of Drug Design 196
2. Molecular Docking 197

2.1 Introduction 197
2.2 Docking Software Description 199
2.3 Molecular Docking Approaches 199
2.4 Types of Docking 200
2.5 Theories of Docking 201
2.6 Calculation of Binding Energy 204
2.7 The Docking Process 205
2.8 Applications of Docking 208
3. Quantitative Structure Activity Relationship (QSAR) 209
3.1 Introduction 209
3.2 QSAR Development Process 210
3.3 Descriptors (or) Parameters 211
3.4 2D QSAR Models 217
3.5 QSAR Model Validation 220
3.6 Advances in QSAR 220
4. Pharmacophore Modelling 221
4.1 Introduction 221
4.2 Pharmacophoric Features 222
4.3 Process of Pharmacophore Model 223
4.4 Applications of Pharmacophore Modelling 224

**12. Combinatorial Chemistry** **225–235**
1. Introduction 225
2. Solid Phase Synthesis 227
2.1 Parallel Synthesis 230
2.2 Mix and Split Technique 230
3. Solution Phase Synthesis 233
4. Screening 234
5. Applications 234

*Index* *235–237*

# Syllabus

## BP601T Medicinal Chemistry III (Theory)

Study of the development of the following classes of drugs, classification, mechanism of action, uses of the drugs mentioned in the course, structure activity relationship of selective class of drugs as specified in the course and synthesis of drugs superscripted by (*)

### Unit I — 10 hrs

**ANTIBIOTICS**

Historical back ground, Nomenclature, Stereochemistry, Structure activity relationship, Chemical degradation, Classification and Important products of the following classes.

**β-Lactam antibiotics:** Penicillins, Cephalosporins, *β-Lactamase inhibitors*, Monobactams.

**Aminoglycosides:** Streptomycin, Neomycin, Kanamycin.

**Tetracyclines:** Tetracycline, Oxytetracycline, Chlortetracycline, Minocycline, Doxycycline.

### Unit II — 10 hrs

**ANTIBIOTICS**

Historical back ground, Nomenclature, Stereochemistry, Structure activity relationship, Chemical degradation, Classification and Important products of the following classes.

**Macrolides:** Erythromycin, Clarithromycin, Azithromycin.

**Miscellaneous:** Chloramphenicol*, Clindamycin.

**Prodrugs:** Basic concept and applications of prodrug design.

**Antimalarials:** Etiology of malaria.

**Quinolines:** SAR, Quinine sulphate, Chloroquine*, Amodiaquine, Primaquine phosphate, Pamaquine*, Quinacrine hydrochloride, Mefloquine.

**Biguanides and dihydro triazines:** Cycloguanil pamoate, Proguanil.

**Miscellaneous:** Pyrimethamine, Artesunate, Artemether, Atovaquone.

### Unit III — 10 hrs

**ANTI-TUBERCULAR AGENTS**

**Synthetic anti-tubercular Agents:** Isoniazid*, Ethionamide, Ethambutol, Pyrazinamide, Para amino salicylic acid*.

## URINARY TRACT ANTI-INFECTIVE AGENTS

**Quinolones:** SAR of quinolones, Nalidixic acid, Norfloxacin, Enoxacin, Ciprofloxacin*, Ofloxacin, Lomefloxacin, Sparfloxacin, Gatifloxacin, Moxifloxacin.

**Miscellaneous:** Furazolidone, Nitrofurantoin*, Methenamine.

## ANTIVIRAL AGENTS

Amantadine hydrochloride, Rimantadine hydrochloride, Idoxuridine, Trifluridine, Acyclovir*, Ganciclovir, Zidovudine, Didanosine, Zalcitabine, Lamivudine, Loviride, Delavirdine, Ribavirin, Saquinavir, Indinavir, Ritonavir.

**Unit IV** **08 hrs**

## ANTIFUNGAL AGENTS

**Antifungal Antibiotics:** Amphotericin-B, Nystatin, Natamycin, Griseofulvin.

Synthetic Antifungal agents: Clotrimazole, Econazole, Butoconazole, Oxiconazole, Tioconazole, Miconazole*, Ketoconazole, Terconazole, Itraconazole, Fluconazole, Naftifine hydrochloride, Tolnaftate*.

**Antiprotozoal Agents:** Metronidazole*, Tinidazole, Ornidazole, Diloxanide, Iodoquinol, Pentamidine isethionate, Atovaquone, Eflornithine.

**Anthelmintics:** Diethylcarbamazine citrate*, Thiabendazole, Mebendazole*, Albendazole, Niclosamide, Oxamniquine, Praziquantel, Ivermectin.

## SULFONAMIDES AND SULFONES

**Historical development, Chemistry, Classification and SAR of sulfonamides:**

Sulfamethizole, Sulfisoxazole, Sulfamethazine, Sulfacetamide*, Sulfapyridine, Sulfamethoxazole*, Sulfadiazine, Mafenide acetate, Sulfasalazine.

*Folate reductase* **Inhibitors:** Trimethoprim*, Cotrimoxazole.

**Sulfones:** Dapsone*.

**Unit V** **07 hrs**

## INTRODUCTION TO DRUG DESIGN

Various approaches used in drug design.

Physicochemical parameters used in quantitative structure activity relationship (QSAR) such as Partition coefficient, Hammett electronic parameter, Taft steric parameter and Hansch analysis.

Pharmacophore modeling and docking techniques.

**Combinatorial Chemistry:** Concept and applications of combinatorial chemistry: Solid phase and solution phase synthesis.

Chapter 1

# ANTIBIOTICS

## 1. INTRODUCTION

Antibiotic (Anti means against; bios means life) is a chemical substance produced by one organism that is destructive to another. It is an agent with biological activity against living organisms; however, the term is commonly used to refer to substances with anti-bacterial, anti-fungal or anti-parasitical activity. They have either a bacteriostatic or a bactericidal effect and can be effective against a small group of bacteria (narrow-spectrum) or a wide range of pathogens (broad-spectrum).

**History:** Infections were the major cause of death during the nineteenth century. The introduction of antibiotics not only helped in the treatment of infections but also have a major role in decreasing mortality and morbidity

In 1909, Paul Ehrlich, a German physician, discovered the first antimicrobial Salvarsan for the treatment of syphilis, a disease that was almost incurable back. This became the first modern antibiotic, although Ehrlich himself referred to his discovery as 'chemotherapy' – the use of a chemical to treat a disease. The drug, which was also effective against other spirochaetal infections, is no longer in use in modern medicine.

In 1932 Prontosil, a sulphonamide antibiotic was discovered and since it was cheap, many companies were encouraged to mass production of many derivatives of Prontosil. The antibiotic properties of *Penicillium spp.* were first described in France by Ernest Duchesne in 1897. However, his work went by without much notice from the scientific community until Alexander Fleming's discovery of Penicillin.

Antibiotics were further developed in Britain following the re-discovery of Penicillin in 1928 by Alexander Fleming. More than ten years later, Ernst Chain and Howard Florey became interested in his work and came up with the purified form of Penicillin. The three shared the 1945 Nobel Prize in Medicine. In the same year,

Dorothy determined the chemical structure of penicillin by x-ray crystallography and in 1950 chemically synthesized. The isolation of 6-aminopenicillanic acid in 1958 led to the semi-synthesis of new penicillins such as Ampicillin, Methicillin and Carbenicillin. In 1953, Newton and Abraham discovered Cephalosporin C; its antibacterial activity was low but was not susceptible to hydrolysis by *penicillinase*. Cephalothin, the first cephalosporin available for clinical use, was introduced in 1964, but it was only available for parenteral use. Later Cephalexin was developed, which was effective upon oral administration and total synthesis of cephalosporin C was accomplished in 1970.

"Antibiotic" was originally used to refer only to substances extracted from a fungus or other microorganism, but has come to include also the many synthetic and semi-synthetic drugs that have antibacterial effects. During 1940's and 50's Streptomycin, Chloramphenicol, and Tetracycline were discovered. Antibiotic agents with large ring systems were also isolated. Erythromycin (1949), was the first macrocyclic compound, is effective against penicillin resistant bacteria. Another large ring system that contains only amino acids is Tyrocidine A, a component of gramicidin antibacterial agents.

The word 'antibiotics' was first used in 1942 by Selman Waksman, who in his lifetime discovered over 20 antibiotics. The search for new antibiotics continues with an emphasis on discovery of drugs that are effective against drug-resistant bacteria. A β-lactam class of antibiotics called Carbapenem (1976) show promise with broad spectrum antibiotic properties. In 2001, Linezolid, the first of the oxazolidinone class was introduced in the market. It is used for the treatment of infections caused by multi-resistant bacteria including S*treptococcus* and methicillin-resistant *Staphylococcus aureus* (MRSA).

## 2. CLASSIFICATION OF ANTIBIOTICS

Antibiotics are classified on the basis of chemical structure, its spectrum of activity and pharmacological activity.

## I. Based on Chemical Structure

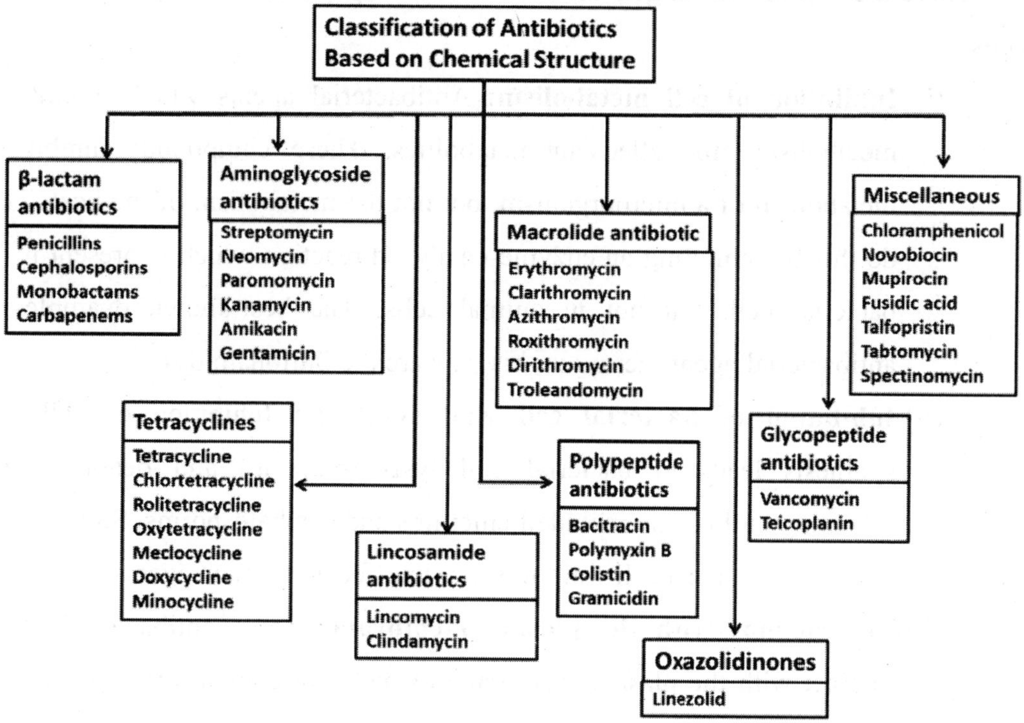


## II. Based on Pharmacological Activity

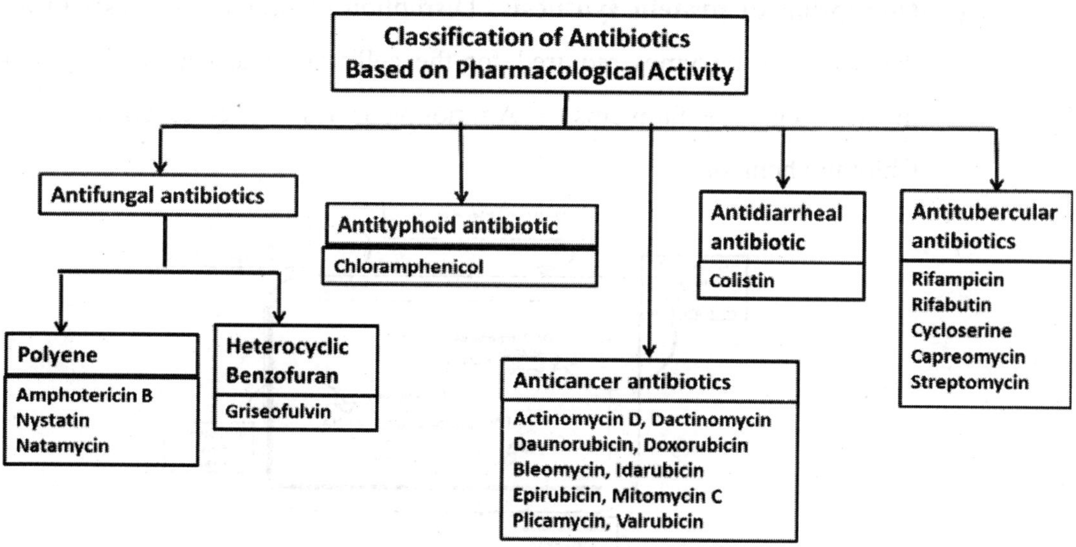

### (a) General Mechanisms of Antibiotics

There are 5 principle targets for antimicrobial agents to work against bacterial cells

(i) **Inhibition of cell metabolism**: Antibacterial agents which inhibit cell metabolism are called antimetabolites. These compounds inhibit the metabolism of a microorganism, but not the metabolism of the host. They do this by inhibiting an enzyme-catalyzed reaction which is present in the bacterial cell, but not in animal cells. The best-known examples of antibacterial agents acting in this way are the Sulfonamides.

(ii) **Inhibition of bacterial cell wall synthesis:** Inhibition of cell wall synthesis leads to bacterial cell lysis (bursting) and death. Agents operating in this way include Penicillins and Cephalosporins. Since animal cells do not have a cell wall, they are unaffected by such agents.

(iii) **Interactions with the plasma membrane:** Some antibacterial agents interact with the plasma membrane of bacterial cells to affect membrane permeability. This has fatal results for the cell. Polymyxins and Tyrothricin operate in this way.

(iv) **Disruption of protein synthesis:** Disruption of protein synthesis means that essential enzymes required for the cell's survival can no longer be made. eg. Rifamycins, Aminoglycosides, Tetracyclines and Chloramphenicol.

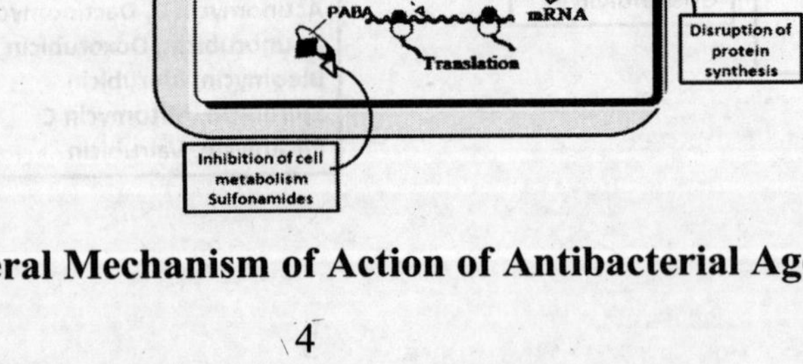


**Fig. 1.1 General Mechanism of Action of Antibacterial Agents**

## 2.1 β - LACTAM ANTIBIOTICS

### 2.1.1 Introduction

β-Lactam antibiotics are antibacterial agents that contain a β-lactam ring in their molecular structure and they include Penicillin derivatives, Cephalosporins, Monobactams and Carbapenems. The groups differ only in the nature of the rings appended to the β-Lactam moiety. Penicillin molecules contain a highly strained 4-membered β-lactam ring fused to a 5-membered thiazolidine ring (penems). Cephalosporins molecules contain a β-lactam ring fused to 6-membered dihydrothiazine ring (cephems). Carbapenems are β-lactams fused to dihydropyrrole rings. β-lactam not fused to any other rings named as monobactam. They are the most widely used group of antibiotics available.

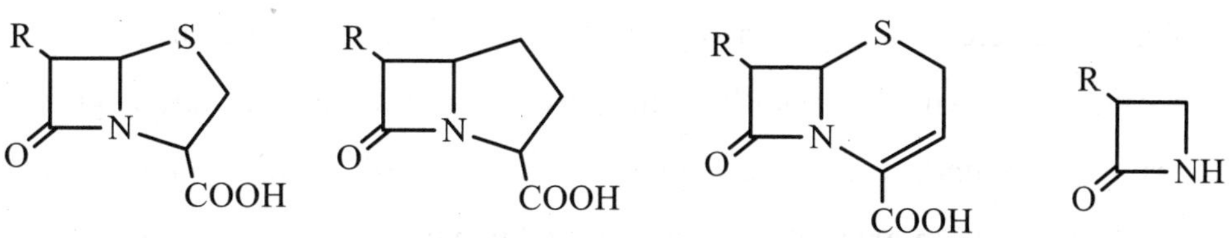

Penam Carbapenam Cephem Monobactam

**2.1.2 Mode of Action:** β-lactam antibiotics are bactericidal and act by inhibiting the synthesis of the peptidoglycan layer of bacterial cell walls. The peptidoglycan layer is important for cell wall structural integrity, especially in Gram-positive organisms. The final transpeptidation step in the synthesis of the peptidoglycan is facilitated by *transpeptidases* known as penicillin binding proteins.

**2.1.3 Clinical Uses:** β-lactam antibiotics are indicated for the prophylaxis and treatment of bacterial infections caused by susceptible organisms. Whilst traditionally β-lactam antibiotics were mainly active only against Gram-positive bacteria, the development of broad-spectrum β-lactam antibiotics active against various Gram-negative organisms has increased their usefulness.

## I. Classification of β - Lactam Antibiotics

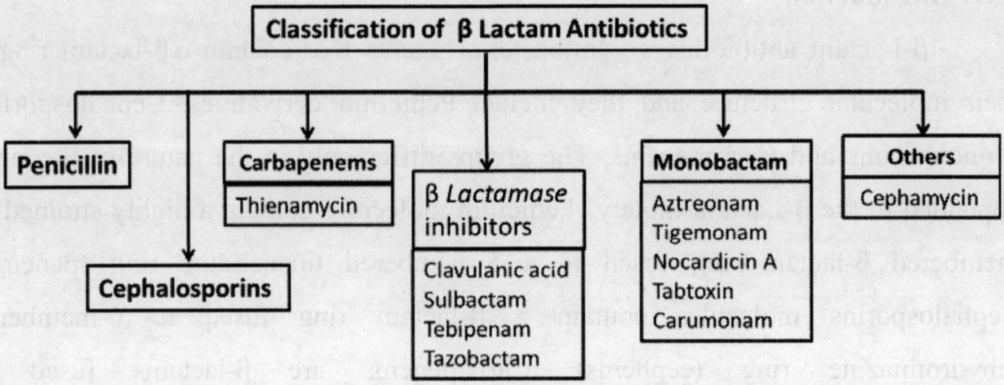


## 2.1.1 PENICILLINS

### 2.1.1.1 Introduction

Penicillin refers to a group of β-lactam antibiotics derived originally from common moulds known as Penicillium moulds; Penicillins are a large group of bicyclic ring compounds which are acylated derivatives of 6-aminopenicillanic acid (6-APA) which /itself an example of a substituted penem.

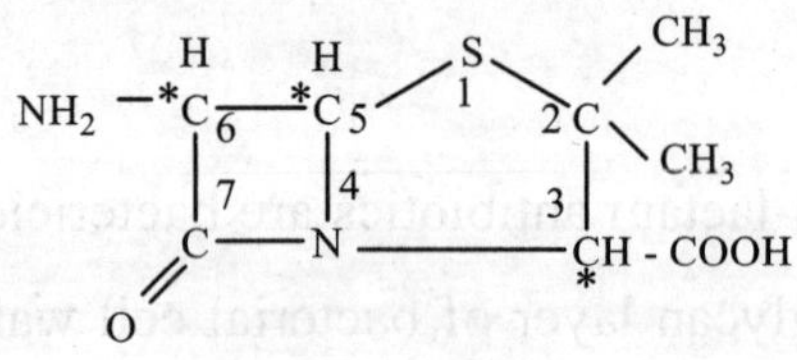
6 - Amino penicillanic acid (6 - APA)

Penicillin was discovered in 1928 by Scottish scientist Alexander Fleming and successfully used in 1942. Penicillin reduced the number of deaths and amputations of troops during World War II. Benzylpenicillin (penicillin G) was the first natural penicillin with potent activity against all Gram-positive pathogens, Gram-negative *Streptococci* and some *Spirochaetes* and *Actinomycetes*. It is the only natural penicillin still in use.

Discovery of the 6-aminopenicillanic acid nucleus has led to considerable manipulation of the basic ring structure, resulting initially in the synthesis of Ampicillin and subsequently the other aminopenicillins analogues, esters and prodrugs. The first major development was Ampicillin, which offered a broad spectrum of activity than either of the original Penicillin. Further development yielded *β-lactamase* resistant penicillin including Flucloxacillin, Dicloxacillin and Methicillin.

The extended-spectrum agents (Mezlocillin and Piperacillin) are unique in that, they have greater activity against Gram-negative bacteria, including *Pseudomonas aeruginosa*, a bacterium that often causes serious infection in people whose immune systems have been weakened. They have decreased activity, however, against *penicillinase* producing *Staphylococcus aureus,* a common bacterial agent in food poisoning. Major adverse effect of Penicillins are hypersensitivity reactions, which range from rash to immediate anaphylaxis.

The semi-synthetic penicillins are produced by growing the mold Penicillium under conditions where by only the basic molecule (6-aminopenicillanic acid) is produced. By adding different acyl chlorides to this molecule, different semi-synthetic penicillins are produced

### 2.1.1.2 Nomenclature

Nomenclature of Penicilln was done in different system.

According to Chemical Abstracts system penicillins are numbered starting form "S". Sulfur atom is assigned $1^{st}$ position and nitrogen atom is assigned $4^{th}$ position.The numbering initates with the sulfur atom and assigns the ring nitrogen the 4-position. Thus, penicillins are named as 4-Aza-1-thiabicyclo [3.2.0] heptanes, according to this system.

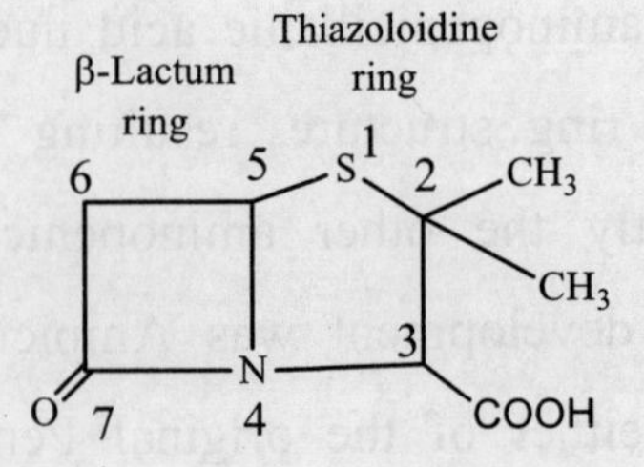


4-aza-1-thiabicyclo[3.2.0]heptanes

The numbering system adopted by the USP is the reverse of the Chemical Abstracts procedure, assigning number 1 to the nitrogen atom and number 4 to the sulfur atom. Thus, penicillins are named as 4-thia-l-azabicyclo[3.2.0]heptanes, according to this system.

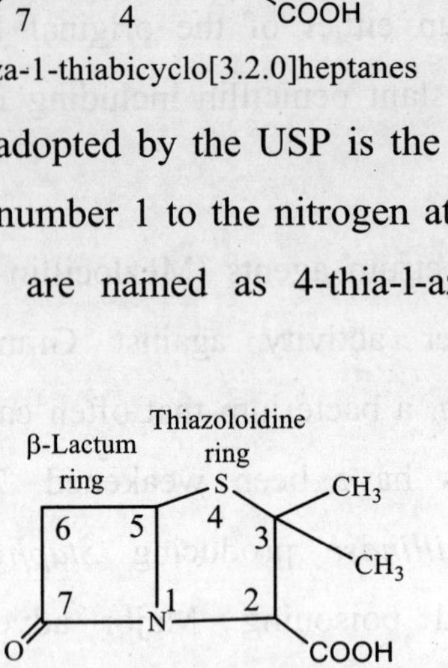


4-thia-l-azabicyclo[3.2.0]heptanes

**(a) As derivative of Penam :** Penam nucleus is used in naming which comprise bicyclic system with the amide carbonyl group. Penicillin is named as 6-acylamino-2,2-dimethylpenam-3-carboxylic acid.

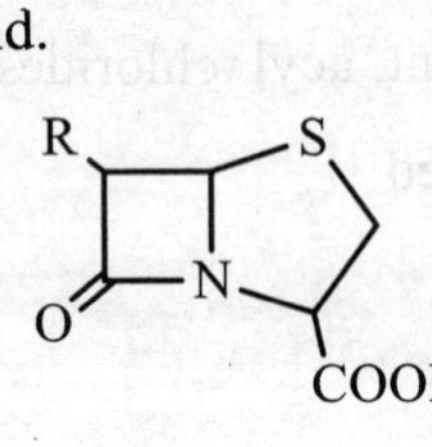


Penam

**(b) As derivative of Penicillanic acid:** Penicillanic acid contains (2,2-Dimethylpenam-3-carboxylic acid) nucleus which includes the 2,2-Dimethyl and 3-Carboxyl groups . Penicillin is named as 6-Carbonylamino penicillanic acid.

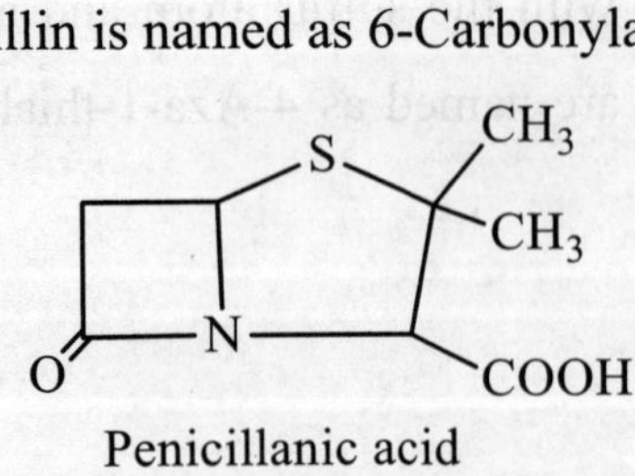


Penicillanic acid

**(c) As derivative of Penicillin:** In this system the 6-Carbonyl amino penicillanic acid portion is named as Pencillin and the different penicillins are named on the basis of the R group attached on the amino acyl side chain. For example Benzyl penicillin - R is benzyl group; Phenoxy methyl Pencillin where R is Phenoxy methyl group. Penicillanic acid is a penam that consists of 3,3-Dimethyl-7-oxo-4-thia-1-azabicyclo[3.2.0]heptane bearing a carboxy group at position 2.

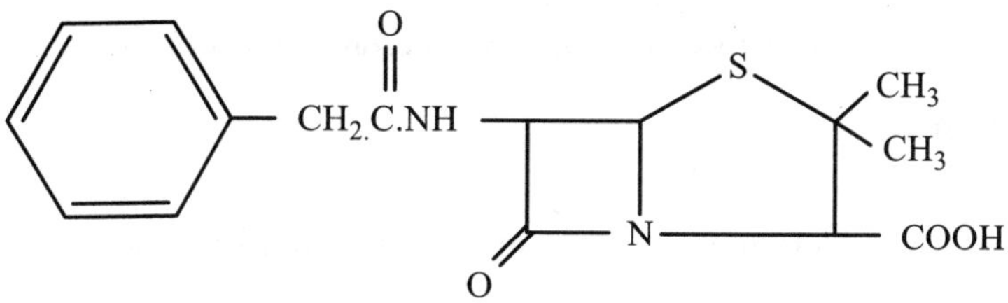


### 2.1.1.3 Chemistry of Penicillin

Penicillin molecules all contain a highly strained 4-membered β-lactam ring fused to a 5-membered thiazolidine ring and acyl substituted side chain at 6$^{th}$ position. The β-lactam ring is unstable and is primarily responsible for the antibiotic potency of these molecules. 6-Amino penicillanic acid (6-APA) is the basic skeleton structure of all penicillins. It contains three chiral carbon atoms ($C_3$, $C_5$ and $C_6$). The absolute stereochemistry of the penicillin was designed as 3S:5R:6R. All natural and synthetic penicillins have the same absolute configuration about these three centers. The 6$^{th}$ carbon atom bearing the acyl amino group has L-Configuration, whereas the carbon to which the carboxyl group was attached has the D-configuration. The acyl amino group and carboxyl group are *trans* to each other with the acyl in α- and amino in β-orientation relative to penam ring.

### 2.1.1.4 Structure Activity Relationship

Penicillin's core structure consists of a fused β-lactam ring with a thiazolidine ring. Basic skeleton essential to show bactericidal activity are the bicyclic ring, free carboxylate group, *Cis* stereochemistry at $C_5$ and $C_6$ and acylamino side chain. (Fig. 1.2). Changing one or more of these results in a loss of activity.

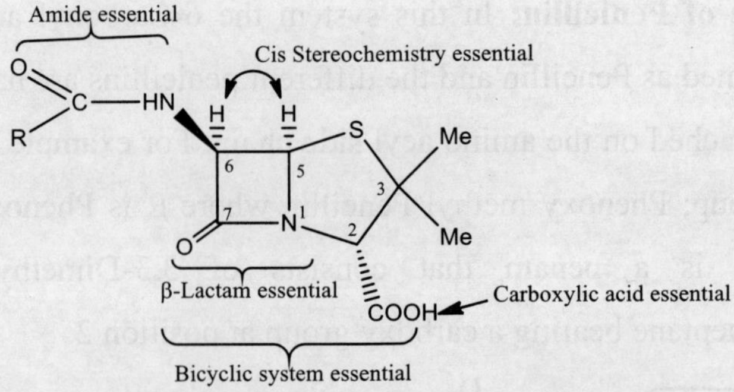


**Fig. 1.2 Essential Structural Features of Penicillins**

## a) Bicyclic system

- The strained β-lactam ring is essential. The greater the strain, the greater the activity and instability of the molecule to other factors.
- β-lactam ring binds with the *pencillinase transpeptidase* is responsible for cross linking of linear peptidoglycan layer.
- β-lactam ring is a good acylating agent for active penicillin binding protein serine.
- The C=O in the $C_7$ position is electrophilic (δ+) and along with adjacent thiazolidine ring confers further strain on the β-lactam ring, making the ring even more reactive to nucleophilic attack.
- Sulfur is not essential. Activity decreases if the sulphur is oxidized to sulphone or sulfoxide but increases the acid stability.
- The N at position 4 is must for antibacterial activity and any modification upon nitrogen will result in lack of activity.
- The germinal dimethyl group at $C_2$ position is a characteristic of the pencillin

## b) Carboxylic acid group

- The free carboxylic acid group at $C_2$ position is essential. The negative charge of carboxlate group directs the drug to positively charged active binding pocket at neutral pH.
- The carboxylate ion binds to the charged ammonium ion of lysine residue in the binding site.

## c) Stereochemistry

- Cis stereochemistry between the two hydrogens at $C_5$ and $C_6$ is essential for activity. Penicillin molecule has 3 chiral carbons, $C_3$, $C_5$ and $C_6$. Modification of these spatial arrangement results in loss of activity.

## d) Acylamino side chain

- The acylamino side chain is a necessary feature. The modification at acylamino side chain is aimed for strengthening of antimicrobial spectrum, stability to stomach acid, resistance, absorption and distribution, cross-hypersensitivity and susceptibility to bacterial degradative enzymes *(β-lactamases)*.

- Natural Penicillins have narrow spectrum of activity and sensitive towards some bacteria, acid and can be hydrolyzed by *β-lactamases* (enzymes produced by Gram-positive and Gram-negative bacteria). Development of semi-synthetic penicillins overcomes these disadvantages. They have various specific properties such as

i. resistance to stomach acids so that they can be taken orally
ii. degree of resistance to *penicillinase* (penicillin destroying enzyme produced by some bacteria)
iii. extended range of activity against some Gram-negative bacteria.

Semi-synthetic penicillins are made by adding different side chains onto the β-lactam ring.

- For penicillin derivatives in general, it has been found that, hydrophobic side chains confer good activity against Gram- positive bacteria, but poor activity against Gram- negative strains. Enhancement of Gram-negative activity is increased by introducing hydrophilic group ($-NH_2$, -OH,

-COOH group) to the carbon α to the carbonyl group on the side chain.eg Ampicillin. The broad spectrum activity was further extended by introducing strong acidic group to the carbon α to the carbonyl group on the side chain.eg. Carbenicillin, Ticarcillin.

- The acyl carbonyl group C=O is rich in electron density and able to attack the neighbouring carbon of β-lactam. Therefore pencillin has self destruction property which can be overcome by using electron withdrawing R group.

- Substitutions of a side chain R on the acylamino group with an electron withdrawing group increases the electron density on the side chain carbonyl group and protect these penicillins from acid degradation result in greater stability and oral availability. eg. Phenoxymethylpenicillin (Penicillin V), Ampicillin (Amino penicillin). Since the amino group and the carboxylic group are ionisable, these compounds are poorly absorbed through the gut. Modifications such as, changing the carboxylic acid to esters were made at the carboxylic group to overcome this problem. **Pivampicillin** and **Bacampicillin** are examples of ester prodrug of Ampicillin.

- Penicillin resistance first became a serious problem in the early 1960s. Penicillin resistant bacterial strains which contained an enzyme *β-lactamases* which deactivated the drug by cleaving the β-lactam ring.

- By placing a bulky group on the acylamino side chain, degradation of the drug by *β-lactamases* would be minimized. However, if a steric shield is too bulky, the penicillin would not be able to bind to *transpeptidase.* Examples of these blocking penicillins are Methicillin and Nafcillin. Both must be administered intravenously, as their side chains are electron releasing, making them too acid sensitive for oral administration.

- Presence of urea group at carbon α to the carbonyl group (ureido penicillins) results in broad spectrum antibiotic. They are used parenterally and are active against *Pseudomonas aeruginosa*. Presence of urea group gives improved penetration into Gram-negative species. They are more active than carboxy pencillins against S*treptococci* and *Haemophilus* species. **Azlocillin** and **Piperacillin** are examples of ureido penicillins.

### 2.1.1.5 Mechanism of Action

β-lactam antibiotics work by inhibiting bacterial cell wall synthesis by binding and inactivating proteins (penicillin binding proteins) present in the bacterial cell wall. Bacteria cells are surrounded by a protective envelope called the cell wall. One of the primary components of the bacterial cell wall is peptidoglycan, a structural macromolecule with a net-like composition that provides rigidity and support to the outer cell wall. In order to form the cell wall, a single peptidoglycan chain is cross-linked to other peptidoglycan chains through the action of the enzyme DD-*transpeptidase* (also called a penicillin binding protein-PBP).

Penicillin have a structural resemblance to two D-alanine residues linked together and are mistaken by the *transpeptidase* enzyme for D-Ala-D-Alanine residue of bacterial peptidoglycan and thus incorporated into the active site. Once bound, the β-lactam carbonyl is attacked by the serine hydroxyl and ring opening occurs to leave the penicillin covalently bound to the enzyme.

The bulky thiazolidine ring now blocks, access to the active site by either a pentaglycine chain or water. As a result, the penicillin becomes irreversibly bound to the *transpeptidase* enzyme, preventing it from functioning properly. This result in incomplete cell walls that are much more fragile and porous and eventually lead to swelling followed by cell lysis and death.

Gram-positive bacteria have thick cell walls containing high levels of peptidoglycan, while Gram-negative bacteria are characterized by thinner cell walls with low levels of peptidoglycan. The cell walls of Gram-negative bacteria are surrounded by a lipopolysaccharide layer that prevents antibiotic entry into the cell. Therefore, penicillin is most effective against Gram-positive bacteria where DD-*transpeptidase* activity is highest. Human and animal cells have no cell wall, which makes it perfect target for internally-used antibiotics.

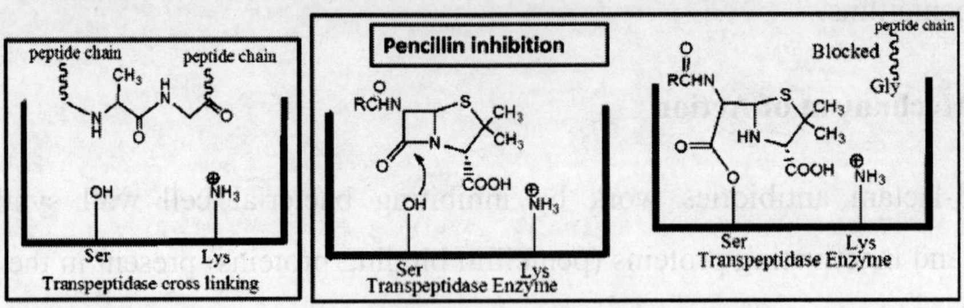


**Fig. 1.3 Mechanism of *transpeptidase* cross-linking and penicillin inhibition**

### 2.1.1.6 General Method of Synthesis of Penicillin

Step I. Synthesis of 6-amino penicillanic acid

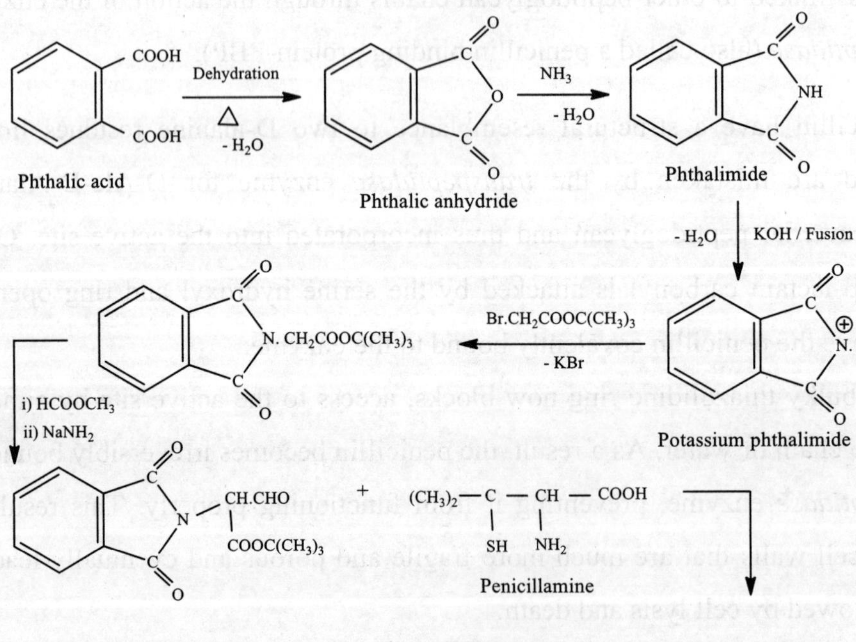

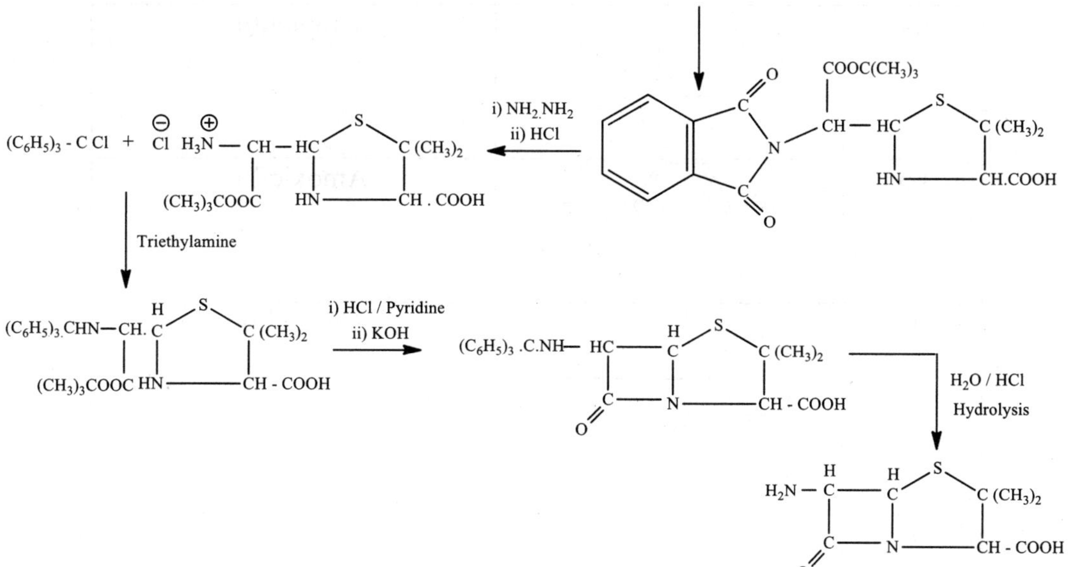

6 - Amino penicillanic acid

## tep 2: Synthesis of Acylsubstituted penicillin

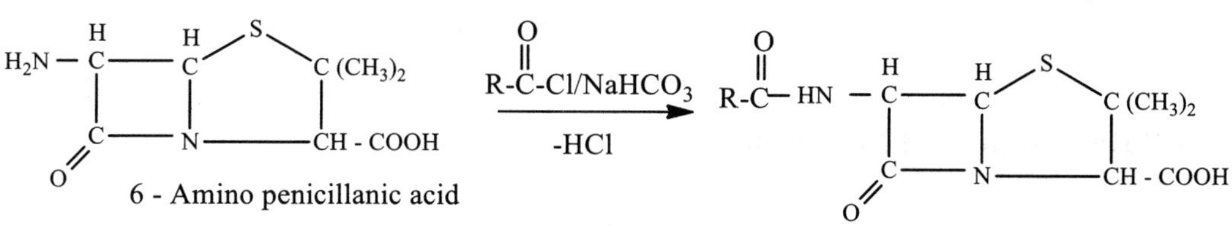

6 - Amino penicillanic acid

Acyl substituted amino penicillins

| S.No. | R Group | Name of the penicillin |
|---|---|---|
| 01 | 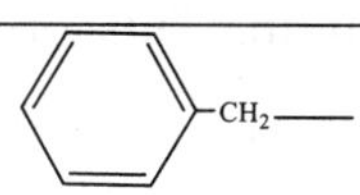 | Benzyl penicillin |
| 02 | 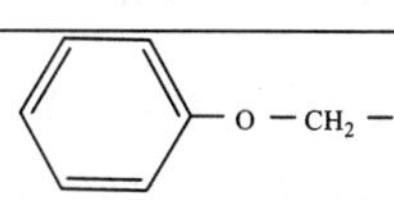 | Phenoxymethyl penicillin |
| 03 | 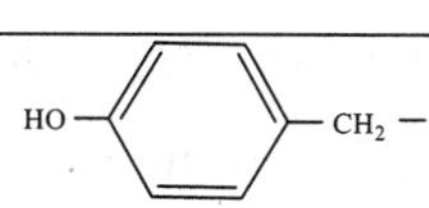 | p-Hydroxy benzyl penicillin |

| 04 | 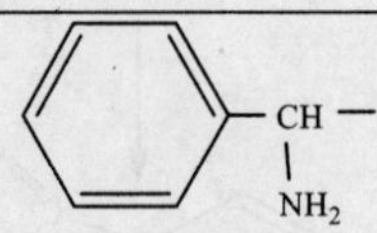 | Ampicillin |
|---|---|---|
| 05 | 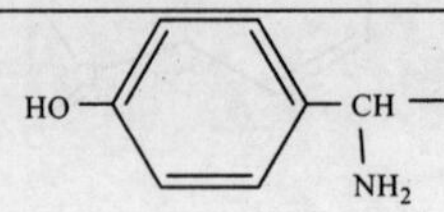 | Amoxicillin |
| 06 | 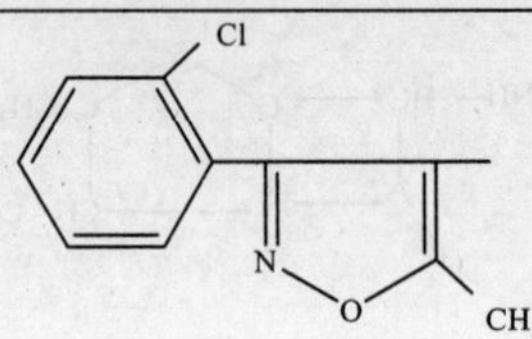 | Cloxacillin |
| 07 | 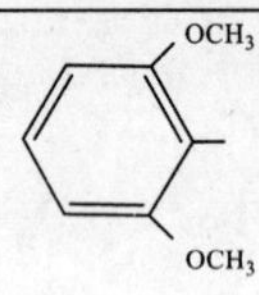 | Methicillin |

### 2.1.1.7 Degradation of Penicillin

The main cause of deterioration of penicillin is the reactivity of the strained lactam ring.

In the 4-membered ring β-lactam system, however, the bond angles are 90° instead of 120°, which results in 30° ring strain. This prevents the overlap of the nitrogen lone pair with the adjacent carbonyl system and thus the β-lactam carbonyl is much more electrophilic than a normal amide and is therefore susceptible to nucleophilic attack. The lone pair of nitrogen is readily protonated under acidic conditions, making the β-lactam ring sensitive to strong acids. Thus, the β-lactam ring system in Penicillins and Cephalosporins are very susceptible to ring-opening under strongly acidic and basic conditions and by strong nucleophiles.

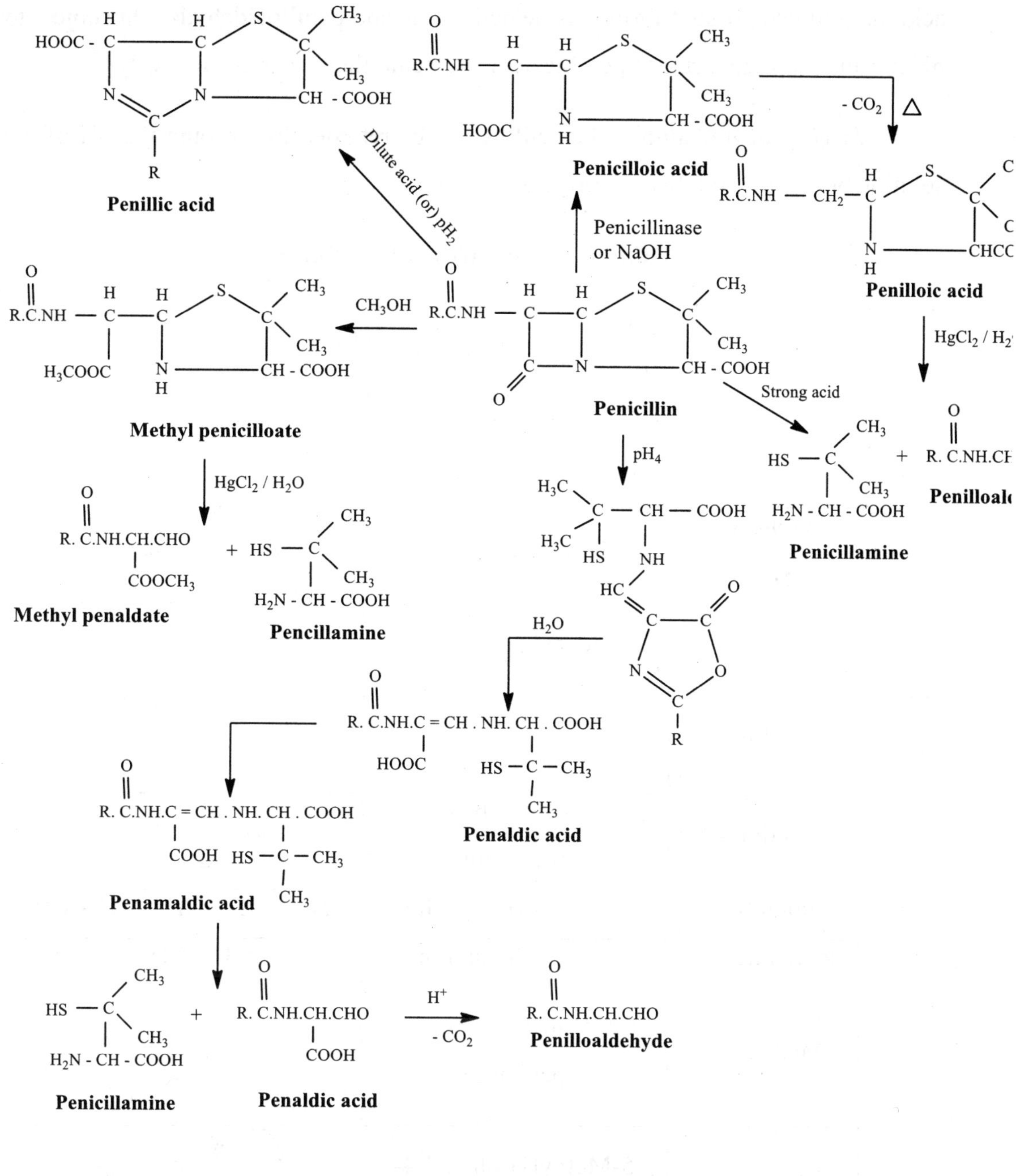


The hydrolysis and the nature of degradation products are influenced by pH of the solution. Thus the β-lactam carbonyl group of penicillin readily undergoes nucleophilic attack by water or hydroxide ion to form inactive penicilloic acid, which on decarboxylation produces penilloic acid. On treatment with strong acid the ultimate product formed is penicillamine and penilloaldehyde. On subject to pH 2.0 and 4.0 it give rise to penillic acid and penicillenic acid respectively.

*In vitro* degradation of Penicillins can be retarded by keeping the pH of the solution between 6 to 6.8 and refrigerating them.

**Table 1.1 Structures of Penicillins**

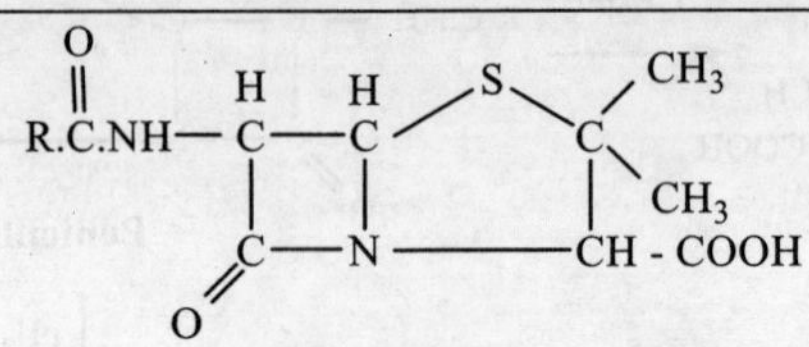

Basic skeletan structure

| S.No. | Generic Name | Chemical Name | R Group |
|---|---|---|---|
| 1. | Penicillin - G | Benzyl penicillin | 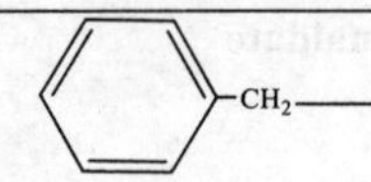 |
| 2. | Penicillin - V | Phenoxymethyl penicillin | 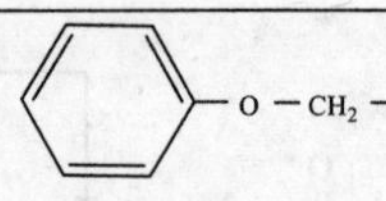 |
| 3. | Penicillin - X | p-Hydroxy benzyl penicillin | 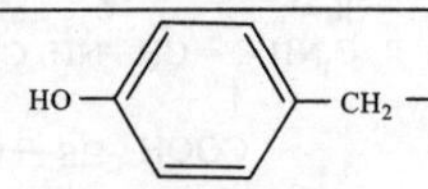 |
| 4. | Penicillin - F | 2- Pentenyl penicillin | $CH_3-CH_2-CH=CH-CH_2-$ |
| 5. | Penicillin - K | n-Heptyl penicillin | $CH_3\ (CH_2)_7-$ |
| 6. | Methicillin | 2,6-Dimethoxyphenyl penicillin | 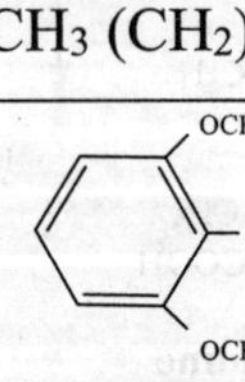 |
| 7. | Oxacillin | 5-Methyl-3-phenyl-4-isoxazolyl penicillin | 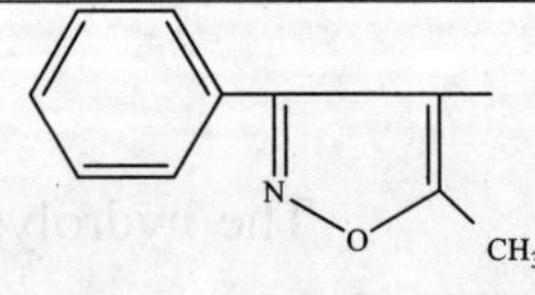 |

| 8. | Cloxacillin | 5-Methyl-3-(2-chlorophenyl)-4-isoxazoly penicillin | 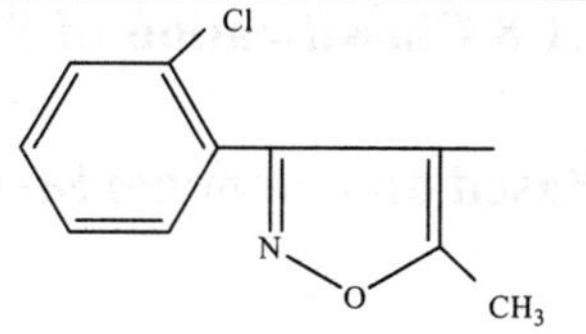 |
|---|---|---|---|
| 9. | Dicloxacillin | 5-Methyl-3-(2,6-dichlorophenyl)-4-isoxazolyl penicillin | 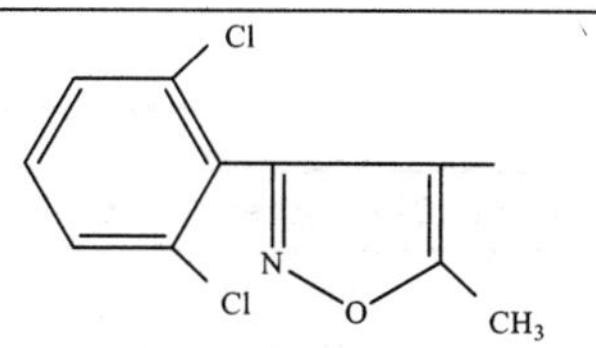 |
| 10. | Ampicillin | D-α-Amino benzyl-penicillin | 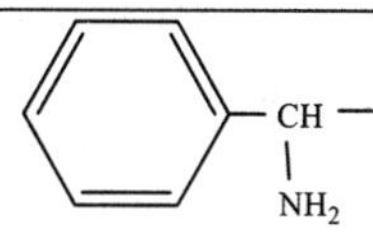 |
| 11. | Amoxicillin | D-α-Amino-p-hydroxy benzyl penicillin | 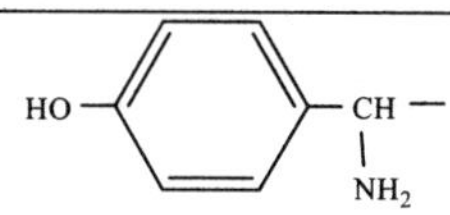 |
| 12. | Carbenicillin | α-Carboxy benzyl-penicillin | 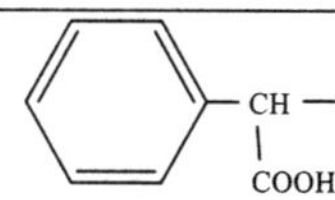 |
| 13. | Ticarcillin | α-Carboxy-3-thienyl-penicillin | 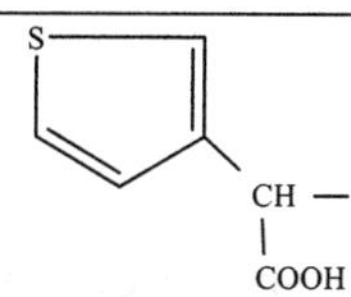 |
| 14. | Piperacillin | α-(4-Ethyl-2,3-dioxo-1-piperazinyl carbonyl-amino) benzyl penicillin | 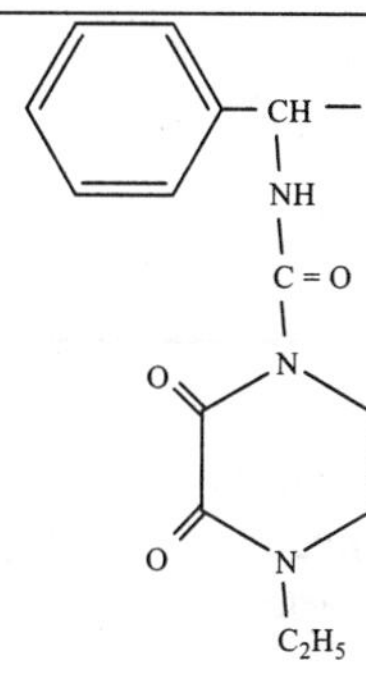 |

### 2.1.1.8 Classification of Penicillins

#### I. Based on Chemical Structure

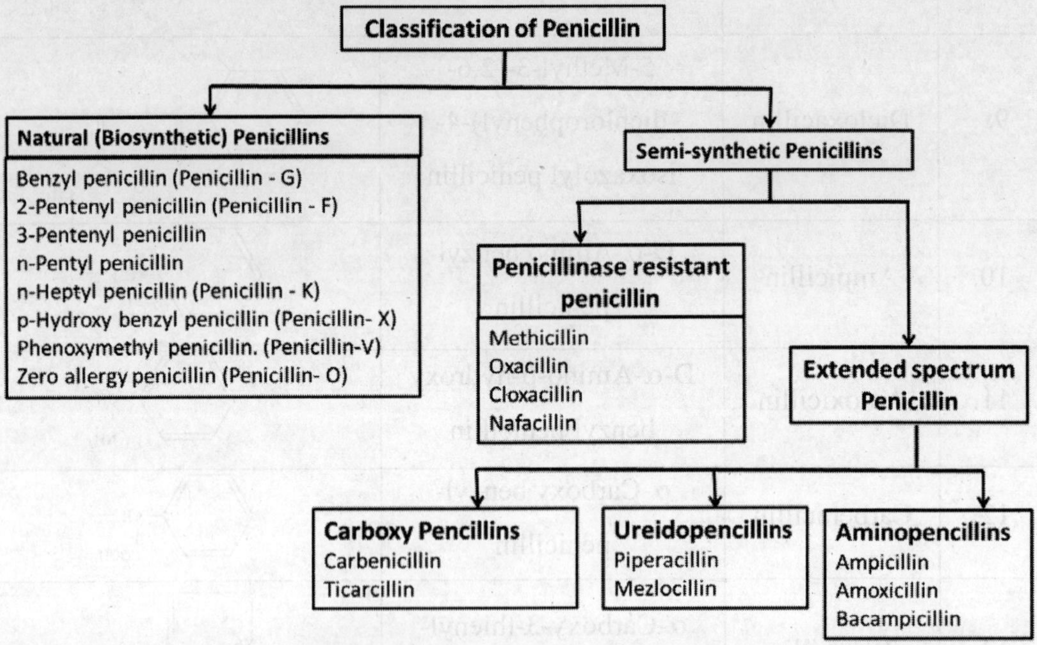


#### II. Based on Spectrum of Activity

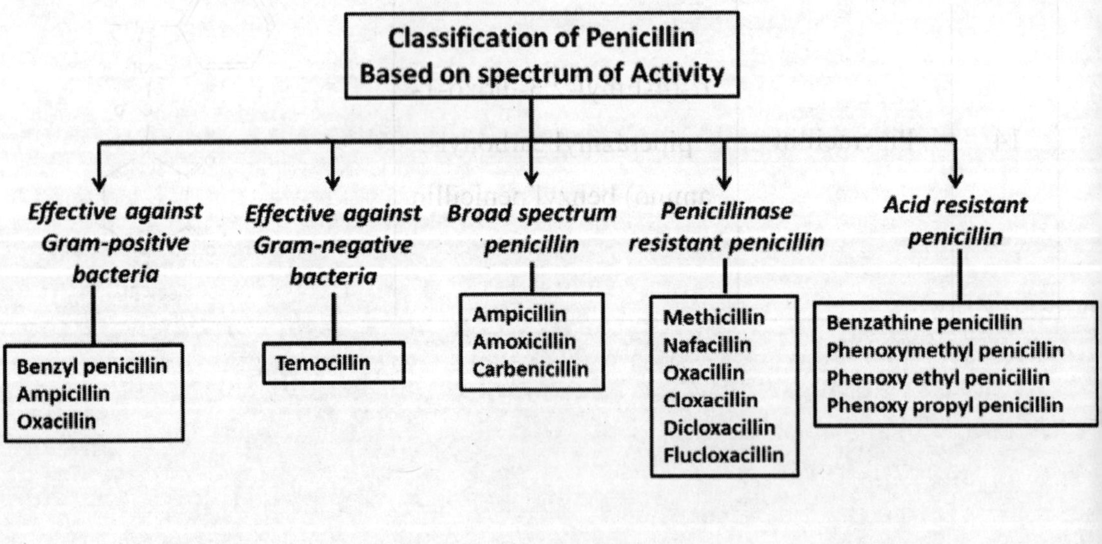

# I. Natural Penicillins

## A. Benzylpenicillin (Pentids)

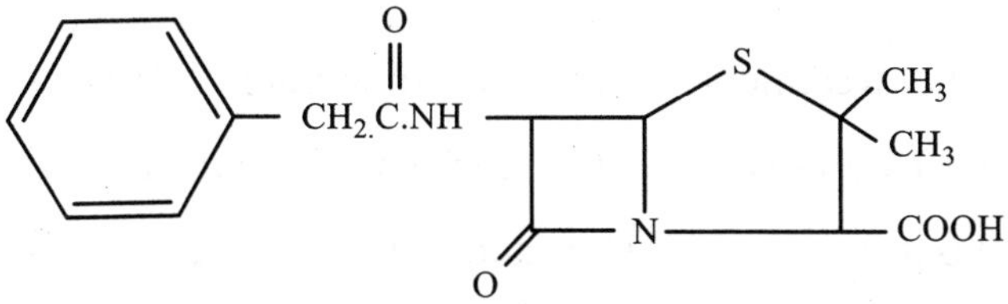

(2S,5R,6R) -3,3 - dimethyl - 7 - oxo - 6 - (phenylacetamido) - 4 - thia - 1- azabicyclo[3.2.0]heptane - 2 - carboxylic acid

Benzyl penicillin or Penicillin G, is the gold standard penicillin, which is obtained biotechnologically using the fungus *Penicillium chrysogenum.* It is a narrow spectrum antibiotic used to treat infections caused by susceptible bacteria. It is administered intravenously or intramuscularly due to poor oral absorption. It is active with respect to Gram-positive bacteria (*Staphylococcus, Streptococcus* and *Pneumococcal*) causative agent of diphtheria and anthrax bacillus. Gram-negative bacteria are resistant to it. Benzylpenicillin is broken down by stomach acid and destroyed by *penicillinase.* It is stored in tightly-closed container in a cool, dry place. It is available as intramuscular or intravenous injection or infusion in divided doses.

**Use:** It is useful for the treatment of strep throat caused by *Streptococcal pharyngitis,* pneumonia, syphilis, diphtheria, leptospirosis, necrotizing enterocolitis, cellulitis and tetanus.

## B. Phenoxymethylpenicillin (Fevospen)

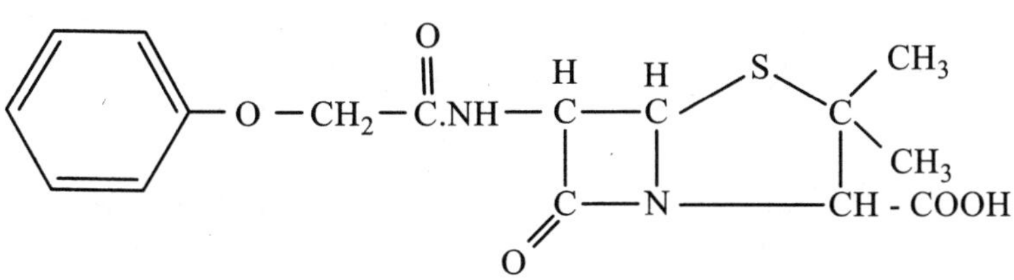

(2S,5R,6R) - 3, 3 - dimethyl - 7 - oxo - 6 - [(phenoxyacetyl)amino] - 4 - thia - 1 -azabicyclo[3.2.0]heptane-2-carboxylic acid

It is a narrow spectrum antibiotic also commonly referred as Penicillin V or Penicillin VK. It is a Phenoxy methyl analogue of Penicillin G. It is an orally active naturally penicillin.

**Use:** It is used for the treatment of mild to moderate infections of the upper respiratory tract caused by *Pneumococcus*, scarlet fever and mild erysipelas caused by *Streptococcus* without bacteremia, skin and soft tissues caused by Penicillin G-sensitive microorganisms.

## II. Semi-synthetic Penicillins

### *II(a). Penicillinase* Resistant Penicillins

### A. Cloxacillin (Cloxapen)

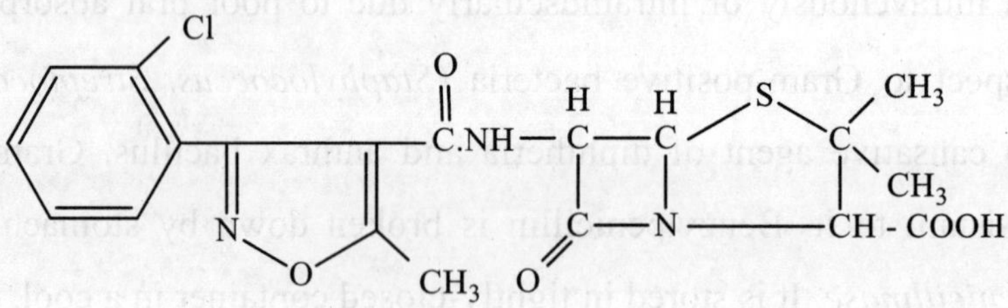


(2S,5R,6R) - 6 - ({[3 - (2 - chlorophenyl) - 5 - methylisoxazol - 4 -yl]carbonyl}amino) - 3,3 - dimethyl - 7 - oxo - 4 - thia - 1 -azabicyclo[3.2.0]heptane - 2 - carboxylic acid

**Use:** It is used for the treatment of infections includes pneumonia, cellulitis, septic arthritis and impetigo.

### B. Methicillin (Dimocillin)

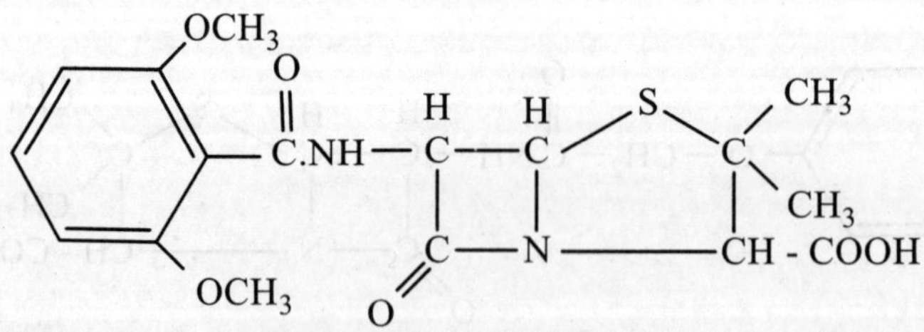


(2S,5R,6R) - 6 - [(2,6 - dimethoxybenzoyl)amino] - 3,3 - dimethyl - 7 - oxo - 4 - thia - 1 -azabicyclo[3.2.0]heptane - 2 - carboxylic acid

It is one of the semi-synthetic, narrow spectrum *β-lactamase*-resistant penicillin with bactericidal and *β-lactamase* resistant activity. It is also known as Staphcillin. Rarely used now, it has been largely superseded by Vancomycin. A strain known as methicillin-resistant *S. aureus* (MRSA) is pandemic, causing infection in thousands of hospital patients and healthy individuals worldwide each year.

**Use:** It is used to treat infections caused by susceptible Gram-positive bacteria, such as *Staphylococcus aureus* that would otherwise be resistant to most penicillins. It is inactivated by gastric acid so administered by injection.

### II. (b). Extended Spectrum Penicillins

### II. (b). i. Aminopenicillins

### A. Ampicillin (Biocilin)

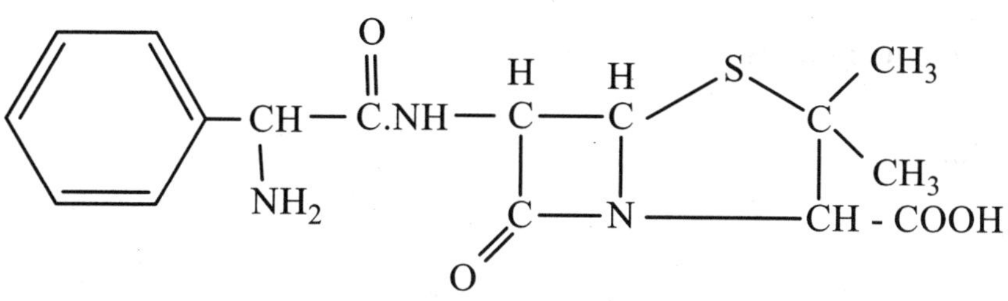

(2S,5R,6R) - 6 - ([(2R) - 2 - amino - 2 - phenylacetyl]amino) - 3,3 -dimethyl - 7 - oxo - 4 - thia - 1 - azabicyclo[3.2.0]heptane - 2 - carboxylic acid

It is orally active semi-synthetic penicillin that functions as broad-spectrum antibiotic. The bactericidal activity of Ampicillin results from the inhibition of cell wall synthesis and is mediated by binding to penicillin binding proteins (PBPs). Ampicillin is stable against hydrolysis by a variety of *β-lactamases*, including *penicillinases* and *cephalosporinases*. The amino group and the carboxylic group in Ampicillins are ionizable, so these compounds are poorly absorbed through the gut.

**Use:** It is used for treatment of infection (Respiratory, GI, UTI and meningitis) due to *Escherichia coli, Proteus mirabilis,* Enterococci, Shigella, *Salmonella typhi* and other Salmonella, *non-penicillinase* producing *Neisseria gonorrhoeae*, *Haemophilus influenzae*, Staphylococci and Streptococci.

**B. Amoxicillin (Lomox)**

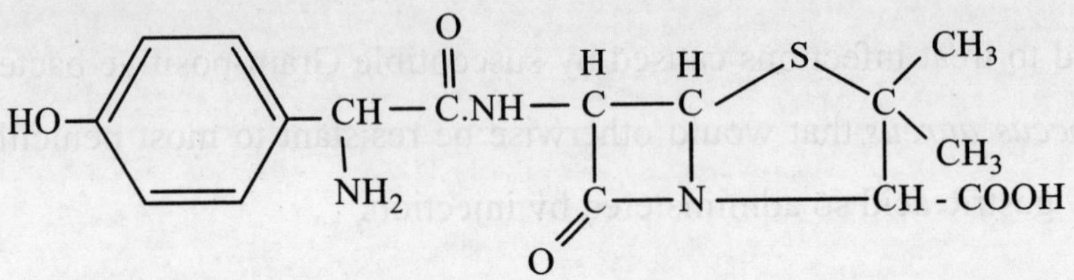

(2S,5R,6R) - 6 - ([(2R) - 2 - amino - 2 - (4 - hydroxyphenylacetyl]amino) - 3,3 - dimethyl - 7 - oxo - 4 - thia - 1 - azabicyclo[3.2.0]heptane - 2 - carboxylic acid

**Use:** It is used to treat infections caused by bacteria, such as tonsillitis, bronchitis, pneumonia, infections of the ear, nose, throat, skin and urinary tract.

**II. (b). ii. Carboxypenicillins**

**A. Carbenicillin**

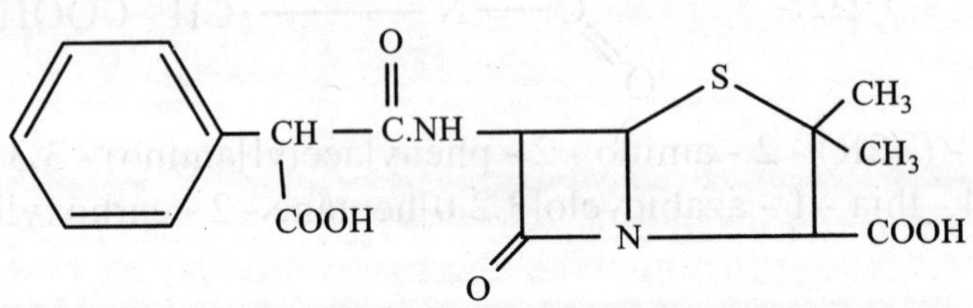

(2S,5R,6R) - 6 - {[ 2 - carboxy (2 - phenyl)acetyl]amino} - 3,3 - dimethyl - 7 - oxo - 4 - thia - 1 - azabicyclo[3.2.0]heptane - 2 - carboxylic acid

**Use:** It is broad-spectrum semi-synthetic penicillin used parenterally for the treatment of acute and chronic infections of the upper and lower urinary tract infections.

## II. (b). iii. Ureidopenicillins

### A. Piperacillin (Ecosette)

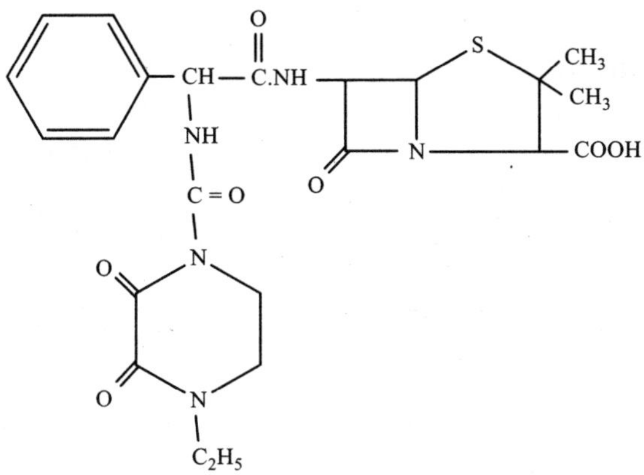

(2S,5R,6R) - 6 - {[(2R) - 2 - {[(4 - ethyl - 2,3 - dioxopiperazin - 1 -yl)carbonyl]amino} - 2 - phenylacetyl]amino} - 3,3 - dimethyl - 7 - oxo - 4 -thia - 1 - azabicyclo[3.2.0]heptane - 2 - carboxylic acid

**Use:** It is one of the semi-synthetic broad-spectrum penicillin used for the treatment of polymicrobial infections.

## III. Penicillin Combinations

### A. Benzathine penicillin (Penidure)

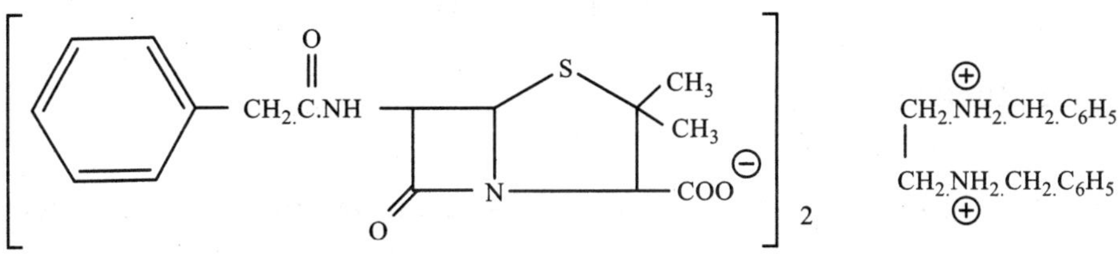

It is a combination of two molecule of Benzyl penicillin with one molecule of Benzathine (N, N'- dibenzyl ethylene diamine). It has low solubility and thus, the drugs are slowly released from intramuscular injection sites. The drugs are hydrolyzed to penicillin G. In should be stored in a tightly-closed container, in a cool and dry place. It is given orally, intramuscularly or intravenously in a divided dose. A single injection is found to be effective for a week.

**Use:** It is useful for the treatment of strep throat caused by *Streptococcal pharyngitis*, diphtheria, syphilis and yaws caused by *Spirochete bacterium* and also used to treat rheumatic fever.

**B. Procaine penicillin (Wycillin)**

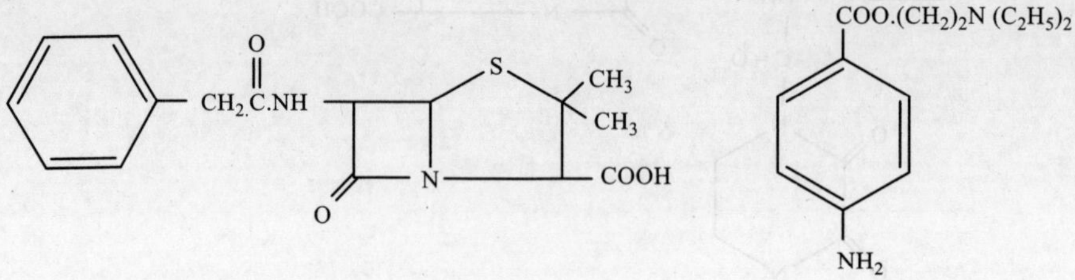

It is a combination of equimolar mixture of one molecule of Benzyl penicillin with one molecule of Procaine. It is a white crystalline powder, slightly soluble in water, sparingly soluble in ethanol (95%). It should be stored in a tightly closed container in a cool and dry place. It is given as intramuscular injection. It is a popular respiratory product which reduces the injection frequency.

**Use:** It is used for the treatment of syphilis, anthrax, mouth infections, pneumonia and diphtheria.

## 2.1.2 CEPHALOSPORINS

### 2.1.2.1 Introduction

Cephalosporins are semi-synthetic β-lactam antibiotic closely related in structure, mechanism of action, spectrum of activity and pharmacology to the penicillins. The first isolated Cephalosporin was Cephalosporin-C from cultures of *Cephalosporium acremonium* from a sewer in Sardinia in 1948 by Italian Scientist Giuseppe Brotzu. Cephalosporins are more stable to acid hydrolysis, *Penicillinase* enzyme, low risk of allergic reactions and good ratio of activity against Gram-positive and Gram-negative compared to penicillin. The clinical use of Cephalosporin C was limited due its weak antibacterial activity and difficulty in isolation. Basic nucleus of Cephalosporin is 7-Amino cephalosporanic acid (7-ACA), which was derived from the hydrolysis of Cephalosporin-C. Modification of the 7-ACA side-chains resulted in the development of useful antibiotic agents and the first agent Cephalothin was launched by Eli Lilly in 1964.

### 2.1.2.2 Chemistry of Cephalosporins

Cephalosporin consists of bicyclic ring system called as cepham, a 4-membered lactam ring fused through the nitrogen and the adjacent tetrahedral carbon atom to a second heterocycle forming a 6-membered dihydrothiazine ring. Other structural features common to all the Cephalosporins are a carboxyl group on the dihydrothiazine ring on the carbon next to the ring nitrogen and a functionalized amino group on $C_7$, the carbon of the β-lactam ring opposite the nitrogen. The fused ring system is designated by Chemical Abstracts as 5-Thia-1-azabicyclo [4.2.0] oct-2-ene.

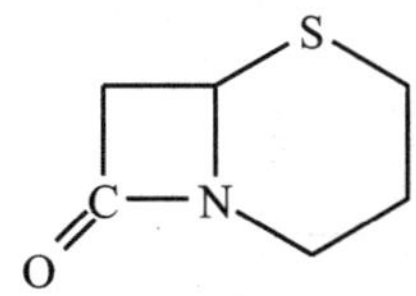


Cepham

Basic nucleus of Cephalosporin is 7-Amino cephalosporanic acid (7-ACA).

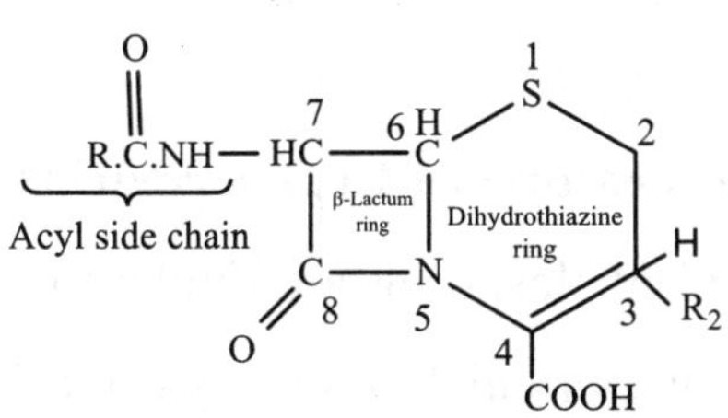


General structure of Cephalosporin

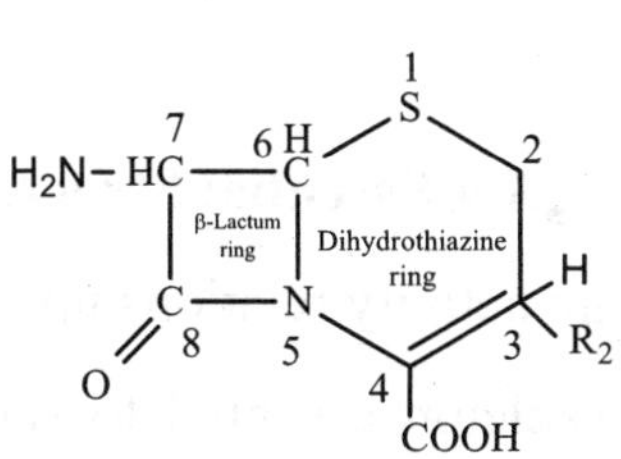


7 -Amino cephalosporanic acid

7-Aminocephalosporinic acid (7-ACA) is used as precursor for many semi-synthetic Cephalosporins. Advantages of semi-synthetic Cephalosporins over natural Caphalosporins are

- increased acid stability
- better oral absorption
- broad antimicrobial spectrum
- increased activity against resistant microorganisms.
- decreased allergenicity
- increased tolerance.

**2.1.2.3 Mechanism of Action:** Cephalosporins are bactericidal and have the same mode of action as other β-lactam antibiotics (such as Penicillins). Cephalosporins disrupt the synthesis of the peptidoglycan layer of bacterial cell walls. The peptidoglycan layer is important for cell wall structural integrity, especially in Gram-positive organisms. The final transpeptidation step in the synthesis of the peptidoglycan is facilitated by *transpeptidases* known as penicillin binding proteins.

**2.1.2.4 Structure Activity Relationship**

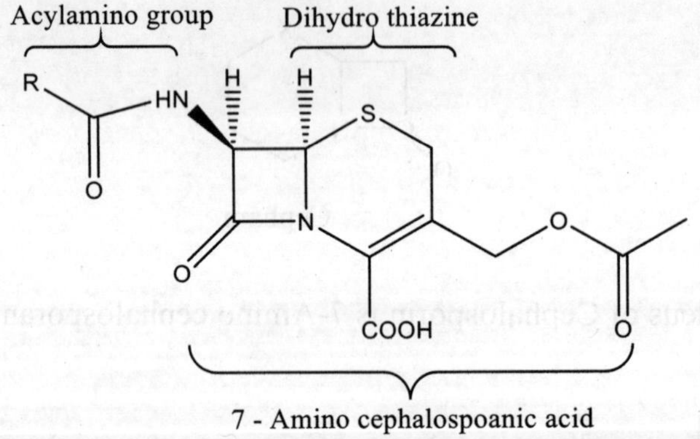


**Fig.1.4 Essential Structural Features of Cephalosporins**

- Structure activity relationships of Cephalosporins are similar to penicillins.
- Basic skeleton essential to show bactericidal activity are the bicyclic ring, free carboxylate group and Cis stereochemistry at $C_6$ and $C_7$. The cephalosporins are derivatives of 7-Aminocephalosporanic acid and are closely related in structure to penicillin.

- They have a β-lactam ring which is vital for activity. Bicyclic ring system, fused β-lactam and dihydrothiazine ring form a bicyclic system which is important for activity.
- The *cis*-stereochemistry at positions 6 and 7 are important.
- They are relatively stable in dilute acid and are highly resistant to *penicillinase.*
- Like penicillin modification can be made in limited position at 7-acylamino side chain and 3-acetoxylmethyl side chain
- The acylamino side chain may be altered.
- Other groups may be substituted for the acetoxy group which may or may not serve as good leaving group. The nature of the leaving group is important for activity.
- Better leaving group tend to give better activity.

**(a) First-Generation Cephalosporins:** Activity is comparably lower than penicillins but possess a broad spectrum of activity. Greater activity for Gram-positive organisms than Gram-negative organisms. The methyl group in Cephalexin is a poor leaving group (less active), but improves absorption. Cephalothin has an acetoxy as a leaving group and 1-(Thiophen-2-yl) propan-2-one in its acylamino side chain. Despite being a good leaving group, the acetoxy moiety is susceptible to enzyme-catalyzed hydrolysis. Cephaloglycin acylamino side chain is same as Ampicillin. Cephaloridine has pyridinium as a leaving group.

**(b) Second-Generation Cephalosporins:** Have increased activity against Gram-negative bacteria, but some have decreased Gram-positive activity. Many can cross the blood-brain barrier. **Cefuroxime** is also an example of an oximino cephalosporin**.** The presence of the imino methoxy group appears to increase stability against certain *β-lactamases*.

**(c) Third-Generation Cephalosporins:** Even better activity against Gram-negative bacteria. Some compounds have the same problem of decreased Gram-positive activity as the previous generation. Improved *β-lactamase* resistance and many can also cross blood-brain barrier.

**(d) Fourth-Generation Cephalosporins:** Better Gram-negative bacteria activity, *β-lactamase* resistance and many can cross blood-brain barrier. Gram-positive activity similar to the first generation. The fourth-generation compound exists as Zwitterion. They are also used against *Pseudomonas aeruginosa*.

**(e) Fifth-Generation Cephalosporins:** It is used to treat bacteria, including methicillin-resistant *Staphylococcus aureus* (MRSA) and Streptococcus species, that are resistant to penicillin antibiotics and Gram-positive bacteria. eg. Ceftaroline, Ceftobiprole.

**(f) Cephalosporin combinations:** eg. Cefadroxil with Clavulanate K, Cefadroxil with Probenecid, Cefalexin with Bromohexine HCl, Cefepime with Tazobactam, Cefepime with Sulbactam, Cefixime with Ornidazole, Cefixime with Azithromycin, Cefixime with Clavulanic acid, Cefixime with Ofloxacin, Cefixime with Clavulanate K, Cefixime with Dicloxacillin, Cefixime with Sulbactam, Cefoperazone with Tazobactam, Cefotaxime with Sulbactam, Cefpirome with Sulbactam, Cefpodoxime with Sulbactam, Cefpodoxime with Clavulanate K, Clavulanate K with Clavulanic acid, Cefpodoxime with Levofloxacin, Cefpodoxime with Dicloxacillin, Cefpodoxime with Azithromycin, Cefpodoxime with Ofloxacin, Ceftazidime with Tazobactam, Ceftriaxone with Sulbactam, Ceftriaxone with Tazobactam, Cefuroxime with Clavulanate K, Cefuroxime with Sulbactam, Cefuroxime with Clavulanic acid and Cefuroxime with Linezoid.

### 2.1.2.5 Clinical Uses

Cephalosporins are indicated for the prophylaxis and treatment of bacterial infections caused by susceptible organisms. First-generation cephalosporins are predominantly active against Gram-positive bacteria and successive generations have increased activity against Gram-negative bacteria.

### 2.1.2.6 Degradation of Cephalosporins

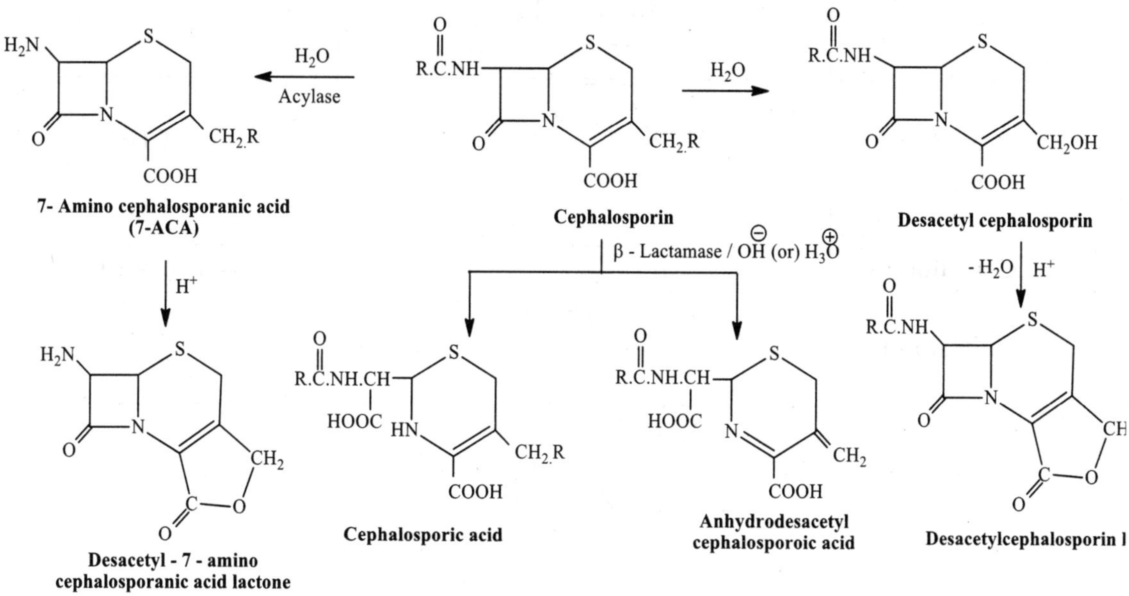


**Table 1.2 Structures of Cephalosporins**

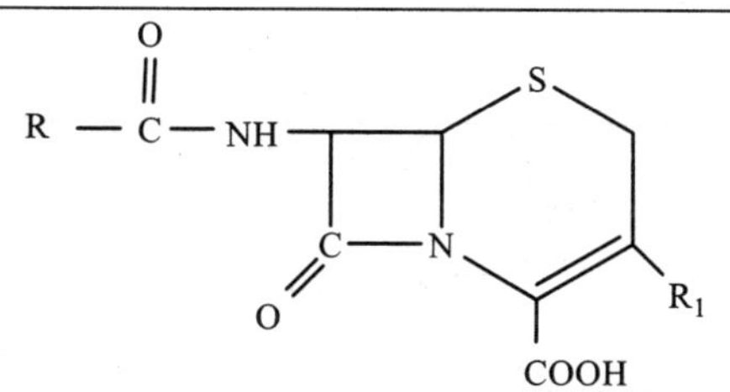


| Generic Name | R | R1 |
|---|---|---|
| | **First Generation** | |
| Cephalexin | 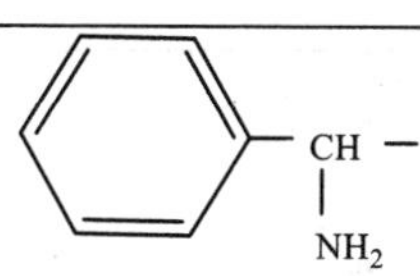 | $-CH_3$ |

| | | |
|---|---|---|
| Cefradine | 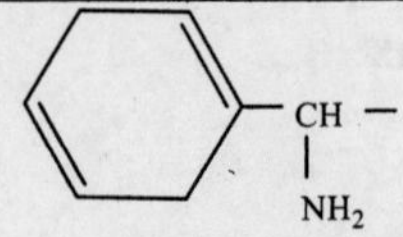 | $-CH_3$ |
| Cefadroxil | 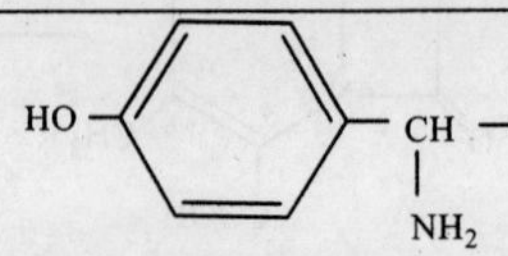 | $-CH_3$ |
| Cephalothin/ Cefalotin | 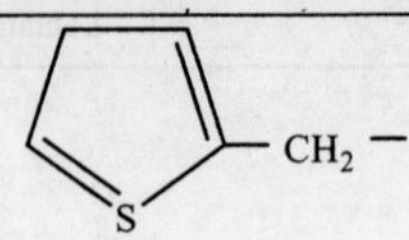 | $-CH_2OC(=O)CH_3$ |
| Cefazolin | 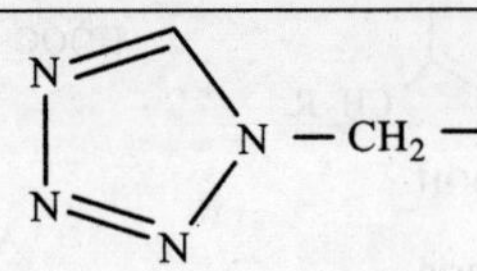 | 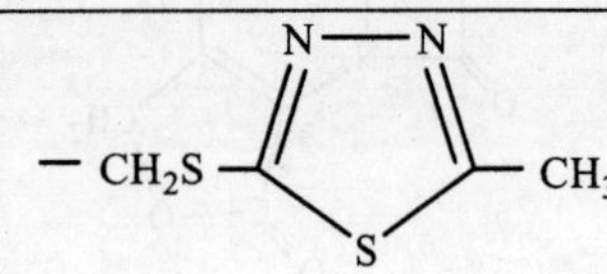 |
| **Second Generation** | | |
| Cefaclor | 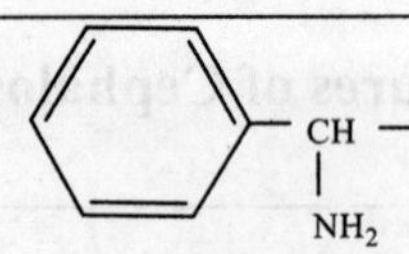 | $-Cl$ |
| Cefprozil | 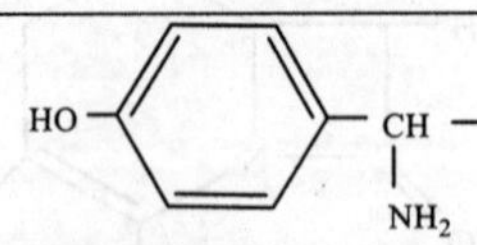 | $-CH=CHCH_3$ |
| Cefamandole | 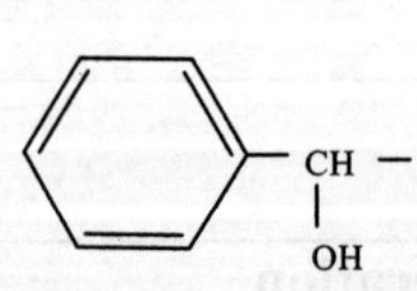 | 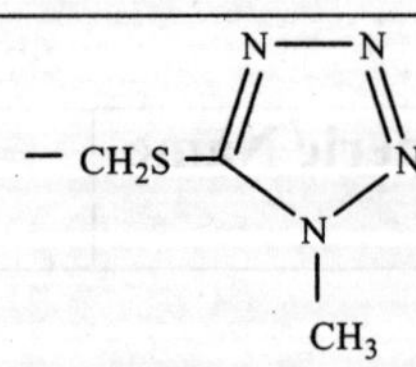 |
| Cefuroxime | 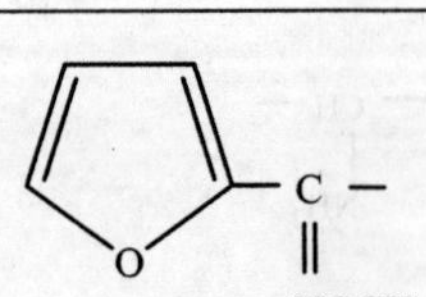 | $-CH_2OC(=O)NH_2$ |

| | | |
|---|---|---|
| Cefoxitin | 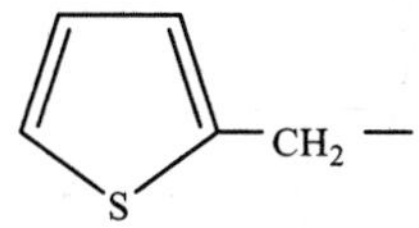 | $-\ CH_2OCONH_2$ (– $OCH_3$ at $C_7$ also) |
| Cefotetan | 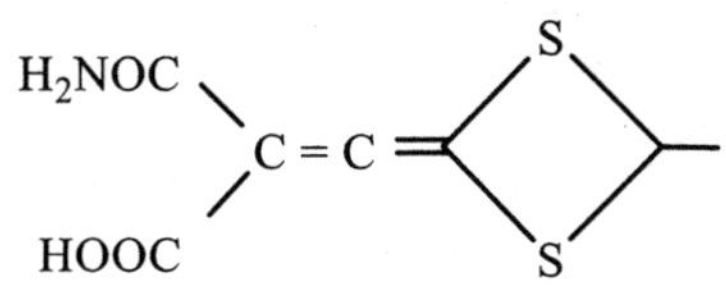 | 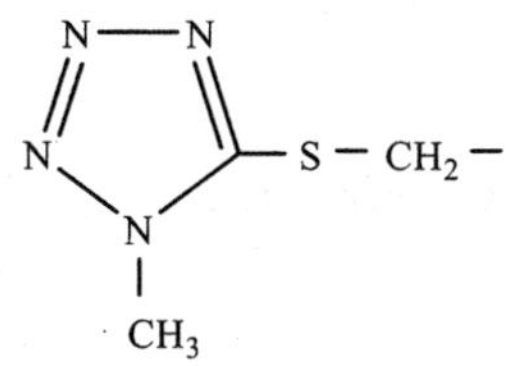 |
| **Third Generation** | | |
| Cefotaxime | 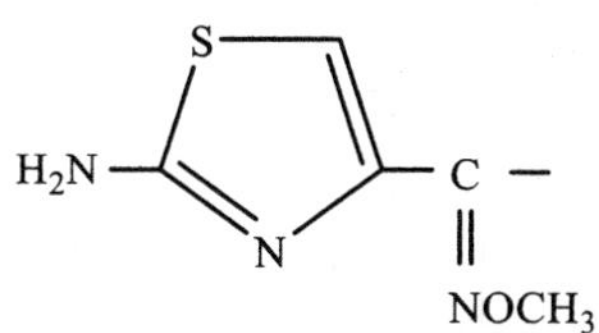 | 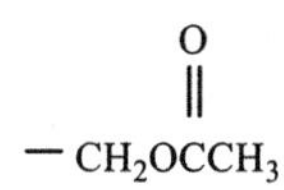 |
| Cefpodoxime | 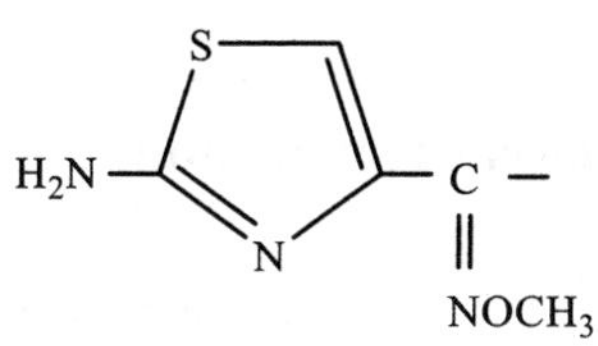 | $-\ CH_2.O.CH_3$ |
| Cefixime | 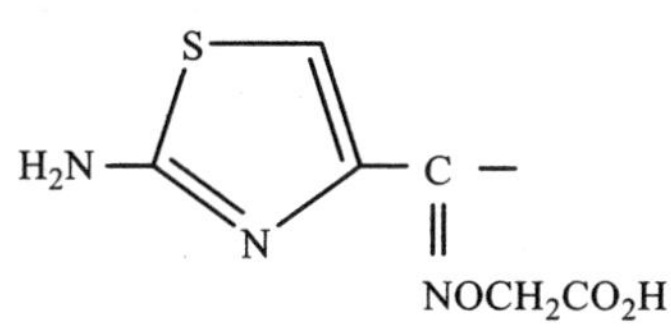 | $-CH=CH_2$ |
| Ceftizoxime | 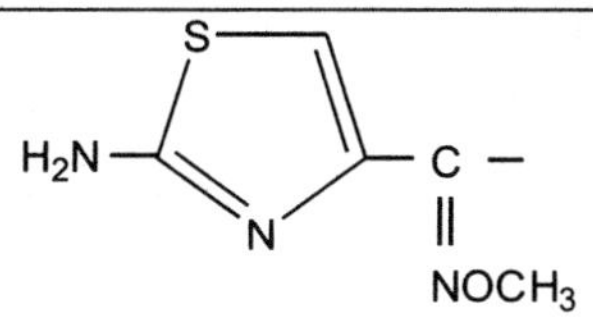 | $-H$ |

<table>
<tr><td>Ceftriaxone</td><td>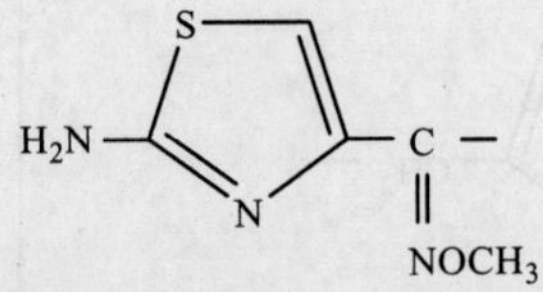</td><td>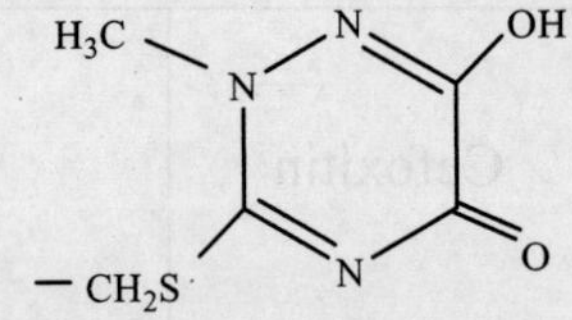</td></tr>
<tr><td>Ceftazidime</td><td>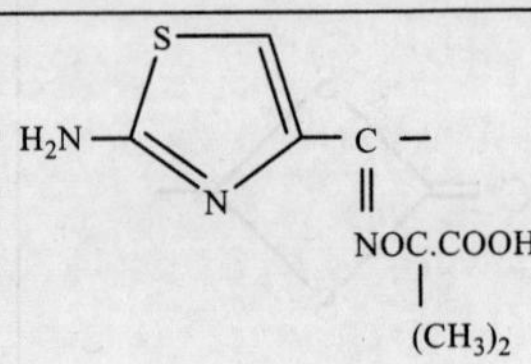</td><td>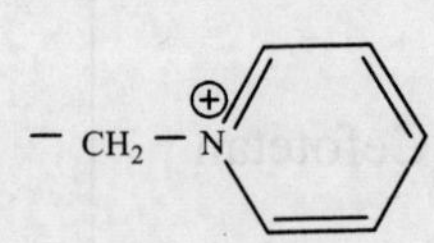</td></tr>
<tr><td>Cefoperazone</td><td>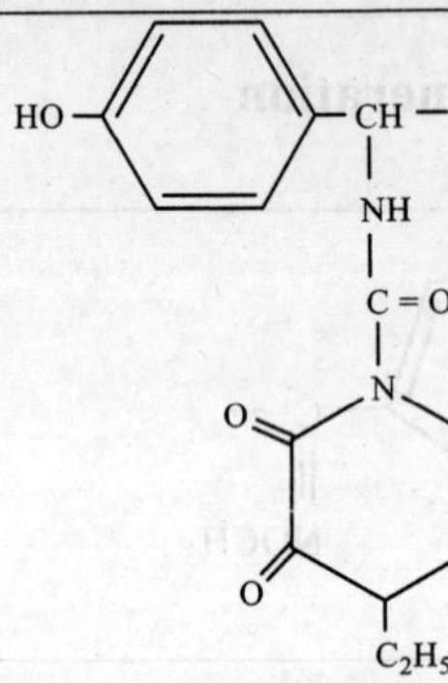</td><td>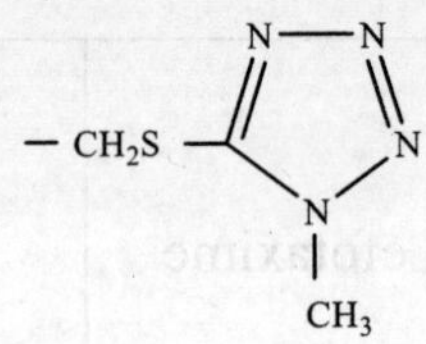</td></tr>
</table>

**Fourth Generation**

<table>
<tr><td rowspan="3">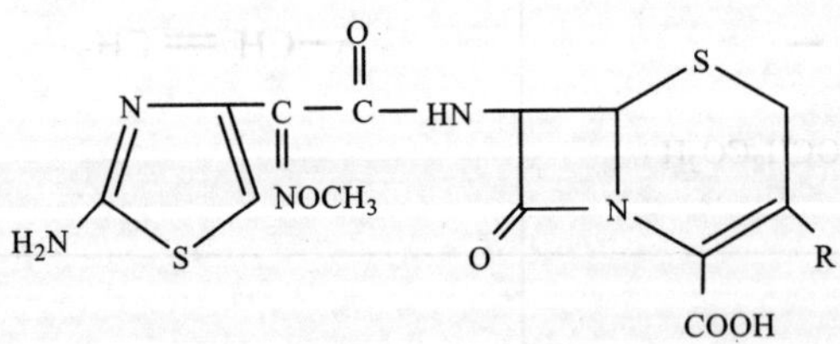</td><td>Generic Name</td><td>R</td></tr>
<tr><td>Cefepime</td><td>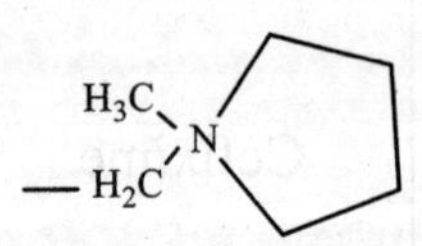</td></tr>
<tr><td>Cefpirome</td><td>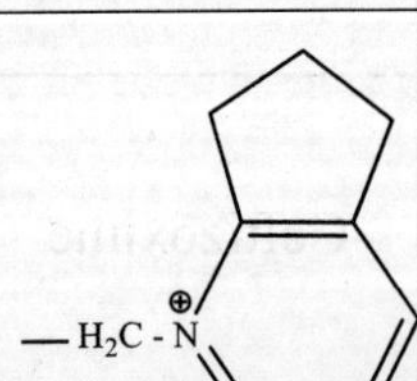</td></tr>
</table>

## 2.1.2.7 CLASSIFICATION

The classification of Cephalosporin into generations is commonly practiced, although the exact categorization of Cephalosporins is often in precise.

### I. Based on Generation

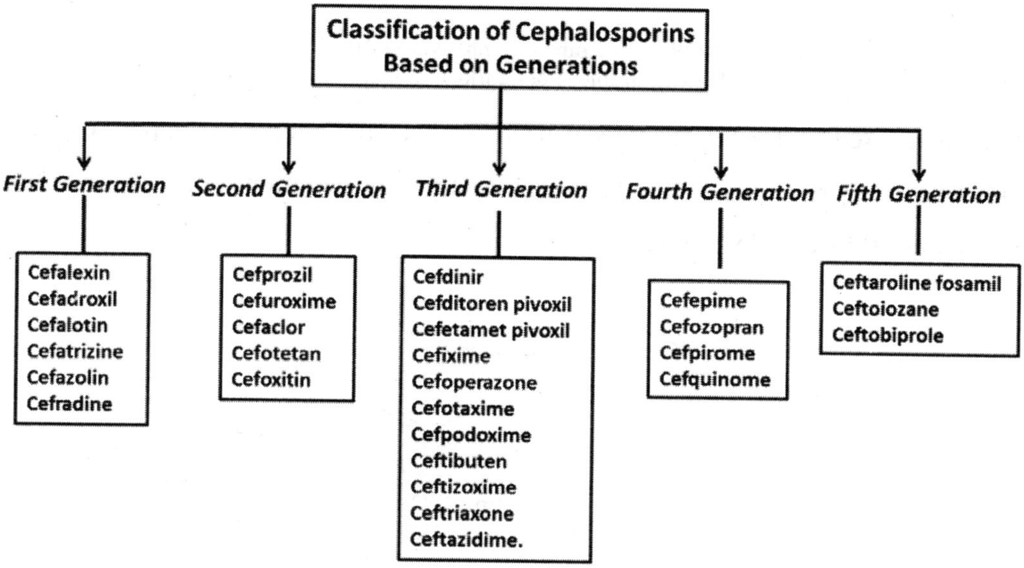


### II. Based on Route of Administration

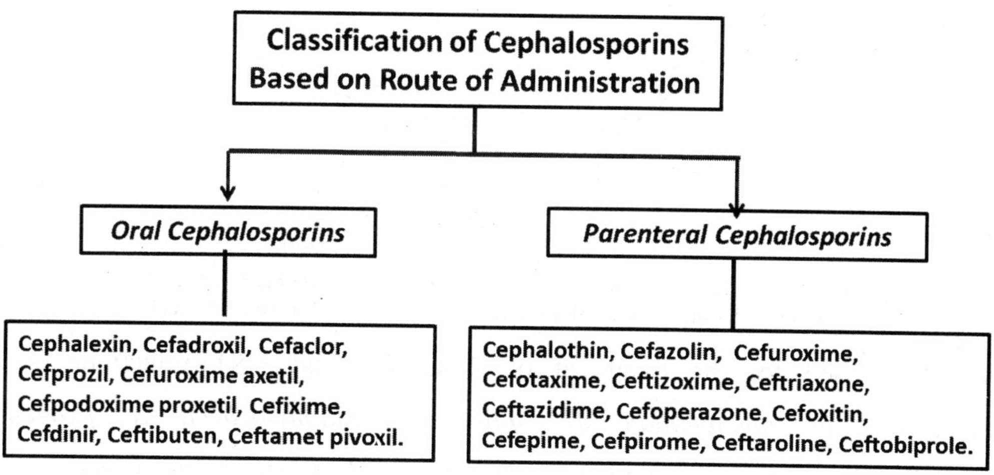

## (I). First Generation

### A. Cefalexin (Biocef)

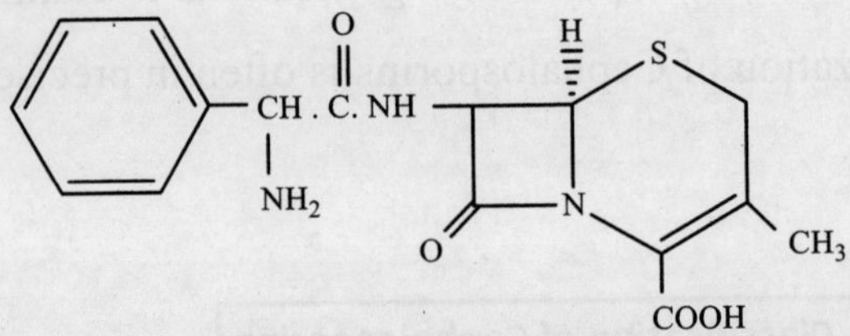

(6R,7R) - 7 - {[(2R) - 2 - amino - 2 - phenylacetyl]amino} - 3 - methyl - 8 - oxo - 5 - thia - 1 - azabicyclo[4.2.0]oct - 2 - ene - 2 - carboxylic acid

**Use:** It is used to treat infections caused by bacteria, including upper respiratory infections, ear infections, skin infections, urinary tract infections and bone infections.

### B. Cephalothin/Cefalotin (Keflin)

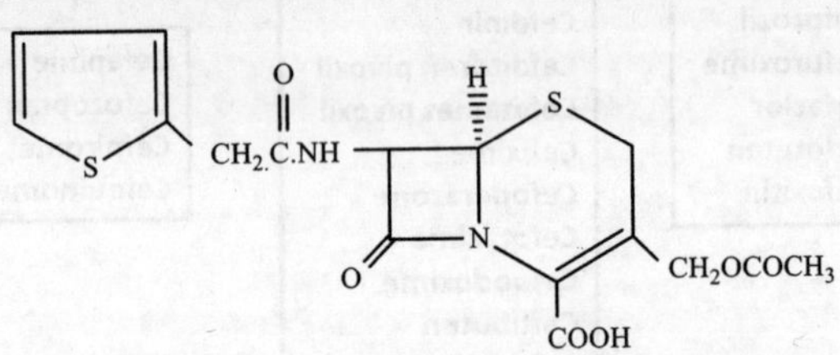

(6R,7R) - 3 - [(acetyloxy)methyl] - 8 - oxo - 7 - [2 - (thiophen - 2 - yl)acetamido] - 5 - thia - 1 - azabicyclo[4.2.0]oct - 2 - ene - 2 - carboxylic acid

**Use:** It is used to treat the infections of the respiratory tract, skin and urinary tract.

### C. Cefadroxil (Duricef)

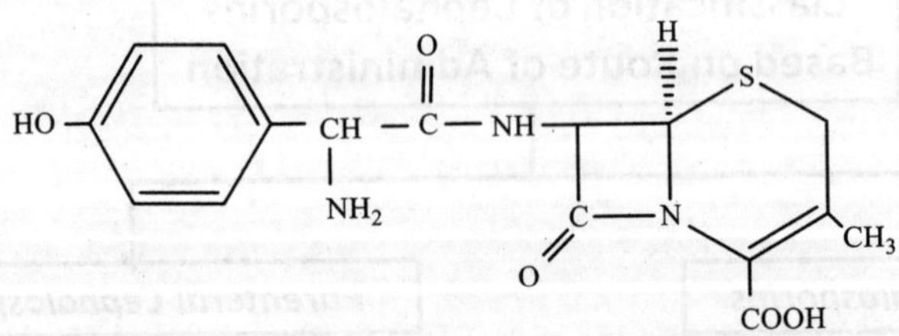

(6R,7R) - 7 - [(2R) - 2 - amino - 2 - (4 - hydroxyphenyl)acetamido] -3 - methyl - 8 - oxo - 5 - thia - 1 - azabicyclo[4.2.0]oct - 2 - ene - 2 -carboxylic acid

**Use:** It is used for the treatment of skin, UTI and ENT infections caused by *Streptococcus pneumoniae*, *H. influenzae*, *Staphylococci*, *S. pyogenes*, *Klebsiella* spp., *coagulase*-negative *Staphylococci* and *Streptococcus pyogenes*.

### D. Cefazolin (Ancef)

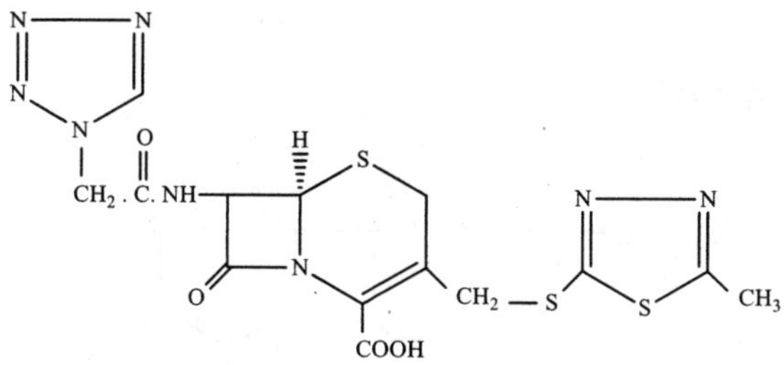

(6R,7R) - 3 - {[(5 - methyl - 1,3,4 - thiadiazol - 2 - yl)sulfanyl]methyl} - 8 - oxo - 7 - [2 - (1H - 1,2,3,4 - tetrazol - 1 - yl)acetamido] - 5 - thia - 1 - azabicyclo[4.2.0]oct - 2 -ene - 2 - carboxylic acid

**Use:** It is used to treat cellulitis, urinary tract infections, pneumonia, endocarditis, joint infection and biliary tract infections.

## (II). Second Generation

### A. Cefuroxime (Zinacef)

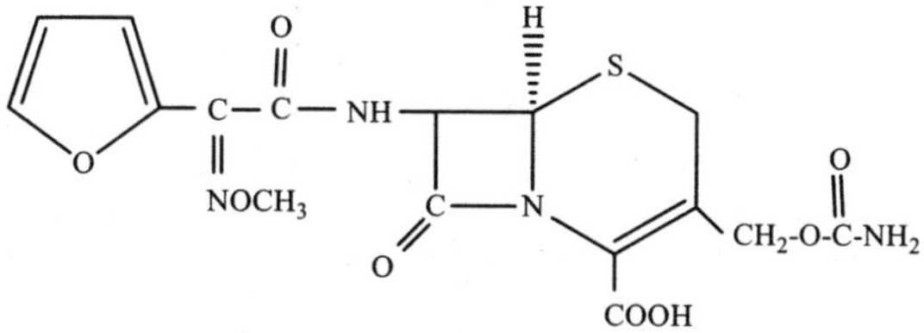

(6R,7R) - 3 - [(carbamoyloxy)methyl] - 7 - {[(2Z) - 2 - furan - 2 - yl - 2 -(methoxyimino)acetyl]amino}- 8 - oxo - 5 - thia - 1 - azabicyclo[4.2.0]oct - 2 - ene - 2 -carboxylic acid

**Use:** It is used for the treatment of many bacterial infections such as bronchitis, sinusitis, tonsillitis, ear infections, skin infections, gonorrhea and urinary tract infections.

## (III). Third Generation

### A. Cefotaxime (Claforan)

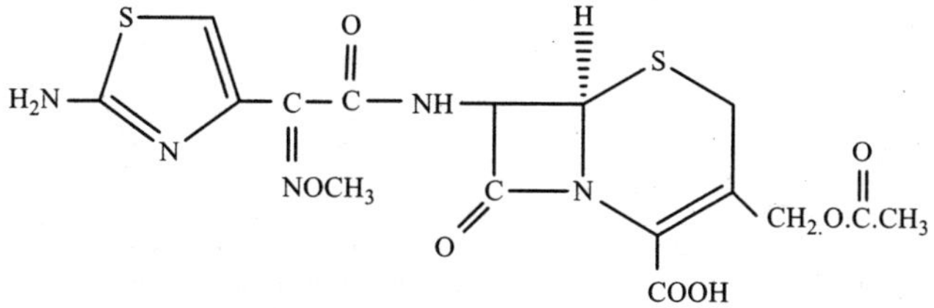

(6R,7R) - 3 - Acetoxymethyl - 7 - {2 - (2 - amino - thiazol - 4 - yl) - 2 - [(Z) -methoxyimino] - acetylamino} - 8 - oxo - 5 - thia - 1 - aza - bicyclo[4.2.0]oct - 2 - ene - 2 - carboxylic acid

**Use:** It is used to treat gonorrhoea, meningitis and severe infections of urinary system.

**B. Cefpodoxime (Cefoprox)**

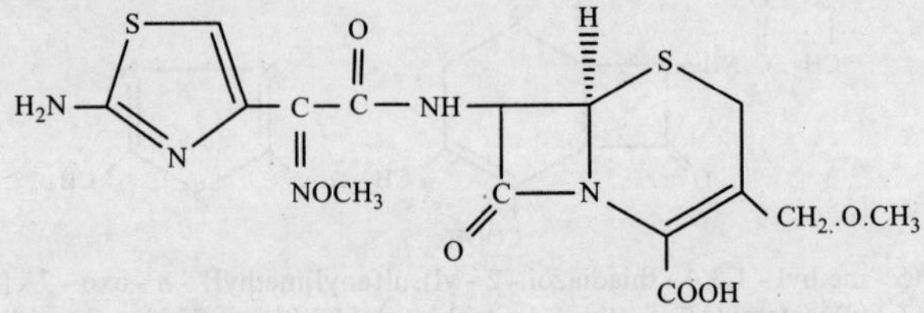

(6R,7R) -7 - [(2Z) - 2 - (2 - amino - 1,3 - thiazol - 4 - yl) - 2 - (methoxyimino)acetamido] - 3 - (methoxymethyl) - 8 - oxo - 5 - thia - 1 -azabicyclo[4.2.0]oct - 2 - ene - 2 - carboxylic acid

**Use:** It is used to treat acute otitis media, pharyngitis and sinusitis.

**C. Cefixime (Eurox)**

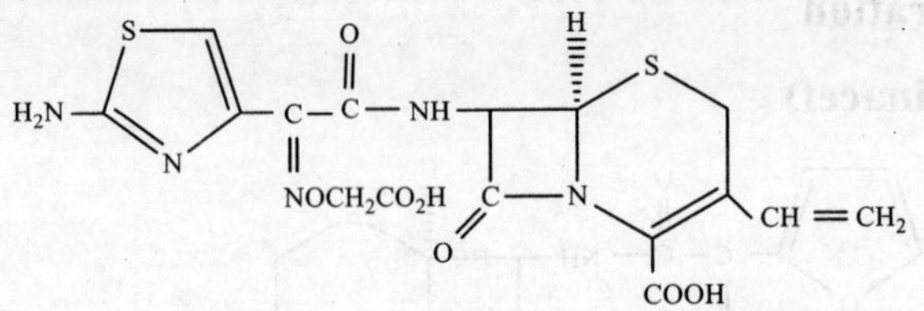

(6R,7R) - 7 - [(2Z) - 2 - (2 - amino - 1,3 - thiazol - 4 - yl) - 2 -[(carboxymethoxy)imino]acetamido] - 3 - ethenyl - 8 - oxo - 5 - thia - 1 -azabicyclo[4.2.0]oct - 2 - ene - 2 - carboxylic acid

**Use:** It is used for the treatment of otitis media, strep throat, pneumonia, urinary tract infections and gonorrhea.

**(IV). Fourth Generation**

**A. Cefpirome (Cefrom)**

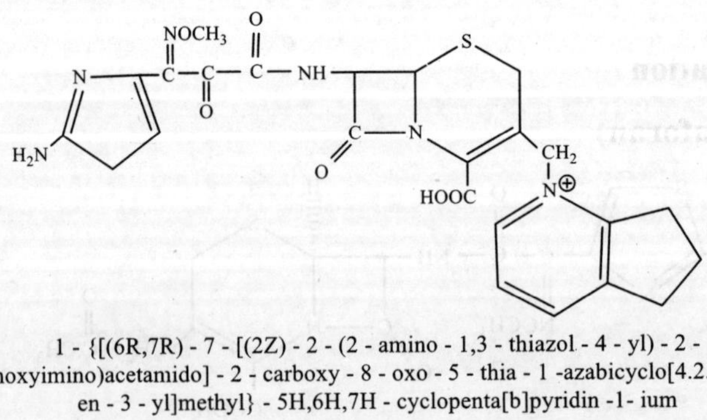

1 - {[(6R,7R) - 7 - [(2Z) - 2 - (2 - amino - 1,3 - thiazol - 4 - yl) - 2 - (methoxyimino)acetamido] - 2 - carboxy - 8 - oxo - 5 - thia - 1 -azabicyclo[4.2.0]oct - 2 - en - 3 - yl]methyl} - 5H,6H,7H - cyclopenta[b]pyridin -1- ium

**Use:** It is active against Gram-negative bacteria, including *P. aeruginosa* and Gram-positive bacteria.

## B. Cefepime (Axepim)

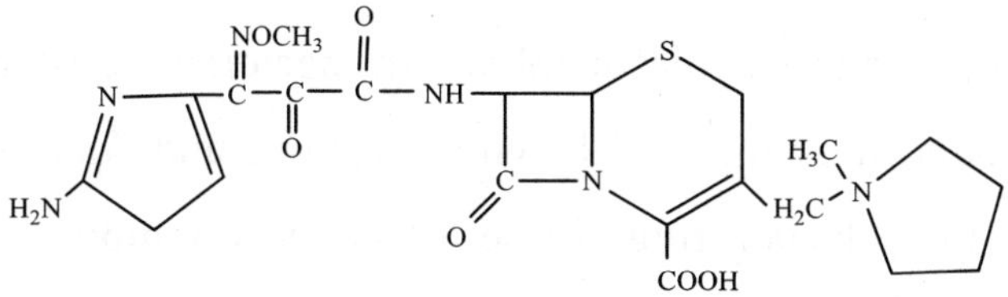

(6R,7R) - 7 - {[(2Z) - 2 - (2 - amino - 1,3 - thiazol - 4 - yl) - 2 - (methoxyimino)acetyl]amino} - 3 - [(1 - methylpyrrolidinium - 1 - yl)methyl] - 8 -oxo - 5 - thia - 1 - azabicyclo[4.2.0]oct - 2 - ene - 2 - carboxylate

**Use:** It is active against Gram-positive and Gram-negative bacteria, usually to treat severe hospital-acquired pneumonia infections caused by multi-resistant microorganisms.

### (V). Fifth Generation

## A. Ceftaroline (Teflaro)

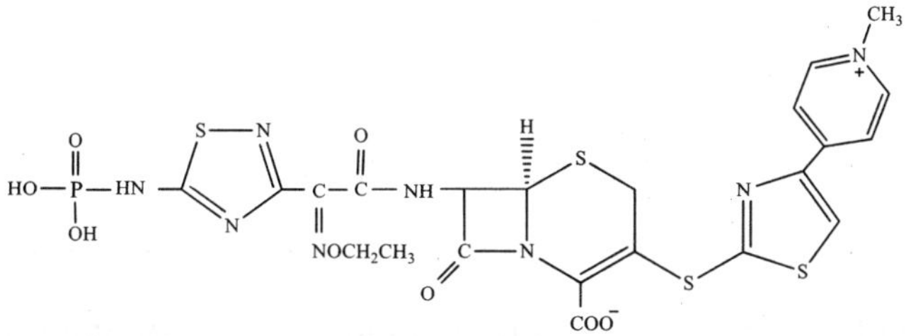

(6R,7R) - 7 - [(2Z) - 2 - ethoxyimino - 2 - [5 - (phosphonoamino) - 1,2,4 - thiadiazol - 3 - yl]acetyl]amino] - 3 - [4 - (1 - methylpyridin - 1 - ium - 4 - yl) - 1,3 - thiazol - 2 - yl]sulfanyl] - 8 - oxo - 5 - thia - 1 -azabicyclo[4.2.0]oct - 2 - e ne - 2 - carboxylate

**Use:** It is active against Methicillin resistant *Staphylococcus aureus* (MRSA) and few Gram-positive bacteria.

## B. Ceftobiprole (Zevtera)

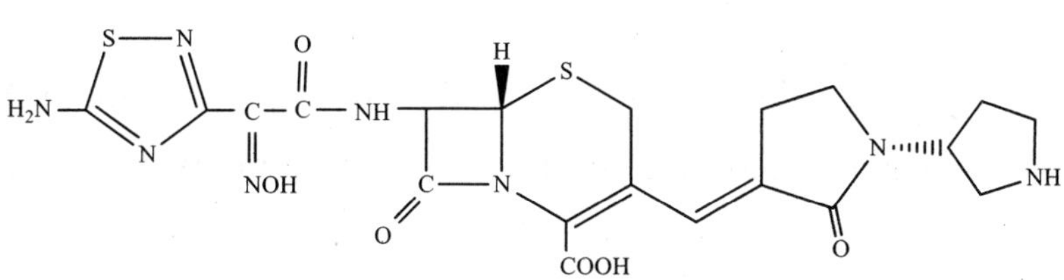

(6R,7R) - 7 - [(2Z) - 2 - (5 - amino - 1,2,4 - thiadiazol - 3 - yl) - 2 - (N - hydroxyimino)acetamido] - 8 - o xo - 3 - {[(3E,3'R) - 2 - oxo - [1,3' - bipyrrolidin] - 3 -ylidene]methyl} - 5 - thia - 1 - azabicyclo[4.2.0]oct - 2 - ene - 2 - carboxylic acid

**Use:** It is active against Methicillin resistant *Staphylococcus aureus* (MRSA).

## 2.1.3. *β-LACTAMASE* INHIBITORS

*β-lactamase* is an enzyme involved in bacterial resistance to β-lactam antibiotics. It is produced by most of the Gram-positive and Gram-negative bacteria which break down the β-lactam ring. These *β-lactamase* inhibitors are used only in combination with either specific penicillins or cephalosporins. eg. Clavulanic acid, Sulbactam, Tazobactam.

**A. Clavulanic acid (Augmentin)**

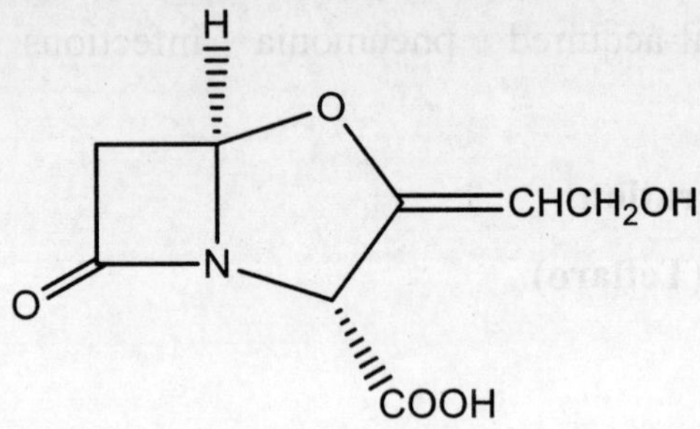


(2*R*, 5*R*, *Z*) - 3 - (2 - hydroxy ethylidene) - 7 - oxo - 4 - oxa - 1- azabicyclo [3.2.0] heptane - 2 - carboxylic acid

Clavulanic acid is derived from the organism *Streptomyces clavuligerus.* It is a *β-lactamase* inhibitor that is frequently combined with Amoxicillin or Ticarcillin to fight antibiotic resistance by preventing their degradation by *β-lactamase* enzymes, broadening their spectrum of susceptible bacterial infections.

**Mechanism of action:** It contains a β-lactam ring and binds strongly to *β-lactamase* at or near its active site, thereby hindering enzymatic activity. This protects other β-lactam antibiotics from *β-lactamase* catalysis, thereby enhancing their antibacterial effects.

**Use:** It is used in combination with Amoxicillin for treatment for skin infection, intra-abdominal and gynaecological sepsis, urinary respiratory tract infection and gonorrhoea.

## B. Sulbactam (Sultacillin)

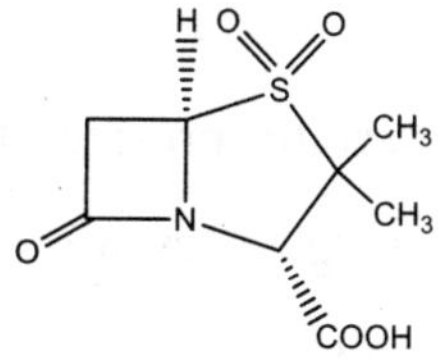


(2S, 5R) - 3, 3 - dimethyl - 7 - oxo - 4 - thia - 1 -azabicyclo (3.2.0) heptane - 2 - carboxylic acid - 4, 4 - dioxide

It is a semi-synthetic *β-lactamase* inhibitor. It is usually given in combination with either Ampicillin or Cefoperazone.

**Mechanism of action:** The β-lactam ring of Sulbactam irreversibly binds to *β-lactamase* at or near its active site, thereby blocking enzyme activity and preventing metabolism of other β-lactam antibiotics by the enzyme.

**Use:** It is currently available in combination with Ampicillin. This combination is used for the treatment of infections of skin caused by *β-lactamase* producing strains of *Staphylococcus aureus, Escherichia coli, Klebsiella pneumoniae, Proteus mirabilis, Enterobacter spp.*, and also for the treatment of gonorrhea, mixed aerobic-anaerobic infections and gynaecological infections.

## C. Tazobactam (Baclin)

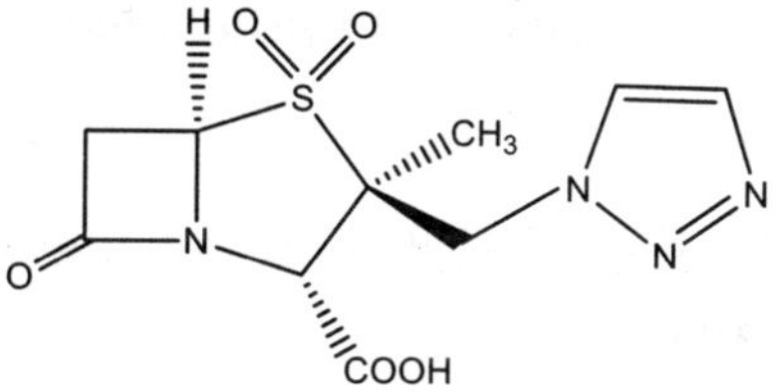


(2S, 3S, 5R) - 3 - methyl - 7 - oxo - 3 (IH- 1,2,3 triazol - 1 - ylmethyl) - 4- thia - 1 - azabicyclo [3.2.0] heptane - 2 - carboxylic acid - 4, 4 - dioxide

It is usually given in combination with Piperacillin and Ceftriaxone

**Mechanism of action:** It contains a β-lactam ring and irreversibly binds to *β-lactamase* at or near its active site. This protects other β-lactam antibiotics from *β-lactamase* catalysis. This drug is used in combination with *β-lactamase* susceptible penicillins to treat infections caused by *β-lactamase* producing organisms.

**Use:** It is combined with Piperacillin for the treatment of infections like peritonitis, pelvic urinary and respiratory infections caused by *β-lactamase* producing bacilli.

## 2.1.4 MONOBACTAMS

They are monocyclic and bacterially produced β-lactam antibiotics. In which β-lactam ring is not fused to another ring. They are effective against Gram-negative bacteria like Neisseria, Pseudomonas etc., eg. Aztreonam, Tigemonam, Nocardicin A, Tabtoxin, Carumonam.

**A. Aztreonam (Azactam)**

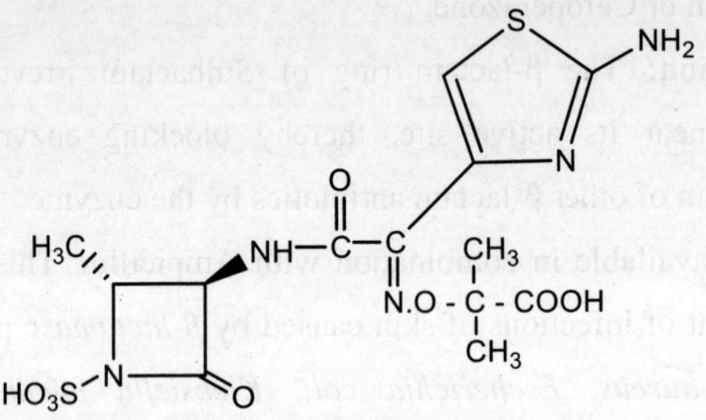

(Z) - 2 - {[(((2 - Amino - 4 - thiazolyl) (((2S,3S) - 2 methyl - 4 - oxo -1 - sulfo - 3 - azetidinyl)carbamoyl) methyene)amino]oxy}- 2 - methyl propionicacid

It is a monocyclic β-lactam antibiotic originally isolated from *Chromobacterium violaceum*. It is resistant to *β-lactamases* and is used in Gram-negative infections.

**Mechanism of action:** It inhibit the bacterial cell wall synthesis by binding with the penicillin binding protein 3 (PBP3).

**Use:** It is used for the treatment of infections caused by susceptible Gram-negative microorganisms, urinary tract infections, lower respiratory tract infections, septicemia, skin and soft tissue infections, intra-abdominal and gynecological infections.

### B. Tigemonam (Tigemen)

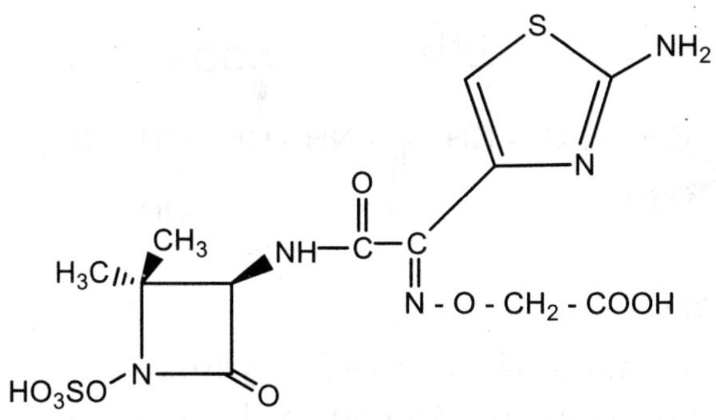


2 - [[1- (2 - Amino -1, 3 - thiazol - 4 - yl) - 2 - [[(3S) - 2, 2 - dimethyl - 4 - oxo - 1 - sulfooxyazetidin - 3 - yl]amino] - 2 - oxoethylidene]amino]oxyacetic acid

**Mechanism of action:** Same as Aztreonam.

**Use:** It is effective against *Escherichia coli* and *Klebsiella pneumonia.*

### C. Nocardicin A

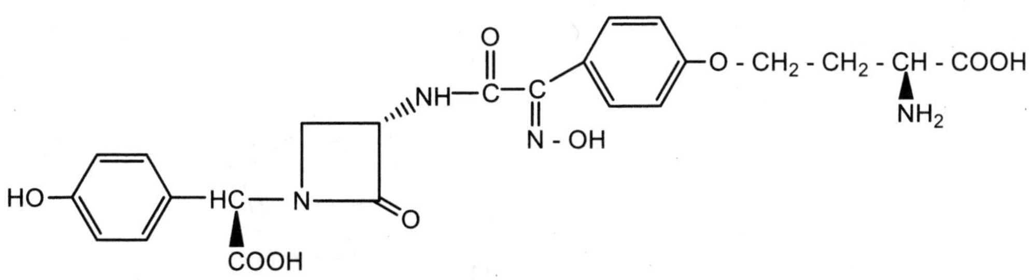


(2R) - 2 - Amino - 4 - [4 - [(Z) - C - [[(3S) - 1 - [(R) - carboxy - (4 - hydroxyphenyl)methyl] - 2 - oxoazetidin - 3 - yl]carbamoyl] - N - hydroxycarbonimidoyl]phenoxy]butanoic acid

It is a monocyclic β-lactam antibiotic obtained from the strains of *Nocardia uniformis*. It is stereo chemically and biologically related to Penicillin and Cephalosporins.

**Mechanism of action:** It acts by inhibiting peptidoglycan biosynthesis.

**Use:** It is effective against *Escherichia coli* and Gram-negative organisms, especially *Pseudomonas aeruginosa* (except *Proteus morganii*) *Serratia marcescens* and the *Neisseria* groups.

**D. Tabtoxin**

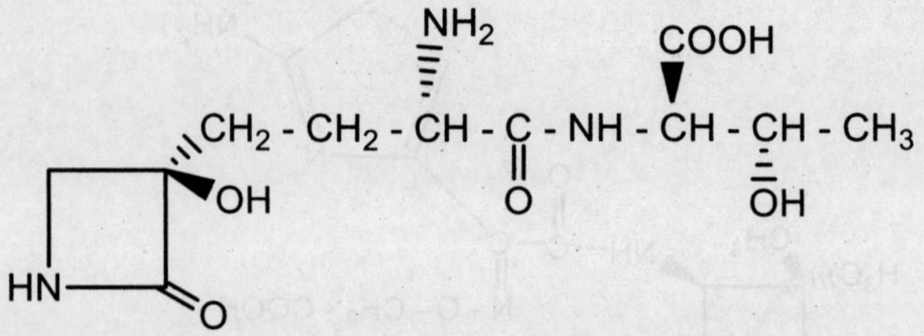

(2S,3R) -2 - [[(2S) - 2 - Amino - 4 - [(3S) - 3 - hydroxy - 2 - oxoazetidin - 3 - yl]butanoyl]amino] - 3 - hydroxybutanoic acid

It is also known as wildfire toxin which is a simple monobactam phytotoxin produced by *Pseudomonas syringae.*

**Mechanism of action:** It acts by inhibiting the enzyme *glutamine synthetase*.

**Use:** It is effective against Gram-negative organism especially *Pseudomonas* spp.

**E. Carumonam**

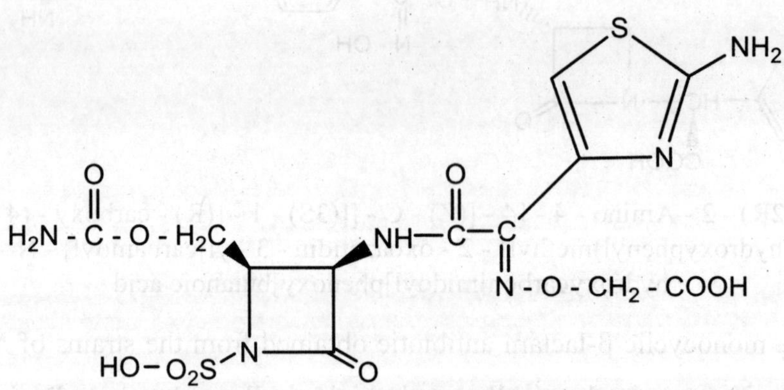

2 - [(Z) - [1 - (2 - amino - 1,3 - thiazol - 4 - yl) - 2 - [[(2S,3S) - 2 - (carbamoyloxymethyl)- 4 - oxo - 1 - sulfoazetidin - 3- yl]amino] - 2 - oxoethylidene]amino]oxyacetic acid

It is an N-sulfonated monocyclic β-lactam antibiotic derived from Sulfazecin.

**Use:** It is used for the treatment of urinary tract infections.

## 2.2 AMINOGLYCOSIDE ANTIBIOTICS

### 2.2.1 Introduction

Aminoglycoside antibiotics are from the *Actinomycetes*, particularly from the genus *Streptomyces*. Among the many antibiotics isolated from the genus, important one is Streptomycin. Several other closely related structures are Kanamycin, Neomycin, Gentamycin, Paromomycin, Tobramycin and Netilmycin. All the structures consist of amino sugars linked glycosidically. All have one amino hexose and some have a pentose. Additionally, each aminoglycoside contains a highly substituted 1, 3 - diamino cyclohexane central ring. They are all basic, water-soluble compounds or mixtures of compounds.

**2.2.2 Mechanism of Action:** They act directly on the bacterial ribosome to inhibit the initiation of protein synthesis and to interfere with translation of the genetic message. They bind to 30s ribosomal subunit to form a complex, that cannot initiate proper amino acid polymerization.

**2.2.3 Spectrum of Activity:** Aminoglycoside antibiotics are broad-spectrum antibiotics, particularly effective against Gram-negative bacilli, Gram-negative and Gram-positive *cocci* except *Staphylococci*, tent to be less sensitive. Streptomycin is particularly active against *Mycobacterium tuberculosis*. Paromomycin is used in amoebic dysentery.

### A. Streptomycin (Cipstryn)

Streptomycin is produced by a culture of *Streptomyces griseus*. It is official as Streptomycin sulfate. Streptomycin is meso (3,5 or 2,4-diguanidin trihydroxy cyclohexyl)-α- glycoside of a disaccharide- 2- (N-methyl-α-L-gluco pyranosamidino) -3-C-formyl-5-deoxy-L-aldopentofuranose. The diguanidino inositol portion is designated as Streptidine. By glycosidic linkage it is bonded to streptose (methyl pentose and streptosamine (N-methyl-L-glucosamine). Both guanido group of streptidine is essential for antibiotic activity.

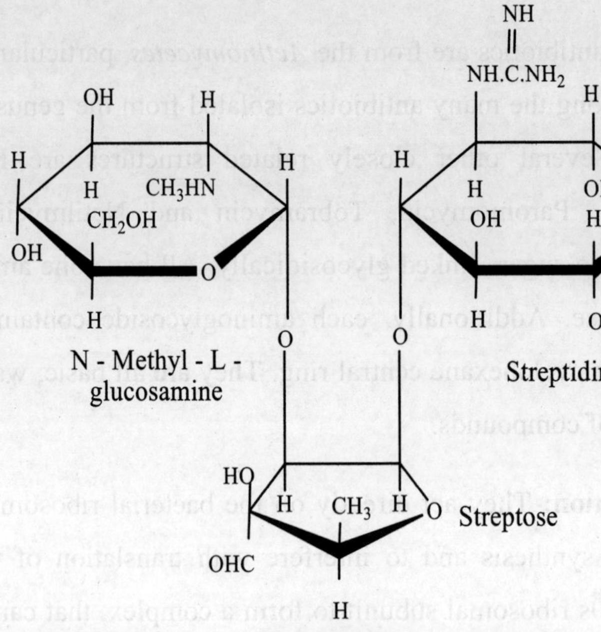


Streptomycin

**Hydrolysis**

Streptomycin —(Acid hydrolysis)→ Streptidine (Diacidic base) + Streptobiosamine (Mono acidic disaccharide)

Streptidine (Diacidic base) —(Hydrolysis)→ Streptamine (Diamino compound)

Streptobiosamine (Mono acidic disaccharide) —(Hydrolysis)→ N - Methyl - L - glucosamine

Streptose cannot be isolated because of its instability

**Use:** It is active against various Gram-positive and Gram-negative bacteria. It is effective against M*ycobacterium tuberculosis*. It is used in the treatment of TB along with other drugs PAS and Rifampicin.

### B. Neomycin B (Neo-Fradin)

Neomycin is a mixture of three substance isolated from *Streptomyces fradiae*. The three components A, B and C have been separated by counter-current distribution technique. Neomycin A is a disaccharide, which is a common degradation product of Neomycin B and C. Neomycin B and C consists of four carbohydrate units and differ only in the configuration of the amino-methyl group in the neosamine ring linked to the ribose unit. Neomycin as a sulfate salt is a white to slightly yellow crystalline hygroscopic and photosensitive powder, freely soluble in water.

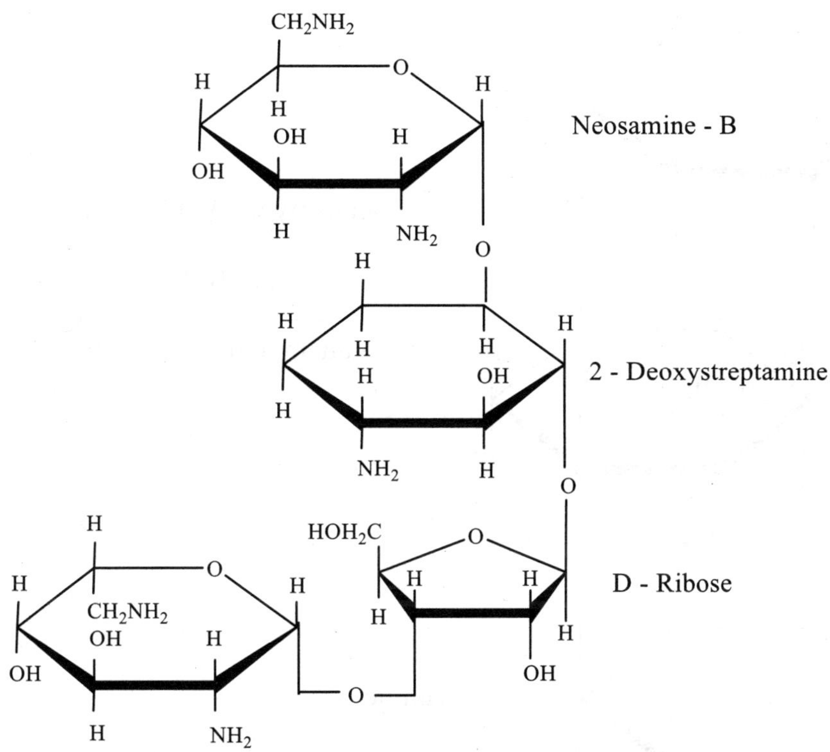


Neomycin B

**Use:** It is used for treatment of gastrointestinal infections, dermatological infections and acute bacterial peritonitis.

### C. Kanamycin (Kancan)

Kanamycin is isolated from a culture of *Streptomyces kanamyceticus*. Kanamycin is a mixture of component. They differ in the substituted D-glucose attached glycosidically to the 4th position of the deoxystreptamine ring. Kanamycin A contains 6-Amino-6-deoxy-D-glucose; Kanamycin B contains 2,6-Diamino-2,6-dideoxy-D-glucose; Kanamycin C contains 2-Amino-2-deoxy-D-glucose. It is basic in nature and forms salts with acids through its amino groups. It is water soluble. It is stable to heat and chemicals.

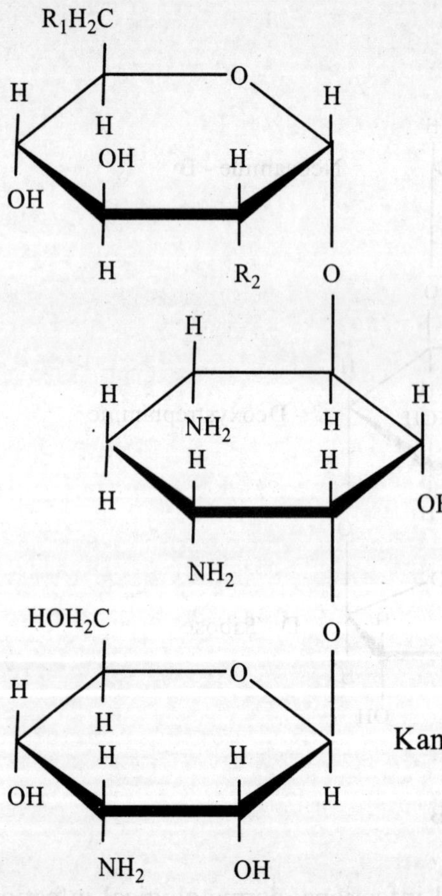


Kanamycin A: $R_1 = NH_2 : R_2 = OH$

Kanamycin B: $R_1 = NH_2 : R_2 = NH_2$

Kanamycin C: $R_1 = OH : R_2 = NH_2$

Kanosamine

**Use:** It is used in the treatment of infections of the intestinal tract and systemic infections.

## 2.3 TETRACYCLINES

### 2.3.1 Introduction

Tetracyclines is a broad spectrum antibiotic obtained by fermentation of *Streptomyces spp.* or by chemical transformation of natural products. They are derivatives of an octahydro-naphthacene, a hydrocarbon system, that comprises of four annulated six membered rings. The group name is derived from this tetracyclic system. The first member of the tetracycline group of antibiotic is Chlortetracycline from a culture of *Streptomyces aureofaciens*. Later Oxytetracycline was isolated from *Streptomyces rimosus*. Tetracycline is a group of antibiotic that include Tetracycline. Volitetracycline, Oxytetracycline, Chlortetracycline, Demeclocycline, Meclocycline, Methacyclin, Doxycycline and Minocycline.

**2.3.2 Chemistry:** The basic tetracycline structure consists of four benzene rings with various substitutions on the ring

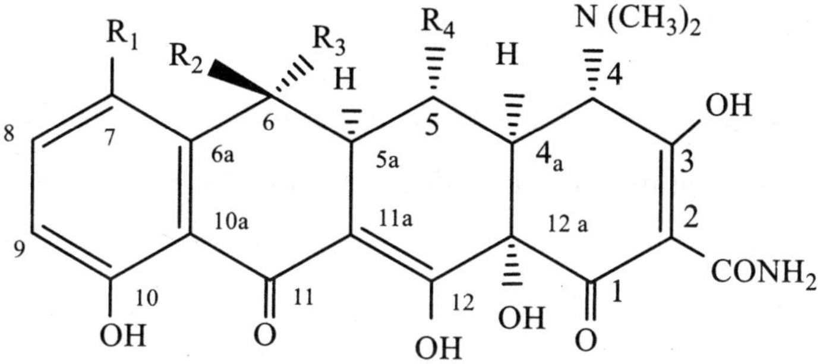


The stereochemistry of the tetracycline is very complex. Carbon atom 4, 4a, 5, 5a, 6 and 12a, are potentially chiral depending on substitution. Oxytetracycline and Doxycycline possess 5α-hydroxy substituent have six chiral carbon and others have only five chiral carbon. The tetracyclines are amphoteric in nature, forming salts with either acids or bases. It exists mainly as Zwitter ions in neutral solutions. They are yellow in color. The hydrochloride salts are used for oral administration and usually given is the form of capsule to mask the bitter taste.

### 2.3.3 Structure Activity Relationship

- Tetracycline and its analogues have basic chemical structure consisting tetracyclic naphthacene carboxamide ring system.

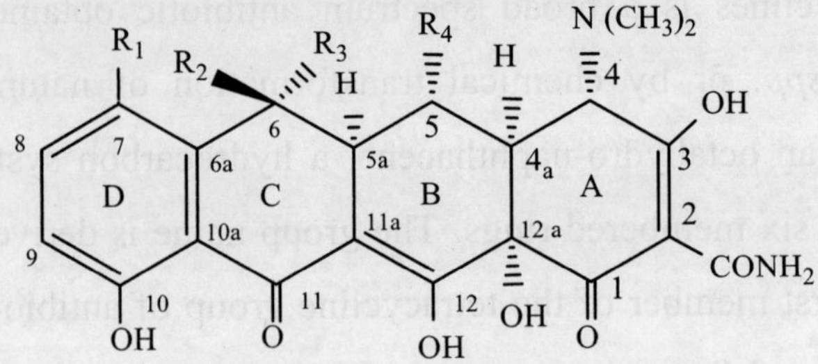


- An active tetracycline (antibacterial activity) must possess a linearly arranged DCBA naphthacene ring system with $C_1$-$C_3$ keto-enolic tautomer substructure and $C_2$ amide group.

- Functional groups at position 5, 6 and 7 or rings B, C and D in tetracyclines can be removed without drastically altering antimicrobial properties.
- All Tetracyclines to inhibit protein synthesis the amino group in position $C_4$ and keto-enolic tautomers in position $C_1$ & $C_3$ of the A ring is essential.

- The amino group at $C_4$ position is essential for the antibacterial activities. A $C_4$-dimethylamino group with its natural 4S isomer is required for optimal antibacterial activity, while epimerization to its 4R isomer decreases Gram–negative activity. It also requires a $C_{10}$-phenol and $C_{11}$-$C_{12}$ keto-enol substructure in conjunction with a 12a-OH group. All those substituents, with the respective tautomeric equilibrium, are indispensable for recognition and bonding in ribosomal subunits, where chemical modification abolishes the activity.

- Modification of the amide in $C_2$ is possible but with loss of potency.
- Chemical modification of the positions $C_5$ to $C_9$ gives various derivatives of tetracyclines with varying antibacterial activities.

- Modification of $R_2$, $R_3$ and $R_4$ groups gives better selectivity to the biological target in antifungal but not for antibacterial activity.
- Substitution of $R_4$ at 5th position with -OH group produces water soluble derivatives which can be administered orally.
- Elimination of -OH group at 6th position increases lipophilicity and more stable to acids. eg. Doxycycline.
- Additional glycylamino substitution at $C_9$ position leads to new class of antibiotics (Tigecyclines)
- The ring D should be always aromatic and changes in this ring leads to inactivation of biological activity.

**2.3.4 Mechanism of Action:** Tetracyclines are specific inhibitors of bacterial protein synthesis. They bind to the 30s ribosomal subunit and thereby prevent the binding of aminoacyl tRNA to the mRNA ribosome complex.

**2.3.5 Spectrum of Activity:** Tetracyclines are broad spectrum antibiotics, active against wide range of Gram-positive and Gram-negative bacteria, *Spirochetes, Mycoplasma, Rickettsia* and *Chalmydiae.* It is used in the treatment of life-threatening infections such as septicemia, endocarditis and meningitis.

**Table 1.3 Structure of Tetracyclines**

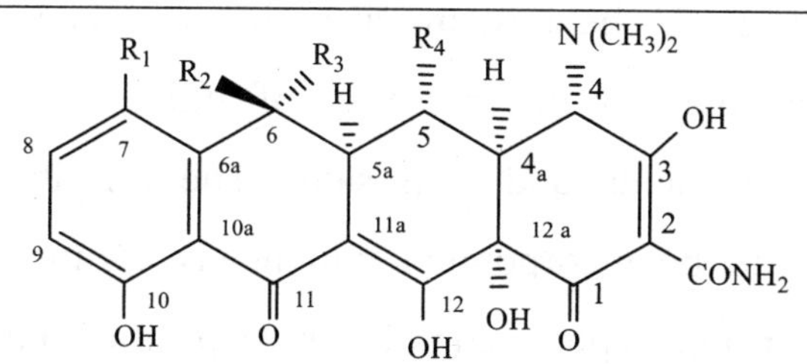


| S.No. | Name | R1 | R2 | R3 | R4 |
|---|---|---|---|---|---|

| 1. | Tetracyclines | - H | - OH | - $CH_3$ | - H |
|---|---|---|---|---|---|
| 2. | Chlortetracycline | - Cl | - OH | - $CH_3$ | - H |
| 3. | Oxytetracycline | - H | - OH | - $CH_3$ | - OH |
| 4. | Demeclocycline | - Cl | - OH | - H | - H |
| 5. | Methacycline | - H | - $CH_2$ | – | - OH |
| 6. | Doxycycline | - H | - $CH_3$ | - H | - OH |
| 7. | Minocycline | - $N(CH_3)_2$ | - H | - H | - H |
| 8. | Meclocycline | - Cl | - $CH_2$ | – | - OH |

The tetracycline is their ability to undergo epimerization at $C_4$ in solutions of intermediate pH range. These isomers are called epitetracycline. They exhibit less activity than the natural isomers.

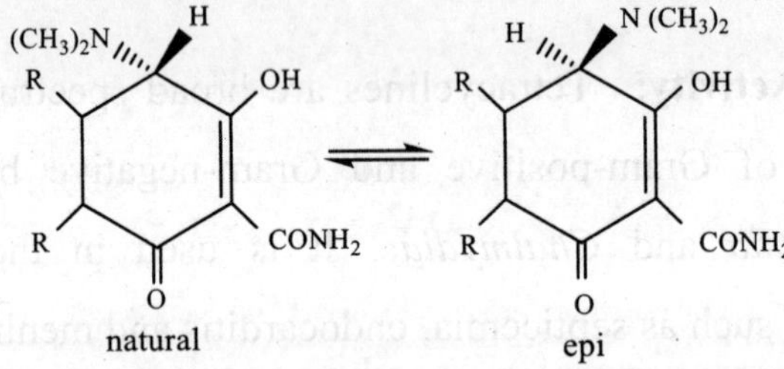


Tetracyclines forms a stable chelate with many metals including calcium, magnesium and iron, such chelates are insoluble in water, leading to impaired absorption of tetracyclines in the presence of milk, calcium, magnesium and aluminium-containing antacids and iron salts. The affinity of tetracyclines for calcium causes them to be incorporated into newly forming bones and teeth as tetracycline-calcium orthophosphate complexes. Deposit of these antibiotics in teeth cause a yellow discoloration that darkens over time. Tetracyclines are distributed into milk of lactating mothers and will cross the placental barrier into the fetus.

## 2.3.6 Degradation of Oxytetracycline

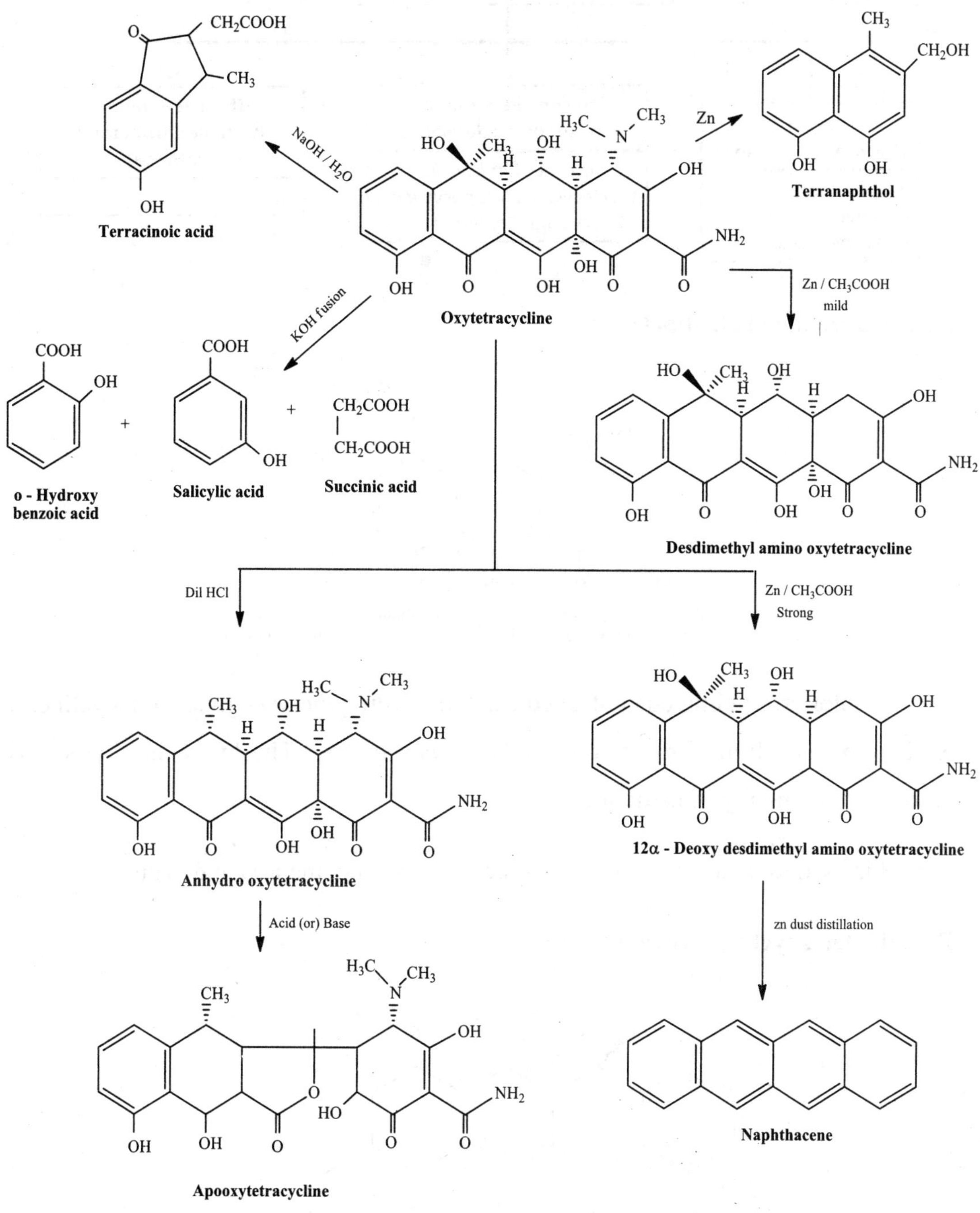

## 2.3.7 Classification

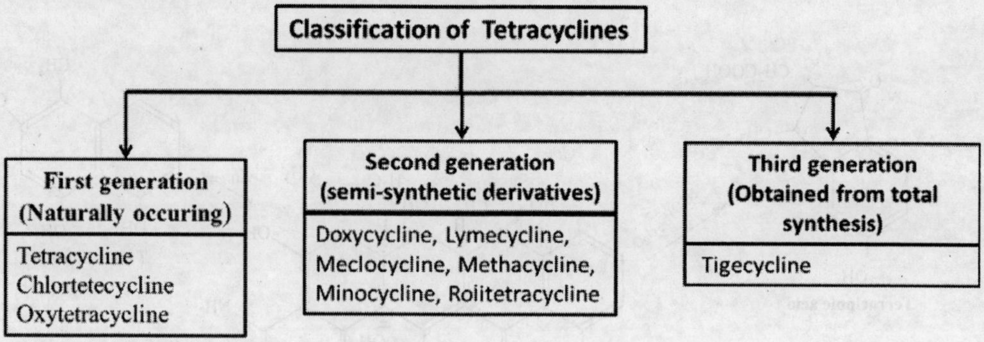


### A. Tetracycline (Tetrabact)

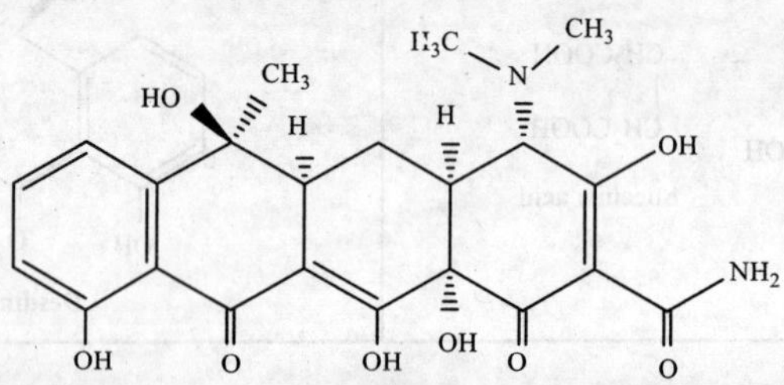


4 - Dimethylamino -1, 4, 4a, 5, 5a, 6, 11, 12a - octahydro - 3, 6, 10, 12, 12a - pentahydroxy - 6 - methyl - 1,11 - dioxo - 2 - naphthacene carboxamide

Chlortetracycline on controlled catalytic hydrogenolysis gives Tetracycline. It is also obtained from fermentation of *Streptomyces spp*. The hydrochloride salt is used most commonly in medicine.

**Use:** It is used to treat acne, cholera, brucellosis, plague, malaria and syphilis.

### B. Chlortetracycline (Aureomycin)

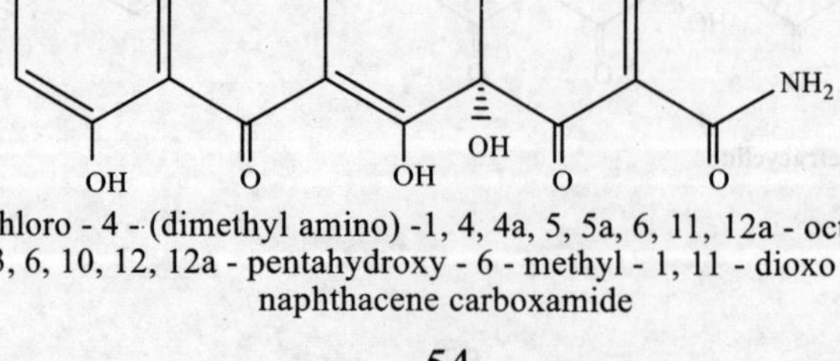


7 - Chloro - 4 - (dimethyl amino) -1, 4, 4a, 5, 5a, 6, 11, 12a - octahydro - 3, 6, 10, 12, 12a - pentahydroxy - 6 - methyl - 1, 11 - dioxo - 2 - naphthacene carboxamide

It is also called Aureomycin and was isolated from *Streptomyces aureofaciens*. Oral and parenteral forms of Chlortetracycline are no longer used because of poor bioavailability.

**Use:** It is used in the form of ointment for ophthalmic and topical use. It is most commonly used in veterinary practice.

## C. Oxytetracyclines (Terramycin)

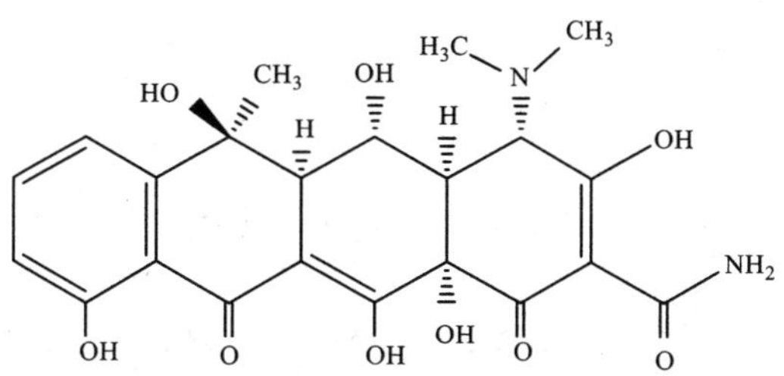

4 - Dimethylamino - 1, 4, 4a, 5, 5a, 6, 11, 12a - octahydro - 3, 5, 6, 10, 12, 12a - hexahydroxy - 6 - methyl - 1,11 - dioxo - 2 - naphthacene carboxamide

It is isolated from *Streptomyces rimosus*. It is used for parenteral administration.

**Use:** It is used to treat systemic bacterial and protozoal infections, such as bronchitis, chlamydial infection, lyme disease, nongonococcal urethritis, rickettsial infection, traveler's diarrhea and urinary tract infections.

## D. Doxycycline (Vibramycin)

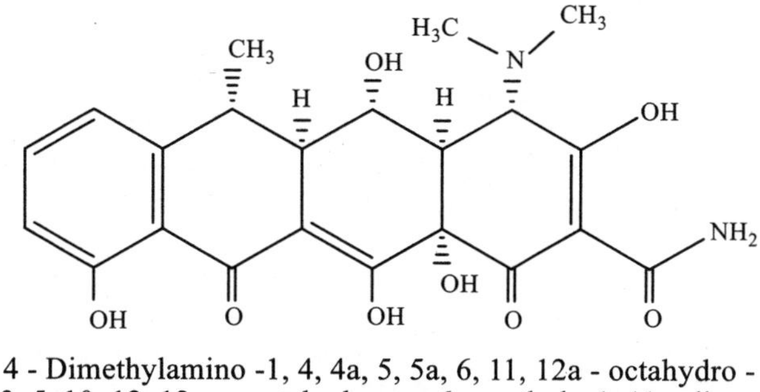

4 - Dimethylamino -1, 4, 4a, 5, 5a, 6, 11, 12a - octahydro - 3, 5, 10, 12, 12a - pentahydroxy - 6 - methyl - 1, 11 - dioxo - 2 - naphthacene carboxamide

It is produced by catalytic hydrogenation of Methacycline. The 6α-methyl epimer is 3 times as active as its β-epimer. It is available in the form of Doxycycline calcium salt.

**Use:** It is used to treat cutaneous, GI or inhalation Anthrax, inflammatory lesions of rosacea, endocervical, rectal and urethral and infections caused by *Chlamydia trachomatis.*

### E. Minocycline (Minocin)

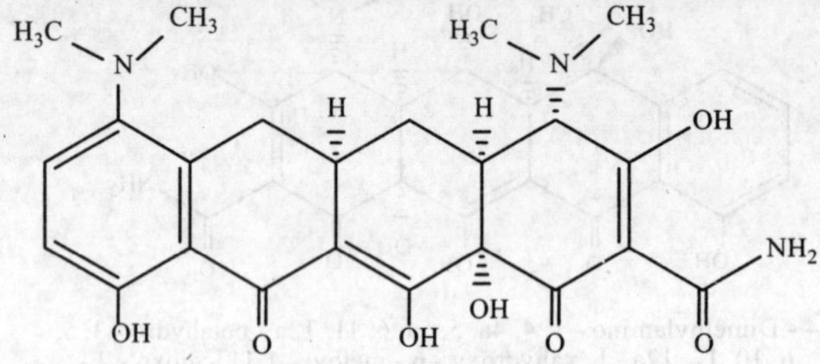


4, 7 - Bis (dimethylamino) -1, 4, 4a, 5, 5a, 6, 11, 12a - octahydro - 3, 10, 12, 12a - tetrahroxy - 1, 11 - dioxo - 2 - naphthacene carboxamide

It is the most potent tetracycline currently used in therapy. It is obtained by reductive methylation of 7-Nitro-6-demethyl-6-deoxytetracycline. It is available in the form of Minocycline hydrochloride.

**Use:** It is used to treat respiratory tract infection including pneumonia, urinary tract infection caused by Gram-negative bacteria. It is also used as adjunct to treat intestinal amoebiasis.

## 2.4 MACROLIDE ANTIBIOTICS

### 2.4.1 Introduction

Macrolide antibiotics are bacteriostatic antibiotics with a broad spectrum of activity against many Gram-positive bacteria. Macrolide antibiotics are produced by various strains of *Streptomyces*. Five macrolide antibiotics are currently available Erythromycin, Clarithromycin, Azithromycin, Fidaxomicin and Telithromycin. Erythromycin was initially isolated in 1952 from *Streptomyces erythreus*; the other macrolide antibiotics are semi-synthetic derivatives. The five macrolide antibiotics have a similar range of activities, being bacteriostatic against many strains of *Streptococci, Staphylococci, Clostridia, Corynebacterium listeria, Haemophilus spp., and Neisseria meningitidis.*

### 2.4.2 Chemistry

They have three common chemical characteristics

- a large non-planar strain less ring
- a keto group
- a glycosidically linked amino sugar

Usually the lactone ring has 12, 14 or 16 atoms in it, unsaturated with an olefinic group conjugated with the ketone function. They may have a neutral sugar also, in addition to the amino sugar, which is linked glycosidically to the lactone ring.

**2.4.3 Mechanism of Action:** Macrolide binds to 50s subunit of the bacterial ribosome, to prevent the translocation step of bacterial protein synthesis. It does not bind to mammalian ribosome.

**2.4.4 Spectrum of Activity:** The spectrum of antibacterial activity of macrolides resembles that of Penicillins. They are effective against most species of Gram-positive bacteria, both *cocci* and *bacillai* and also Gram-negative *cocci* especially *Neisseria spp*. They are also active against *Treponema palladium*, *Mycoplasma, Chalmydia, Compylobacter and Legionella spp.*

**A. Erythromycin (Erycin)**

Erythromycin was isolated from the culture of *Streptomyces erythreus*. It is a mono-acidic base, which on hydrolysis gives a basic sugar desosamine and a neutral sugar cladinose. It is a very bitter, white or yellow white crystalline powder. It is insoluble in alcohol, but only slightly soluble in water. It is degraded in acid medium. It consists of 14-membered lactone ring along with 10 asymmetric centers, two sugars, L-Cladinose on $C_3$ and D-Desoamine.

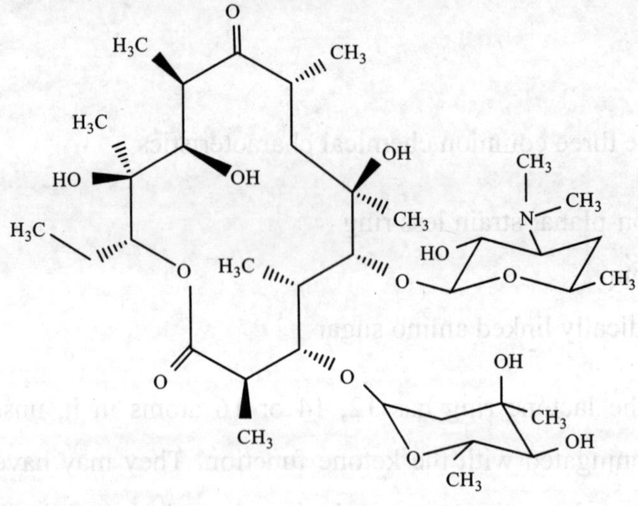


**Mechanism of action:** It binds to 50s ribosomal subunit of the 70s ribosome in many types of aerobic, anaerobic, Gram-positive and Gram-negative bacteria. This action inhibits RNA dependent protein synthesis in bacterial cells, causing them to die.

**Use:** The spectrum of activity resembles penicillin. It is the drug of choice in the treatment of infections caused by *Campylobacter, Chalmydia, Corynebacterium diptheriae, Bordetella pertussis, Legionella pneumophila, Mycoplasma pneumoniae* *and Ureoplasma ureolyticum.* It is effective against Gram-positive cocci, *Streptococci, Pneumococci and Staphylococcus aureus, Neisseria meningitidis, Gonorrhoea, Listeria, H. influenzae and Acnes.*

## B. Clarithromycin (Clear)

Chemically Clarithromycin is 6-Methyl ether of Erythromycin. It is prepared by simply methylation of Erythromycin at 6-hydroxyl group. This semi-synthetic derivative fully retains the antibacterial activity of Erythromycin with increased acid stability and oral bioavailability and reduced gastrointestinal side effects. It inhibits *Cytochrome* p*450 oxidase* and thus potentiates the actions of drugs metabolized by these enzymes. It occurs as white crystalline solid, practically insoluble in water, but sparingly soluble in alcohol, freely soluble in acetone.

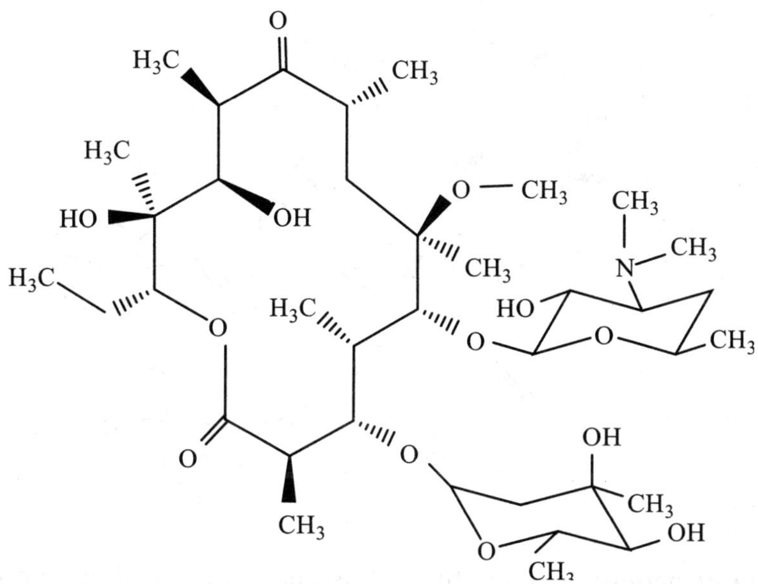

**Mechanism of action:** It inhibits RNA-dependent protein synthesis in many types of aerobic, anaerobic, Gram-positive and Gram-negative bacteria. By binding with the 50s ribosomal subunit of the bacterial 70s ribosome, Clarithromycin causes bacterial cells to die.

**Use:** It exhibit greater potency against *Chalmydia pneumoniae*, *H. influenza*, *M. pneumoniae*: *Legionella spp* and *M. catarrhalis*. It is significantly more active than Erythromycin against *Streptococci* and *S. pneumoniae*, but it is more expensive than Erythromycin.

### C. Azithromycin (Azithrol)

It is a semi-synthetic derivative of Erythromycin. It is a prototype of a series of nitrogen-containing, 15-membered ring macrolide known as azalides. It is more stable than other macrolide antibiotics. It possess N-methyl amino methylene group, which cause 15-membered ring instead 14-membered ring as in Erythromycin. The nitrogen is responsible for higher basicity and reveals higher acid stability.

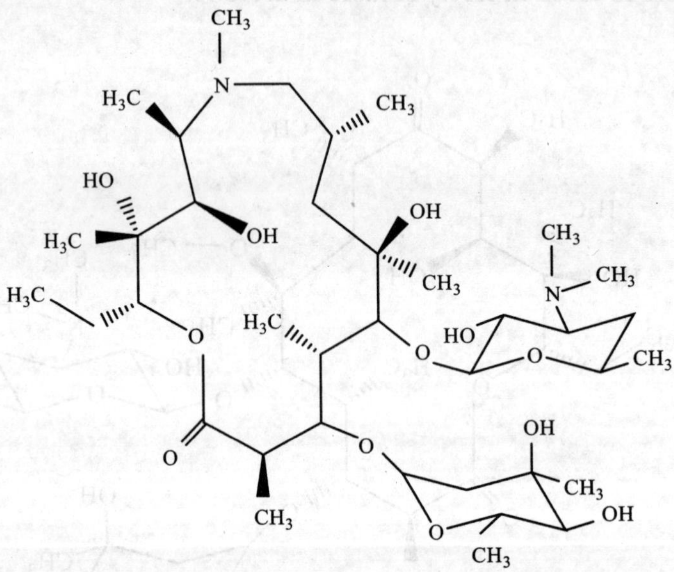

**Mechanism of action:** It binds to a ribosomal subunit of susceptible bacteria, blocking peptide translocation and inhibiting RNA-dependent protein synthesis leading to death of the microbes.

**Use:** Spectrum of antimicrobial activity is similar to Erythromycin and Clarithromycin. It is more active against Gram-negative bacteria and less active against Gram-positive bacteria.

## 2.5 LINCOMYCIN

Lincomycins are sulfur-containing antibiotics isolated from *Streptomyces lincolensis*. Lincomycin is the most active and medicinally useful compounds. Structural modification of Lincomycin resulted in 7-Chloro-7-deoxy derivative called Clindamycin. Clindamycin possess great antibacterial potency, when compare to Lincomycin. Lincomycin resembles macrolide in antibacterial spectrum. They are active against Gram- positive bacteria, particularly *cocci* and also effective against non-spore forming anaerobic bacteria namely *Actinomycetes, Mycoplasma* and *Plasmodium spp*. Lincomycin binds to 50s ribosomal subunit to inhibit protein synthesis.

### A. Clindamycin (Clincin)

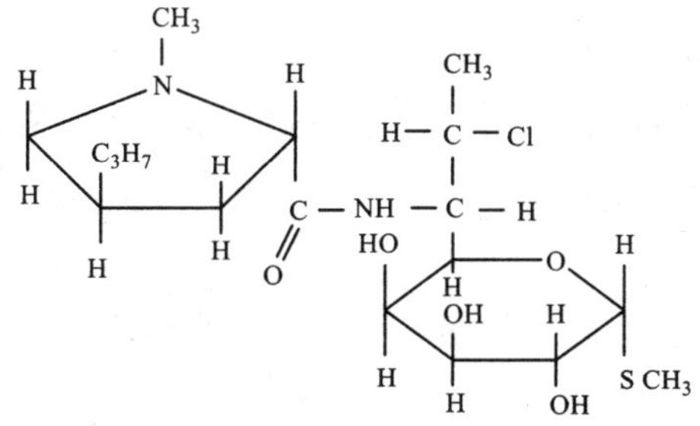

Replacement of 7(R) - hydroxy group of Lincomycin with chlorine gives Clindamycin with enhanced antibacterial activity. Chemically it is called 7(S) - chloro -7- deoxy lincomycin. Clindamycin palmitate hydrochloride salt in oral dosage form as wells as Clindamycin phosphate ester in solution for intramuscular or intravenous injection is also available.

**Mechanism of action:** It inhibits protein synthesis in susceptible bacteria by binding to the 50s subunits of bacterial ribosome and preventing peptide bond formation, which causes bacterial cells to die.

**Use:** It is used in the treatment of a wide variety of upper respiratory, skin and tissue infection. It is active against S*treptococci*, *Staphylococci* and *Pneumococci*.

## 2.6 MISCELLANEOUS

### A. Chloramphenicol (Paraxin)

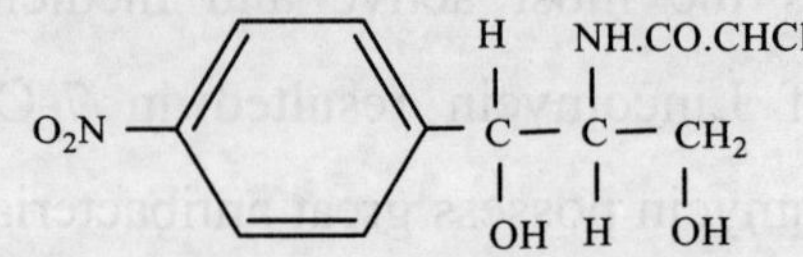

D - *threo* - 2 - Dichloro acetamido - 1 - (p - nitro phenyl) -1, 3 - propanediol

Chloramphenicol was isolated from a culture of *Streptomyces venezuelae.* Hydrolysis (acid or alkali) yielded dichloro acetic acid and a base called 2-Amino-p-nitro phenyl-1,3-propanediol. This base contains two chiral carbon give rise to *threo* and *erythro* forms. By relating the structure to L-Norphedrine, L-Pseudo norephedrine and D-series, it was assigned to D (-) *threo* configuration.

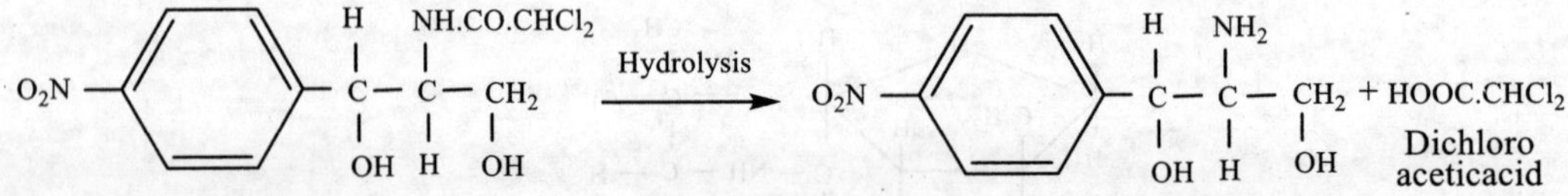

Chloramphenicol D - *threo* - 2 - Amino - 1 - (p - nitro phenyl) - 1, 3 - propanediol

Chloramphenicol is a yellowish-white needle-like crystal, slightly soluble in water, very soluble in alcohol. It has no odor, but has a very bitter taste. It possesses two chiral carbon atoms in the acylamido propanediol chain. Biological activity resides almost exclusively in the *D-threo* isomer, the *L-threo* and D and *L-erythro* isomers are virtually inactive. It is relatively a simple compound possessing aromatic nitro group previously unknown in a natural product. Because of this nitro functional group, it can be reduced, diazotized and coupled with β-naphthol to give a red azo-dye. This reaction is useful for the quantification of chloramphenicol.

Synthesis

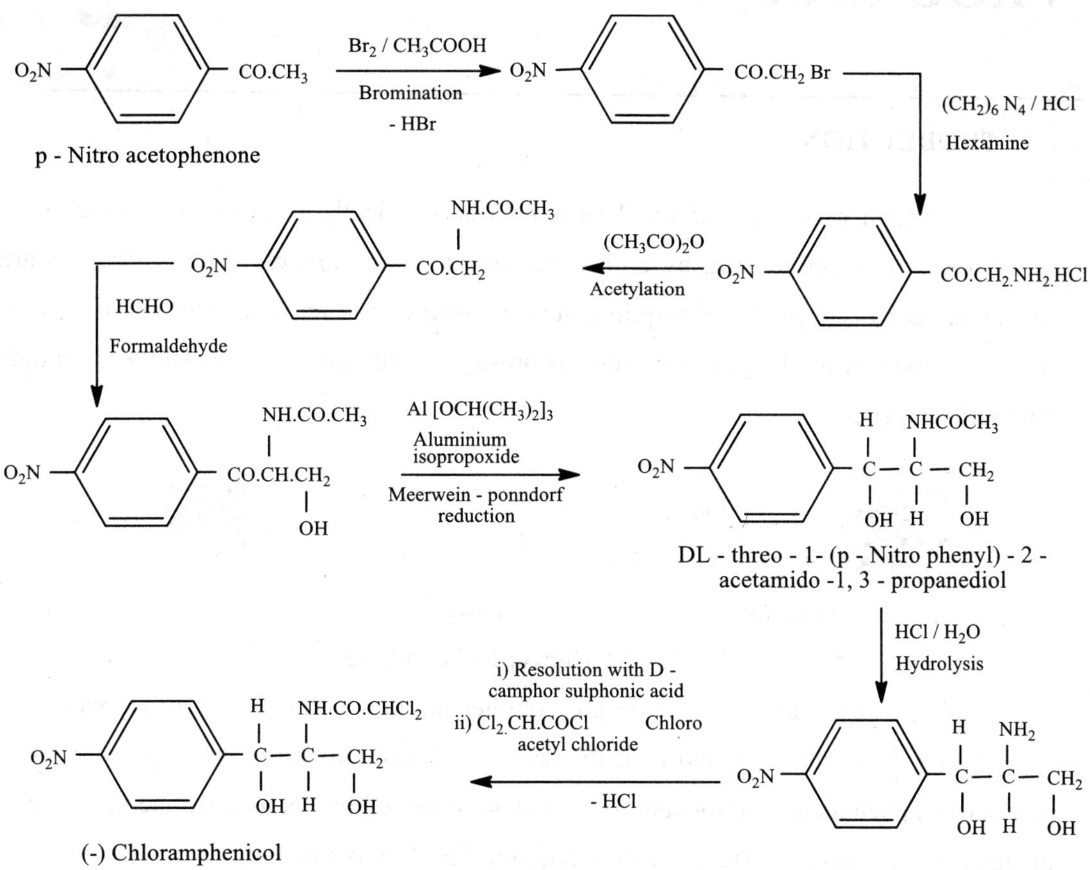


**Mechanism of action:** It inhibits protein synthesis in bacteria. It acts primarily by binding reversibly to the 50s ribosomal subunit and appears to prevent the binding of the amino acid containing end of aminoacyl tRNA to the acceptor site on the 50s ribosomal subunit.

**Use:** Chloramphenicol is an important drug of choice for the treatment of typhoid fever caused by *Salmonella typhi.* It is also effective against most bacteria, *Hemophilus influenza* and *Neisseria meningitidis.*

Chapter

# 2

# PRODRUGS

## 1. INTRODUCTION

The term prodrug is defined as a pharmacologically inactive compound that is converted into an active drug by a chemical or enzymatic process. The prodrug to drug conversion can occur before absorption, during absorption, after absorption or at a specific site in the body. A prodrug is also called as pro-agent, bio-reversible derivative, latentiated drug and congeners.

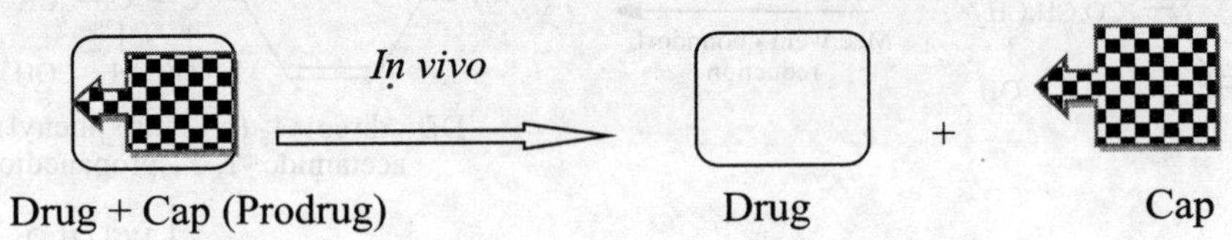


**Fig. 2.1 Concept of Prodrug**

The earliest example of prodrug is Arsphenamine which is used for the treatment of syphilis. Later on, it was found that, the activity of this compound was due to metabolic product Oxophenarsine. Arsphenamine was later replaced by Oxophenarsine in therapy as the metabolite was less toxic at the dose required for effective therapy.

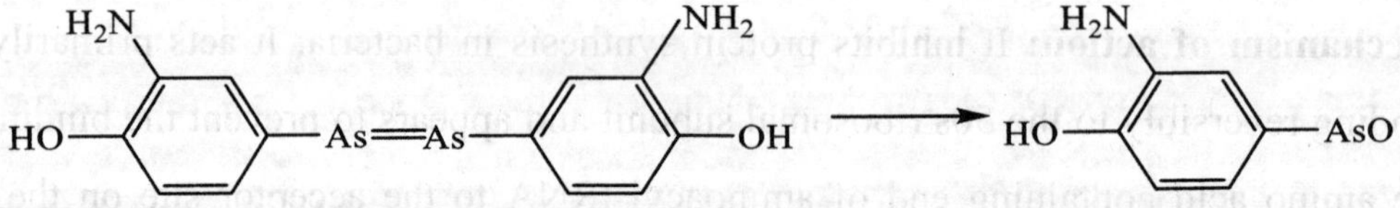


Azo-dye Prontosil had antibacterial activity, is a prodrug for sulphonamide which led to subsequent development of wide range of therapeutically superior sulfonamides through the modification of amino benzene sulfonamide.

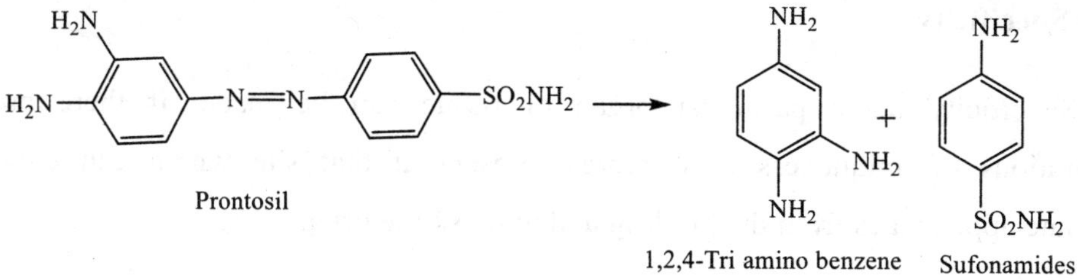


Phenacetin, an analgesic and antipyretic agent is mainly metabolized in the body to active metabolite N-acetyl-p-amino phenol (Paracetamol). Paracetamol has replaced Phenacetin therapy, because it is free from toxic effects associated with Phenacetin (Methemoglobin formation).

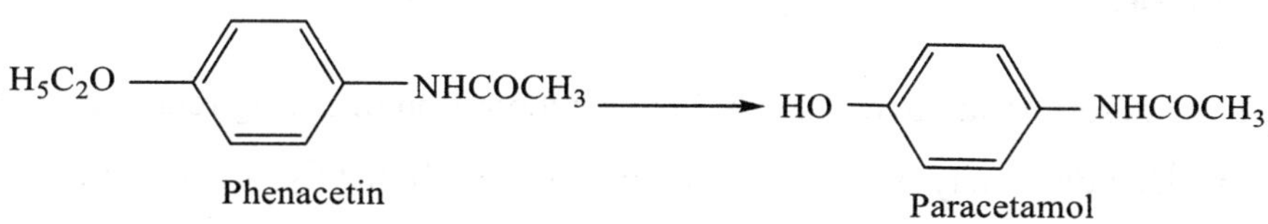


## 2. PRODRUGS STRATEGY IN DRUG DESIGN

There are numerous reasons why one may wish to utilize a prodrug strategy in drug design. Few examples are

### i) Solubility

Consider an active drug that is insufficiently soluble in water, so that it cannot be injected in a small dose. A water-soluble group could be attached which could be metabolically released after drug administration.

### ii) Absorption and Distribution

If the drug is not absorbed and transported to the target site in sufficient concentration it can be made more water soluble or lipid soluble, depending on the desired site of action. Once absorption occurred or when the drug is at the appropriate site of action, the water or lipid soluble group is removed enzymatically.

**iii) Site Specificity**

Specificity for a particular organ or tissue can be made, if there are high concentrations of uniqueness of enzymes, present at that site which can cleave the appropriate appendages from the prodrug and unmask the drug.

**iv) Instability**

A drug may be rapidly metabolized and rendered inactive, prior when it reaches the site of action. The structure may be modified to block that metabolism until the drug is at the desired site.

**v) Prolonged Release**

It may be desirable to have a steady low concentration of a drug released over a long period of time. The drug may be altered, so that it is metabolically converted to the active form slowly.

**vi) Toxicity**

A drug may be toxic in its active form and would have a greater therapeutic index if it were administered in a nontoxic, inactive form that can be converted to the active form only at the site of action.

**vii) Poor Patient Acceptability**

An active drug may have an unpleasant taste or odor, produces gastric irritation, or causes pain, when administered (eg. when injected). The structure of the drug can be modified to alleviate these problems, but once administered; the altered drug can be metabolized to the active drug.

**viii) Formulation Problems**

If the drug is a volatile liquid, it would be more desirable to prepare it in a solid form, so that it could be formulated as a tablet. An inactive solid derivative could be prepared which would be converted in the body to the active drug.

## 3. IDEAL REQUIREMENTS OF PRODRUGS

An ideal prodrug must meet the following requirements

i) The prodrug should be inactive or less active than the parent compound.

ii) It should not have intrinsic pharmacological activity.

iii) The linkage between the drug and the carrier must be cleared *in vivo.*

iv) The carrier molecule released *in vivo* must be non-toxic.

## 4. TYPES OF PRODRUG

Depending upon the constitution, lipophilicity, method of bio-activation and catalyst involved in bio-activation, prodrugs are classified into two types

a. Carrier linked prodrugs

b. Bio-precursors

### 4.1 Carrier Linked Prodrug

Carrier linked prodrug is a compound that contains an active drug linked to a carrier group that can be removed enzymatically, such as ester which is hydrolyzed to active carboxylic acid containing drug. The bond to the carrier drug must be labile enough to allow the active drug to be released efficiently *in vivo* and the carrier must be non-toxic and biologically inactive when detached from the drug. Carrier linked prodrug can be further subdivided into bipartate, tripartate and mutual prodrug.

A bipartate prodrug is a prodrug comprised of one carrier attached to the drug. When a carrier is connected to a linker that is connected to the drug is called a tripartate prodrug. (Fig. 2.2)

$$\text{Carrier—Linker—Drug} \xrightarrow{\text{Enzyme}} \text{Carrier} + \text{Linker—Drug} \xrightarrow{\text{Spontaneous}} \text{Linker} + \text{Drug}$$

**Fig. 2.2 Tripartate Prodrug**

Bipartate prodrug may be ineffective because the prodrug linkage is too labile or too stable. In order to overcome this problem, tripartate prodrugs are designed. The drug-linker connection must be designed in such a way that it cleaves spontaneously after the carrier detached. One approach to accomplish this, has been termed as double prodrug (Fig. 2.3)

$$\text{Drug - X - CH}_2\text{COOR} \xrightarrow{\textit{Esterase}} \text{Drug - X - CH}_2\text{O + RC}\bar{\text{O}}\text{OH} \xrightarrow{\text{Fast}} \text{Drug - X + HCHO}$$

**Fig. 2.3 Concept of Double Prodrug**

Example for double ester is Bacampicillin or Pivampicillin an ester of Ampicillin. The β-lactam antibiotic Ampicillin is poorly absorbed when administered orally, so 2.5 times more drug must be administered orally than by injection. The extra dosage of the drug may lead to more rapid onset of resistance and may destroy the important intestinal bacteria. A lipid-soluble prodrug of Ampicillin would be a useful approach to increase the absorption of this drug. The various simple alkyl or aryl ester of thiazolidine carboxyl group of Ampicillin are stable and therapeutically useful. But steric hindrance occurs at ester carbonyl group of the thiazolidine ring with enzyme. This problem is overcome by double ester acyloxy methyl ester such as Bacampicillin or Pivampicillin which would extent the carbonyl group away from thiazolidine ring and steric hindrance with the enzyme. Hydrolysis of terminal ester gives an unstable hydroxy methyl ester, which spontaneously decomposes to Ampicillin and either acetaldehyde (Bacampicillin) or formaldehyde (Pivampicillin). Bacampicillin is absorbed to the extent of 98%, so only one half to one-third of Ampicillin dose is required orally.

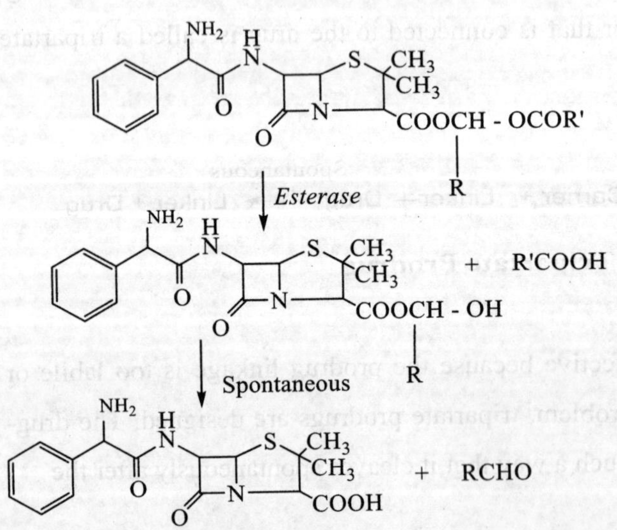


Ampicillin

| Prodrugs | R | R' |
|---|---|---|
| Bacampicillin | $CH_3$ | $C_2H_5$ |
| Pivampicillin | H | t-butyl |

### 4.1.1 Carrier Linkage for Various Functional Groups

#### a) Carboxylic Acids and Alcohols

Prodrugs of carboxylic acid and alcohol functionalities can be prepared by conversion to esters. The esters can be easily hydrolyzed by esterase enzymes *(lipase, cholesterol esterase, acetylcholine esterase, carboxy peptidase)* present in plasma and other tissues to give active drug. Alcohols containing drugs can be acylated with aliphatic or aromatic acid to decrease water solubility (increases lipophilicity) or with carboxylic acids containing amino or additional carboxylate groups to increase water solubility and also conversion to phosphate or sulfate esters increases water solubility.

Carboxylic acid containing drugs can be esterified with various alcohols. The pKa of a carboxylic acid can be raised by conversion to choline ester or amino ester.

Drug - COO promoiety $\xrightarrow{\textit{Esterase}}$ Drug - COOH + HO promoiety

Drug O - CO - promoiety $\xrightarrow{\textit{Esterase}}$ Drug - OH + HO - CO promoiety

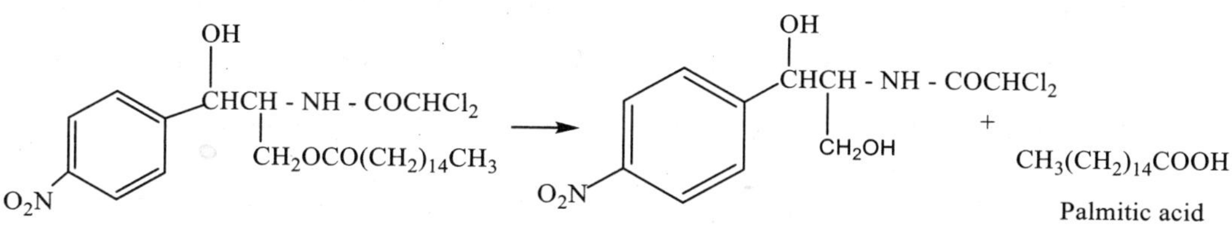


Chloramphenicol palmitate — Chloramphenicol — Palmitic acid

#### b) Amines

Derivatization of amines to give amide has not been widely used as a prodrug, because of high chemical stability of amide and lack of amidase enzyme necessary for hydrolysis. A more common approach is to use Mannich bases as prodrug form of amines. This lowers the basicity of amines, so that at physiological pH few of the prodrug molecule are protonated, thereby increases its lipophilicity. Hetacillin is a prodrug form of Ampicillin in which amide nitrogen and α-amino functionality have been allowed to react with acetone to give a Mannich base [imidazolidine ring system]. This decreases the basicity and increases the lipophilicity and absorption. Another approach to lower the pKa of amine is making them more lipophilic by converting in to imines (Schiff's base).

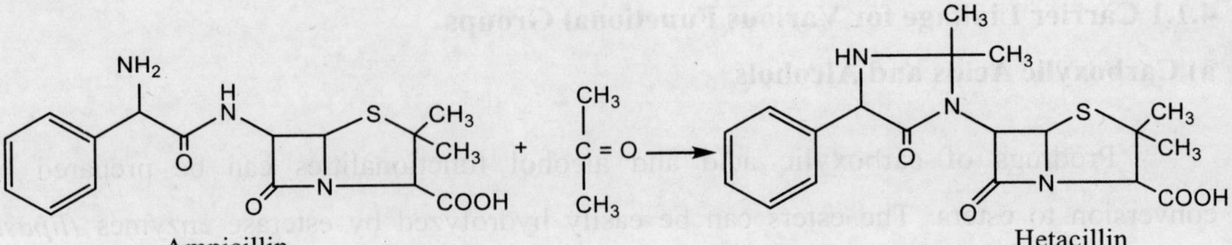

Ampicillin Hetacillin

## c) Azo Linkage

Amines are derivatized to azo linkage prodrug occasionally. Sulfasalazine by the action of *azo reductase* releases the amino salicylic acid and Sulfapyridine. The generation of anti-inflammatory amino salicylic acid prior to absorption prevents the systemic absorption of the agents and concentrates it in active site. Sulfasalazine is an example of mutual prodrug. A mutual prodrug consists of two usually synergistic drugs attached to each other *i.e.*, one drug carrier for the other and vice versa. It is a bipartate or tripartate prodrug in which the carrier is a synergistic drug with the drug to which it is linked. A mutual prodrug is well absorbed, both components are released concomitantly and quantitatively after absorption, the maximal effect of the combination of the two drugs occurs and distribution and elimination of the two components are similar.

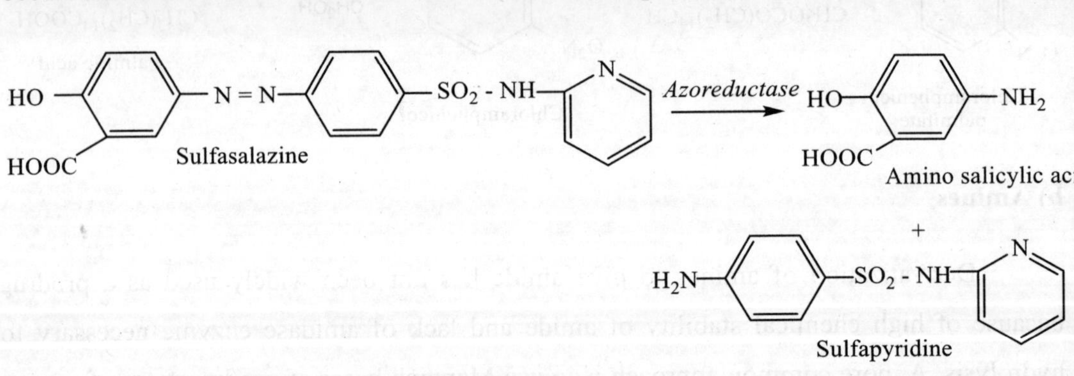


Sulfasalazine Amino salicylic acid Sulfapyridine

## d) Carbonyl Moiety

Carbonyl functionalities such as aldehyde and ketones conversion to prodrug have not found wide clinical utility. These are converted into derivatives in which the $sp^2$ carbonyl carbon is converted to a $sp^3$ hybridized carbon attached to hetero atoms. These prodrugs are reconverted to carbonyl compound by hydrolysis. The most important prodrug form of aldehydes and ketones are oximes, acetals, enol esters, oxazolidines, Schiff base and thiazolidines. For example, hexamine releases formaldehyde in the urine (acidic pH), which acts as an antibacterial agent.

$$\underset{\text{Hexamine}}{(CH_2)_6N_4} \xrightarrow{\overset{+}{H}} \underset{\text{Formaldehyde}}{6\ HCHO} + \underset{\text{Ammonia}}{4\ NH_3}$$

**Table 2.1 Carrier linkage for various functional groups**

| Functional groups | Prodrug | Name of groups |
|---|---|---|
| **-COOH** | -COOR | Ester |
| | -CONHR | Amide |
| | $-COOCH(R_1)OCOR_2$ | α- Acyloxy alkyl esters |
| **-NH₂** | -NHCOR | Amide |
| | -NHCOOR | Carbamates |
| | $-N{=}C(R_1)(R_2)$ | Imines |
| | $-NHCH_2N(R_1)COR_2$ | N-Mannich bases |
| | $-NHC(R){=}C(R_1)(R_2)$ | Enamines |
| | $R_1O{-}C{-}OR_2$ | Ketals |

| Functional group | Prodrug | Name |
|---|---|---|
| 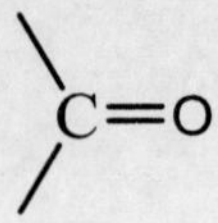 | 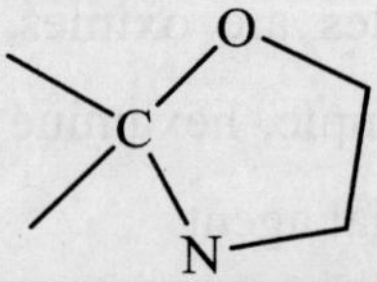 | Oxazolidines |
| | 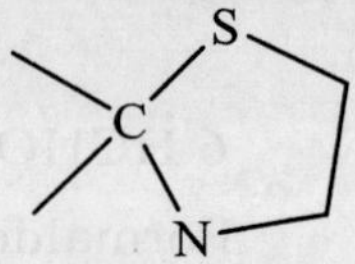 | Thiazolidines |
| **-OH** | -OCOR | Esters |
| | $OPO_3H_2$ | Phosphate ester |
| | $-COOCH(R_1)OCOR_2$ | α-Acyloxy alkyl esters |
| | -OR | Ethers |
| $-SO_2NH_2$ | $RSO_2N=C(R_1)(O-R_2)$ | N-Sulphonyl imides |
| | $-SO_2NHCH_2OR$ | N-Sulphonyl imides |
| **-SH** | -S-CO-R | Thioesters |
| | $-S-CH(R_1)-O-CO-R_2$ | α-Acyloxy alkyl thioethers |
| | -S-S-R | Disulfides |
| 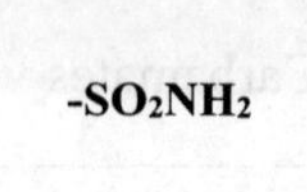 | 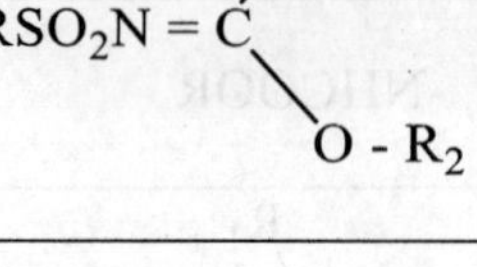 | N-Acyloxy alkyl derivatives |

## 4.2 Bio-precursor Prodrug

Bio-precursors are inert molecule obtained by chemical modification of the drugs but do not contain a carrier. For example, if the drug contains carboxylic acid group, the bioprecursor may be primary amine, which is metabolized by oxidation to aldehyde which is further metabolized to carboxylic acid drug.

Bio-precursor prodrug does not contain a carrier or promoiety, but rather contains a latent functionality that is metabolically or chemically transformed to active drug molecule. The types of activation involve oxidation, reduction, phosphorylation or chemical activation. The examples given below are arranged according to the type of metabolic activation reaction involved.

### a) Oxidative Activation

Nabumetone is an anti-inflammatory drug. NSAIDs normally produce stomach irritation. This is due to the presence of carboxylic acid group present in the drug. This functional group is essential for activity. Nabumetone contains no acidic functionality and so it passes through the stomach without producing irritation. After absorption the drug is metabolized in the liver to active substance.

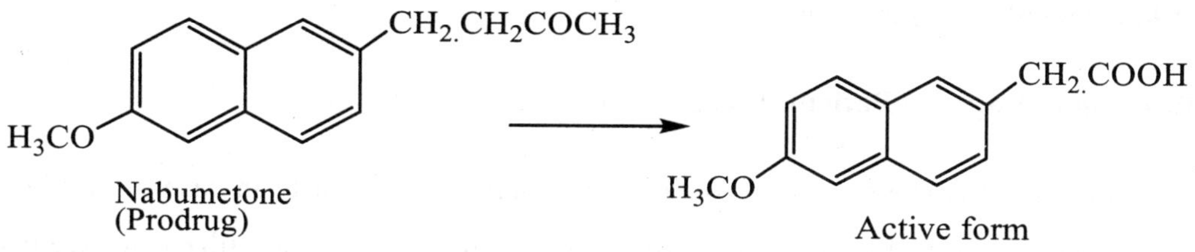


### b) Reductive Activation

Thiamine is a quaternary ammonium salt, it is poorly absorbed into CNS and from gastro intestinal tract. To increase the lipophilicity of Thiamine, tetrahydro furfuryl disulphide was designed as a prodrug. The prodrug permeates rapidly through red blood cell membranes and reacts with glutathione to produce Thiamine.

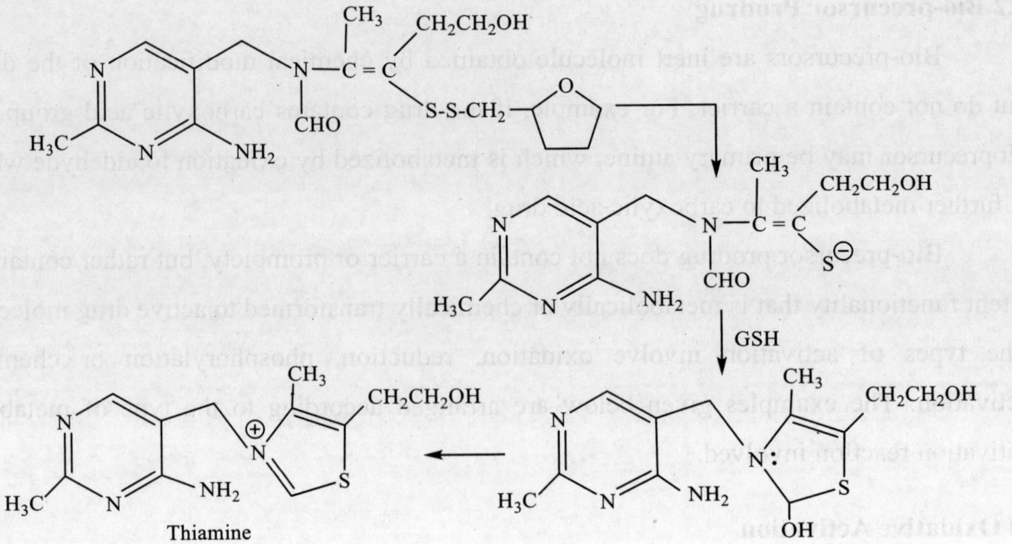


# 5. APPLICATIONS OF PRODRUGS

There are three main reasons for drug action, namely the pharmaceutical, pharmacokinetic and pharmacodynamic phases. Problems exist in all the three phases, but prodrug formation seeks to the problem in pharmaceutical and pharmacokinetic phases.

## 5.1 Pharmaceutical Applications

### a) Prodrug to Improve Patient Acceptability

One of the reasons for poor patient compliance, particularly in case of children is bitterness, acidity or causticity of the drug. Two approaches can be utilized to overcome the bad taste of drug. The first is reduction of drug solubility in saliva and the other is to lower the affinity of drug towards taste receptor. Chloramphenicol has a bitter taste, so it is not well accepted by children. The palmitate ester of it is less soluble in saliva, so it masks the bitter taste. Some other examples are given in Table 2.2.

**Table 2.2 Examples of Drugs and their Prodrugs**

| S. No | Parent Drug | Prodrug |
|---|---|---|
| 1 | Clindamycin | Clindamycin phosphate |
| 2 | Sulfisoxazole | N-acetyl sulfisoxazole |
| 3 | Erythromycin | Erythromycin estolate |
| 4 | Sulfamethoxy-pyridazine | N-acetyl sulfamethoxy-pyridazine |
| 5 | Metronidazole | Benzoyl metronidazole |

The odor of a compound depends upon its vapor pressure; a liquid with high vapor pressure will have a strong odor. For example Ethyl mercaptan is a foul smelling liquid used in the treatment of leprosy. This is converted to phthalate ester, diethyl dithio-isophthalate which has higher boiling point and is odorless. The odourless inactive prodrug is metabolized to the active parent drug by *thioesterase*.

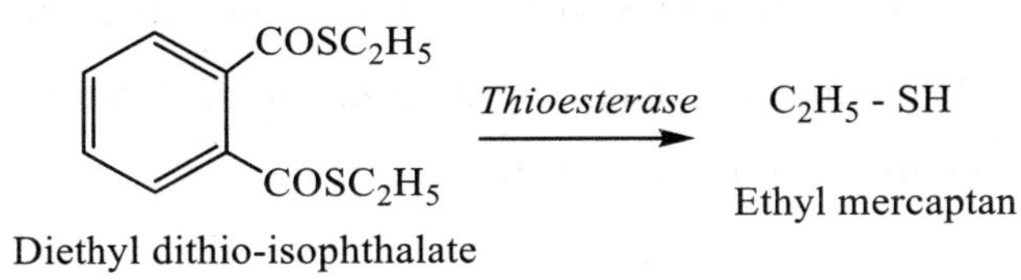


Several drugs (NSAIDS, Nicotinic acid, Kanamycin, Diethylstilboestrol) cause irritation and damage to gastric mucosa. Examples of prodrug designed to overcome such problems of gastric distress are given below (Aspirin & INH).

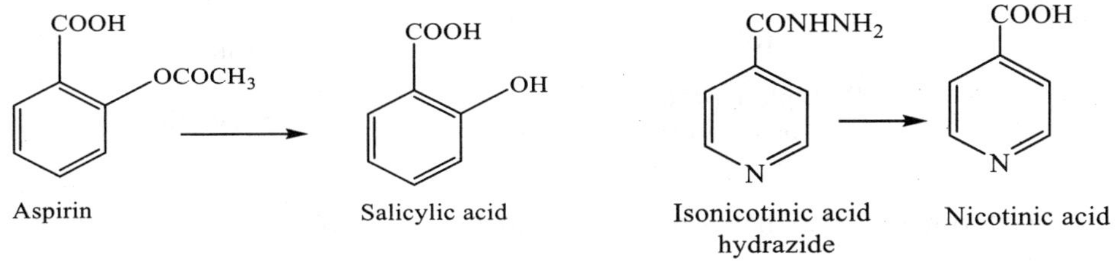

Intramuscular injection is particularly painful when drug precipitates or penetrates into the surrounding cell or when the solution is strongly acidic, alkaline or alcoholic. For example, Clindamycin hydrochloride causes irritation when given by intramuscular route. This can be overcome by use of more water-soluble prodrug Clindamycin - 2' - phosphate.

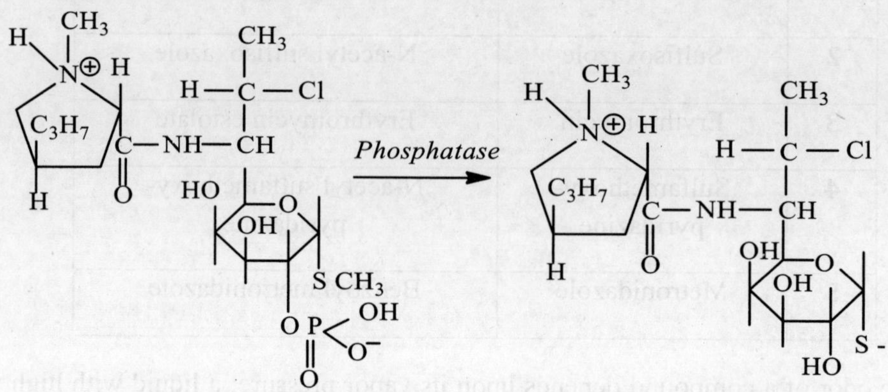

Clindamycin - 2' - phosphate    Clindamycin

**b) Prodrug to Improve Stability**

Many drugs are unstable and may either breakdown on prolonged storage or are degraded rapidly on administration. Several drugs may decompose in GIT when used orally. Although enteric coatings may be used, it is also possible to utilize prodrug design to overcome this problem. An antineoplastic drug Azacytidine hydrolyses readily in acidic pH, but the bisulfite prodrug of it is more stable.

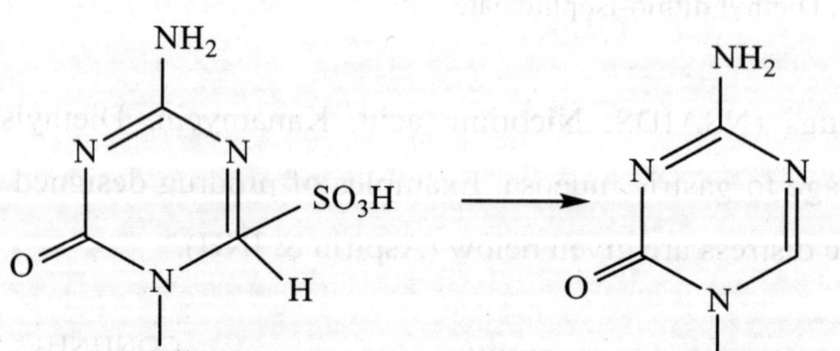

Bisulphite prodrug of azacytidine    Azacytidine

Erythromycin also has similar acid instability problem. Its stearate and estolate ester prodrugs are stable and hydrolyzed in stomach

### c) Prodrug to Overcome Formulation Problem

Formaldehyde is a flammable, colourless gas which could not be used directly as medicine so a stable solid Hexamine (Methenamine) is used. In acidic pH, Hexamine (pH of urine in the bladder is mildly acidic) hydrolyzed to formaldehyde and ammonia which acts as urinary antiseptic. Another example is the topical fungistatic prodrug Triacetin owes its activity to acetic acid, the product of skin *esterase* hydrolysis to acetic acid.

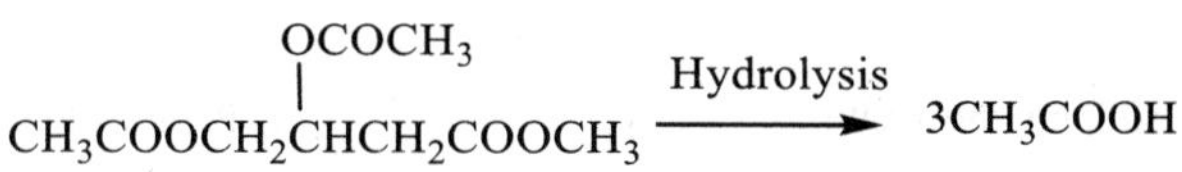


Triacetin Acetic acid

Some drug exists in a form which is unsuitable for formulation. For example, Methyl dopa is a Zwitterion and although charged, its crystal structure causes it to be only poorly water soluble. In order to formulate this drug for injection, it is converted into ethyl ester which may be formulated as hydrochloride salt.

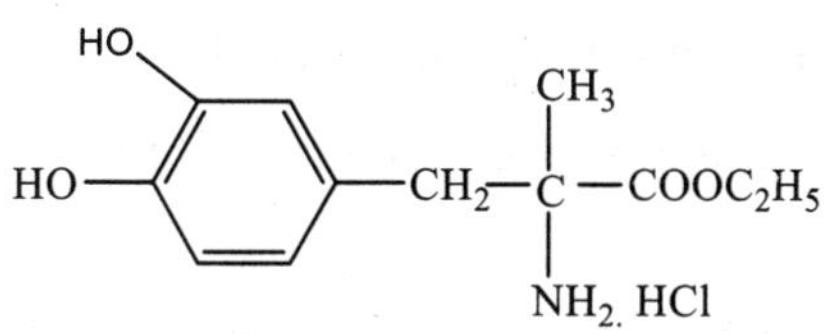


Methyl dopate hydrochloride

Hydrophilicity or water-soluble drugs are desired when parenteral or ophthalmic formulation of such agent is desired. Drugs with hydroxyl functional group can be converted to their hydrophilic form by use of half ester such as hemi-glutarate or hemi-phthalates; the other half of this acid carries sodium, potassium or amine salts and renders the moiety more soluble. Prednisolone and Methyl prednisolone are poor water-soluble corticosteroid drugs. Prednisolone phosphate is a water-soluble prodrug of Prednisolone that is activated *in vivo* by *phosphatase*.

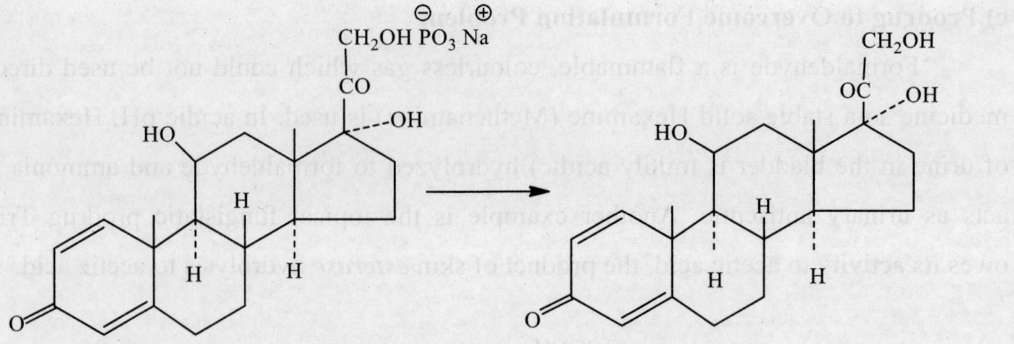

Prednisolone sodium phosphate Prednisolone

### 5.2 Pharmacological Applications

Pharmacological problems may be either related to pharmacokinetic, pharmacodynamic or toxic properties of the drug.

#### a) Prodrug to Improve Absorption

Therapeutic agents have to permeate one or more biological membranes in order to reach the target site. Although drugs are administered by a number of quite different routes, prodrugs designed to solve delivery problems related to some of the mostly used route of administration e.g. oral, dermal and ocular delivery system.

**(i) Oral Absorption**

For orally administered drugs one major challenge of reaching their site of action is that, they have to cross the intestinal epithelial cells to enter the systemic circulation. Poor transport properties may lead low bioavailability, which may also result from low water solubility, low stability in gastro intestinal juices or extensive first-pass metabolism. Prodrug design has been utilized in a number of cases to optimize the absorption of such drugs, thereby improving their bioavailability.

Well known example of prodrug to enhance absorption of polar drug modification is Ampicillin derivative (Discussed in tripartate prodrug). Ampicillin a wide spectrum antibiotic is readily absorbed orally as the inactive prodrug, Pivampicillin, Bacampicillin and Talampicillin which are then converted by enzymatic hydrolysis to Ampicillin.

The low absorption of antiviral Acyclovir is increased by orally active prodrug Valacyclovir, the L-valyl ester of Acyclovir, which is rapidly hydrolyzed by first pass intestinal metabolism. The prodrug is converted into Acyclovir in human by the hydrolase enzyme present in the liver and gut.

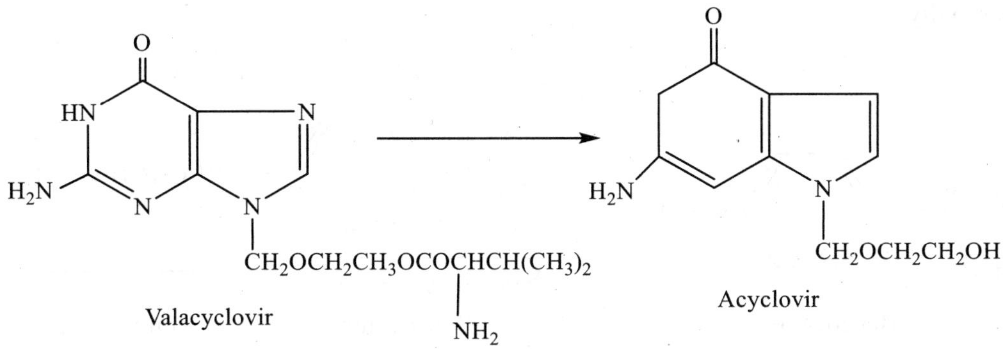


In antihypertensive drug Enalaprilat oral absorption has been improved by conversion to more efficiently absorbed ethyl ester Enalapril. The prodrug Enalapril is converted *in vivo* to an active Enalaprilat by hydrolysis in the liver.

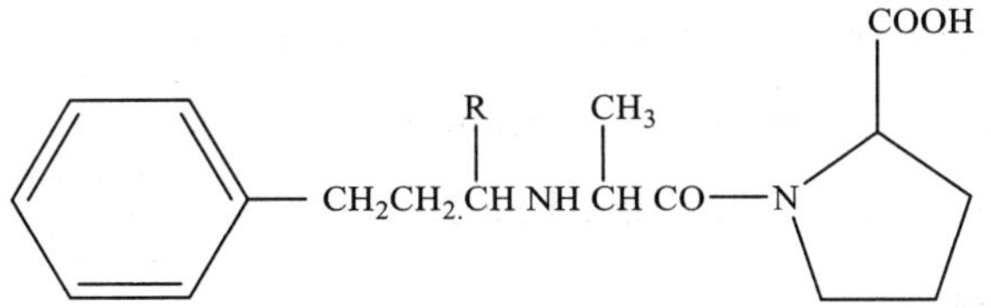


| Name | R |
|---|---|
| **Enalapril** | $-COOC_2H_5$ |
| **Enalaprilat** | -COOH |

Several drugs show poor and variable oral absorption characteristics as a result of insufficient water solubility leading to dissolution rate-limited absorption. The antitumor drug Etoposide is toxic due to its poor water solubility. Conversion to corresponding phosphate ester, Etoposide phosphate allows the drug to be delivered in a more concentrated form over a much shorter period to time.

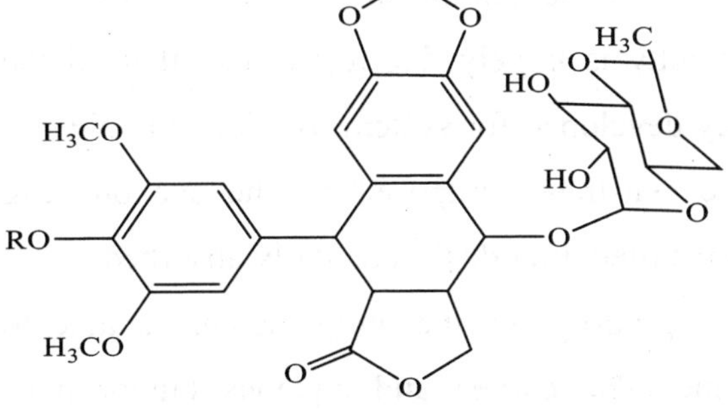


| Name | R |
|---|---|
| **Etoposide** | -H |
| **Etoposide phosphate** | $-PO_3H_2$ |

The local anesthetic Benzocaine has been converted into water soluble amide prodrug form with various amino acids; *amidase*-catalyzed hydrolysis in human serum occurs rapidly.

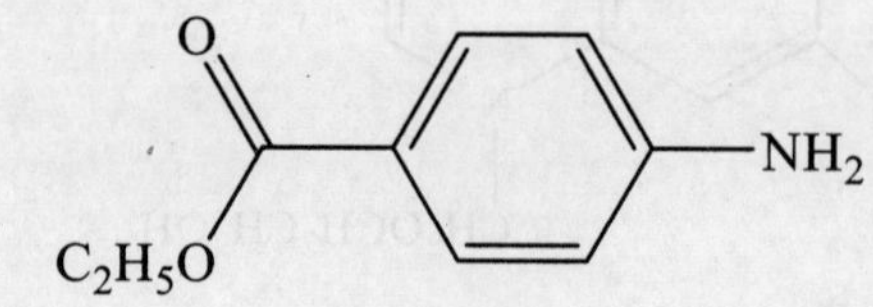

Benzocaine

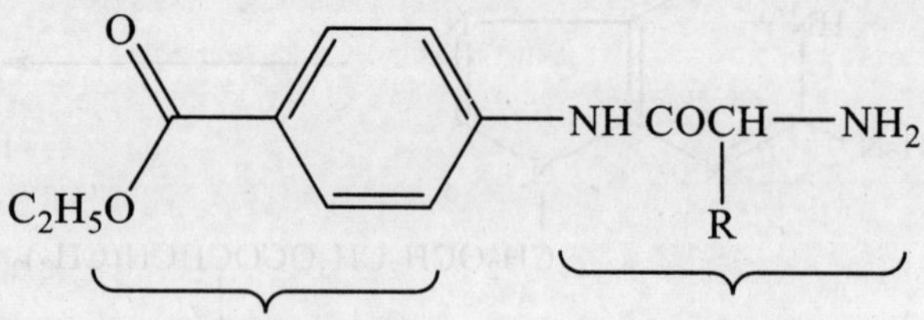

Benzocaine Amino acids

### (ii) Dermal Absorption

The skin is designed to maintain the body fluids and prevent absorption of xenobiotics into the general circulation. Consequently, drugs applied to the skin are poorly absorbed. Corticosteroids for the topical treatment of inflammatory, allergic and pruritic skin conditions can be made more suitable for topical absorption by esterification or acetonidation. For example, both Fluocinolone acetonide and Fluocinonide are prodrugs used for inflammatory and pruritic manifestations.

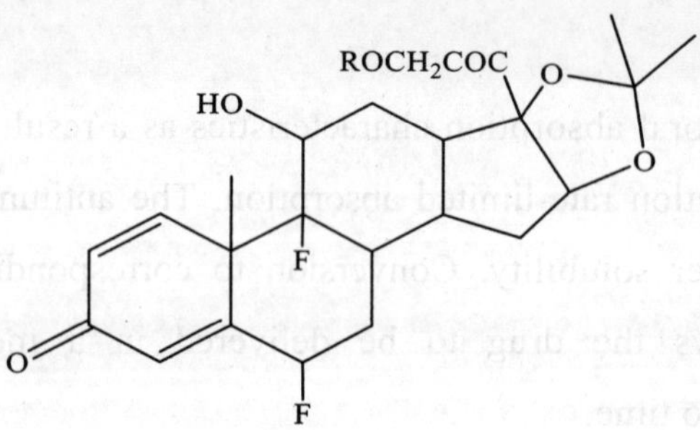

| Name | R |
|---|---|
| Fluocinolone acetonide | -H |
| Fluocinonide | $-COCH_3$ |

### (iii) Ocular Absorption

A major problem in ocular therapeutic is the attainment of an optional drug concentration at the site of action. The difficulty is largely due to the fact that all the existing drugs, many of which were originally developed for system use, lack the physio-chemical properties to overcome the severe constraints imposed by the eye on drug absorption. The net result is 1% or less of the instilled drug dose is ocularly absorbed.

Dipivaloyl epinephrine (Dipivefrin) a prodrug for the antiglaucoma is able to penetrate the cornea better than Epinephrine. The cornea and aqueous humor have significant esterase activity.

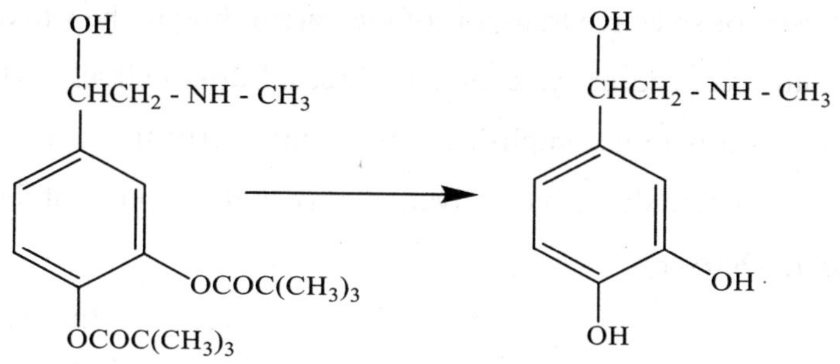

Dipivaloyl epinephrine Epinephrine

The approach of “soft” quaternary salt is utilized to achieve improved bio-availability of Pilocarpine on ocular administration. Pilocarpine is rapidly drained from the eye resulting in a short duration of action. The “soft” quaternary salt has a lipophilic side chain which has been shown to improve absorption in rabbits and gives a more prolonged effect at one tenth of the concentration of Pilocarpine. The “soft” quaternary salt is formed by reaction between α-chloromethyl ester and amino group of the drug. The quaternary salt formed is termed as “soft” quaternary salt since unlike normal quaternary salt it can release the active basic drug on hydrolysis. “Soft” quaternary salt increases the absorption since it has surfactant property and capable of forming micelles and unionized pair with bile acid etc., which are able to penetrate the intestinal epithelium more effectively. The prodrug after absorption rapidly releases the parent drug by hydrolysis process.

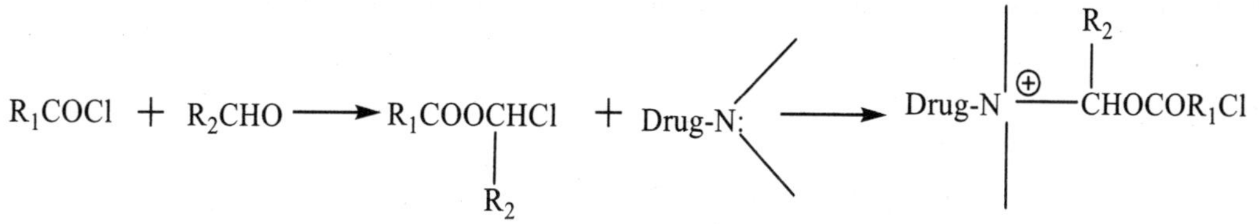

α- Chloromethyl ester Basic drug "Soft" quaternary salt

**(b) Prodrug for Site Specific Drug Delivery**

Targeting of drug for a specific site in the body by conversion to a prodrug are designed to ensure that, the release of active drug only occurs at its site of action thereby reducing toxic side effects due to high plasma concentration of the drug or non- specific update by other body tissues. Site specific drug delivery might achieve by site directed drug delivery or site-specific bio activation. Site directed delivery relates to design prodrug that affords an increased or selective transport of the parent drug to the site of action. It can be further divided into localized or systemic site directed drug delivery. The objective of site-specific bio-activation is to accomplish bio-reversible derivatives, that are distributed throughout the organism but undergo bio-activation only in the vicinity of the target area.

**(i) Site Directed Drug Delivery**

Successful site-directed drug delivery has been achieved in the field of localized drug delivery. Compared to localized drug delivery, systemic site-directed delivery constitutes a much more difficult task, since the drug has to be transported via the systemic circulation to the desired organ or tissue, passing various complex and not easily predictable on the way. Drug targeting in cancer chemotherapy, an interesting approach to obtain site-directed delivery to the brain has been investigated.

One important membrane that must be trans-versed for drug delivery into the brain is the blood-brain barrier, a unique lipid-like protective barrier that prevents hydrophilic compounds from entering the brain unless they are actively transported. They also contain active enzymes to protect the central nervous system further. Anticonvulsant activity can be achieved by increasing concentration of γ-aminobutyric acid (GABA) in the brain which results in neurotransmission inhibition. GABA is too polar to cross blood brain barrier, so it's effective lipophilic analog of GABA that crosses the blood-brain barrier, releases GABA inside the brain and shows anticonvulsant activity. In the above example, the lipophilicity was increased, so that they could diffuse through the membranes.

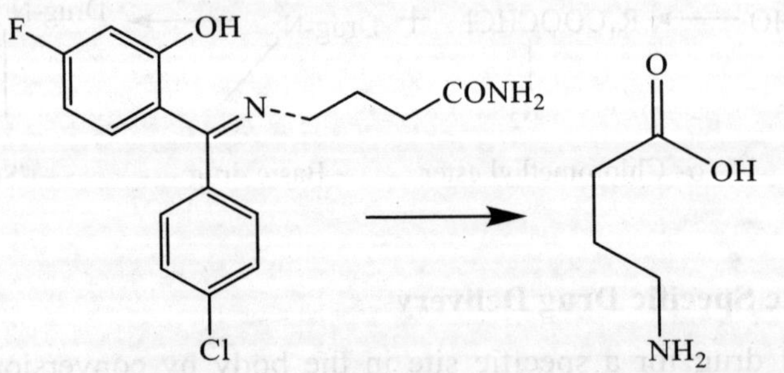


Probabide γ - Amino butyric acid

Although lipophilic prodrug may be used, but increased lipid solubility may enhance uptake in other tissue with a resultant increase in toxicity. Furthermore, therapeutic levels of such lipophilic prodrug can only be maintained if there is a constant plasma level. These problems may be overcome by utilizing a dihydropyridine-pyridine-pyridinium salt type redox system. (Fig.2.4). The drug (D) which is aimed to be delivered to the brain, is coupled to a quaternary carrier (i.e. N-methyl nicotinic acid) $QC^+$ to yield $D\text{-}QC^+$ which is reduced to neutral, lipophilic dihydro from (D-DHC).

After administration, this compound is distributed throughout the body including the brain. D-DHC is then enzymatically oxidized back to the original quaternary entity ($D\text{-}QC^+$). The later hydrophilic compound is prevented from passing through the blood-brain barrier. Thus, the ionic form is trapped in the brain and undergoes slow enzymatic cleavage releasing the active agent. Because of the facile elimination of $D\text{-}QC^+$ from the circulation, only small amount of the free drug is released in the blood. This concept has been applied to several drugs including Dopamine, Phenytoin and Penicillin.

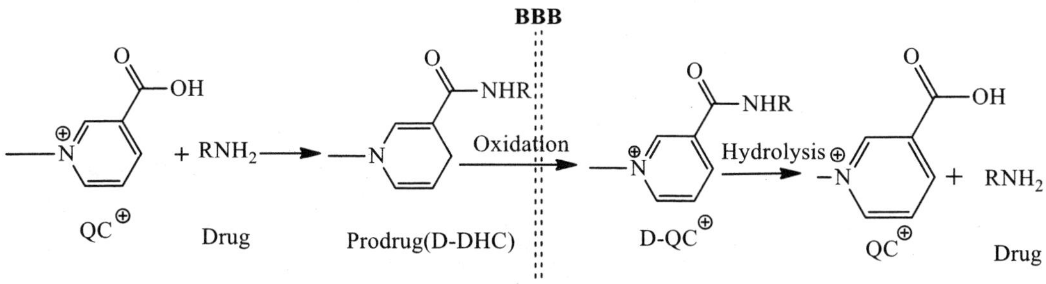


**Fig. 2.4 Quaternary Ammonium Carrier Prodrug**

### (ii) Site Specific Bio-activation

Quantitative or qualitative difference between the target and non-target sites might be exploited in prodrug design to activate or release the active agents in the vicinity of the target area. Difference in pH or more often in enzyme levels have founded the platform for the synthesis of bio-reversible derivatives, which after the distribution phase are selectively activated in the desired organ within the body.

Site specific bio-activation can be explained by action of Acyclovir as antiviral agent. The herpes virus encoded *thymidine kinase* converts Acyclovir to its mono phosphate, which by the action of cellular enzyme results in the formation di and tri phosphorylated species. The Acyclovir triphosphate is active one. The triester formation takes place much greater extent in the herpes-infected cells, than the uninfected host cells.

The selectivity of action is manifested in the fact that, a 3000-fold higher concentration of Acyclovir is needed to inhibit uninfected cell multiplication.

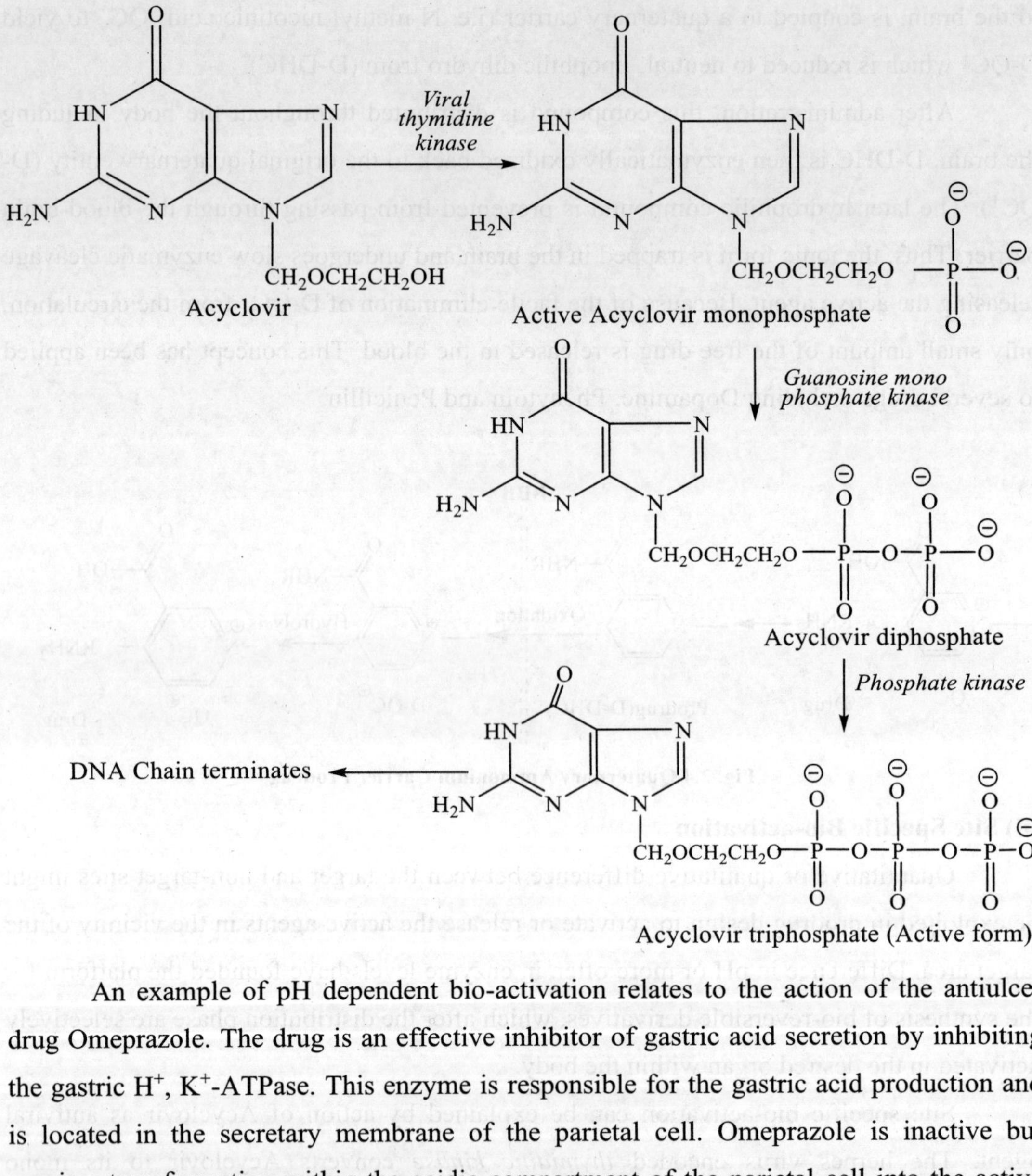


An example of pH dependent bio-activation relates to the action of the antiulcer drug Omeprazole. The drug is an effective inhibitor of gastric acid secretion by inhibiting the gastric $H^+$, $K^+$-ATPase. This enzyme is responsible for the gastric acid production and is located in the secretary membrane of the parietal cell. Omeprazole is inactive but requires transformation within the acidic compartment of the parietal cell into the active inhibitor a cyclic sulfonamide. This intermediate reacts with thiol groups in the enzyme forming a disulphide complex thereby inactivating the enzyme (Fig. 2.5).

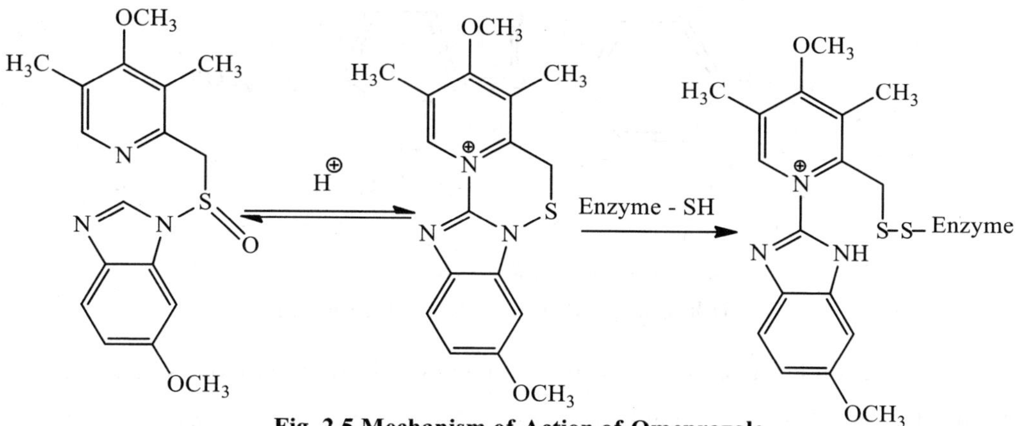

**Fig. 2.5 Mechanism of Action of Omeprazole**

### (c) Prodrug for Slow and Prolonged Release (Sustained Release Action)

A common strategy in the design of slow-release prodrug is to make long-chain aliphatic esters, because these esters hydrolyze slowly and to inject them intramuscularly. The phenothiazine group of drugs acting as tranquillizer has been converted into long acting prodrug which is administered by intramuscular injection. Not only the frequency of administration reduced, but also the problem associated with patient compliance is also eliminated. For example, Fluphenazine has shorter duration of action (6-8h), but prodrugs Fluphenazine decanoate have duration of activity about month.

Conversion of non-steroidal anti-inflammatory drug Tolmetin sodium to corresponding glycine conjugate increases the potency and extend the peak concentration of Tolmetin from 1hr to about 9hr because of the slow hydrolysis of the amide linkage.

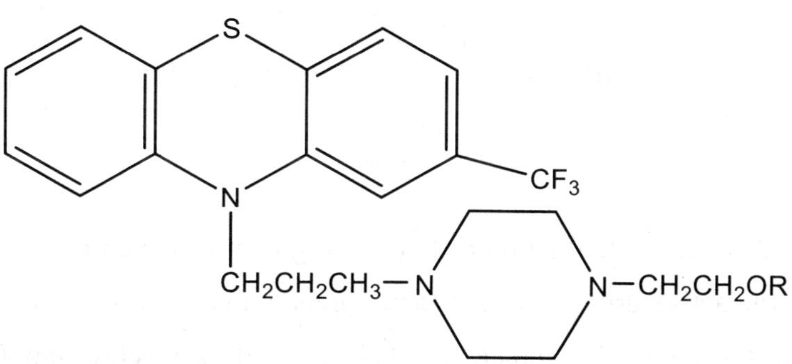

Fluphenazine R = H

Fluphenazine decanoate R = CO $(CH_2)_8CH_3$

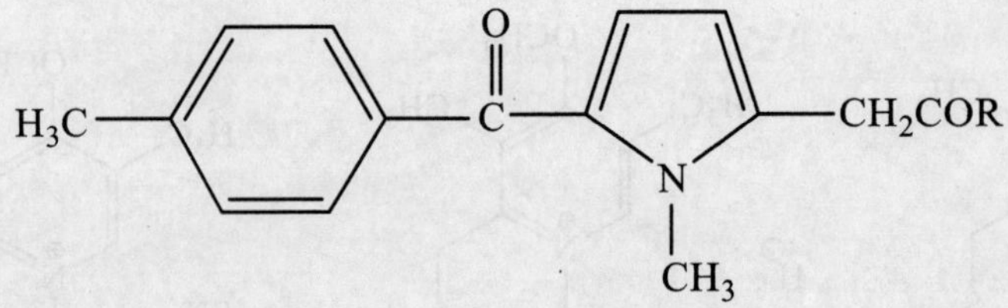

Tolmetin sodium R = $\overset{\ominus\ \oplus}{ONa}$
Tolmetin prodrug R = $NHCH_2CO\overset{\ominus\ \oplus}{ONa}$

Vasopressin has been used for the treatment of bleeding varicose veins in the lower end of the esophagus a condition that affects 1000 individuals annually. The vasoconstrictor action of the drug stops the bleeding, but the action is of short duration and cannot be prolonged by the use of higher doses due to the development of toxic side effects. Glypressin, Gly-Gly-Gly-Lys-Vasopressin is an inactive prodrug of Vasopressin. After injection the glycyl of Vasopressin is obtained, which is sufficient to produce the required vasoconstriction effect on the portal blood pressure, while minimizing the possibility of unwanted effects caused by high blood pressure.

**d) Prodrug to Improve Membrane Transport**

Interference with transport characteristic can serve many purposes. The introduction of a hydrophilic moiety can restrict a drug to the gastro intestinal tract and prevent its absorption. For example, Succinyl sulfathiazole.

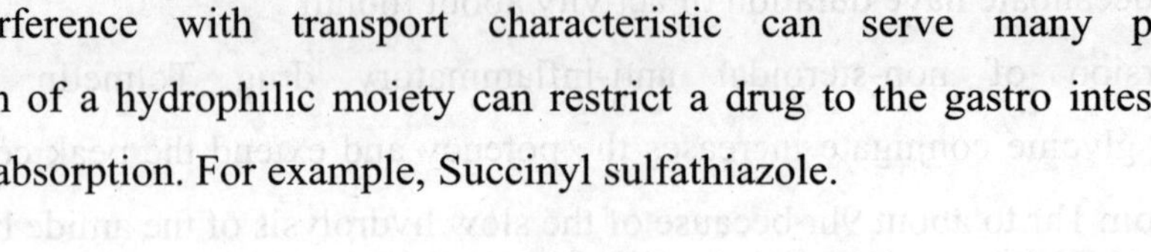

Succinyl sulfathiazole

On the other hand introduction of lipophilic group decreases the rate of hydrolysis, which liberates the active drug slowly, in depot preparation for a period of days or weeks. The antimalarial Cycloguanil pamoate can deliver the drug Cycloguanil for longer time (for several months). The membrane transport characteristic of the neurotransmitter Dopamine used for the treatment of Parkinson's disease can be improved by administering its prodrug 3, 4-dihydroxy phenyl alanine (Levodopa). This derivative has better blood-brain permeation characteristic, since it uses amino acid channels for transportation. Once it enters the cell, decarboxylase enzyme removes the acid group to generate dopamine.

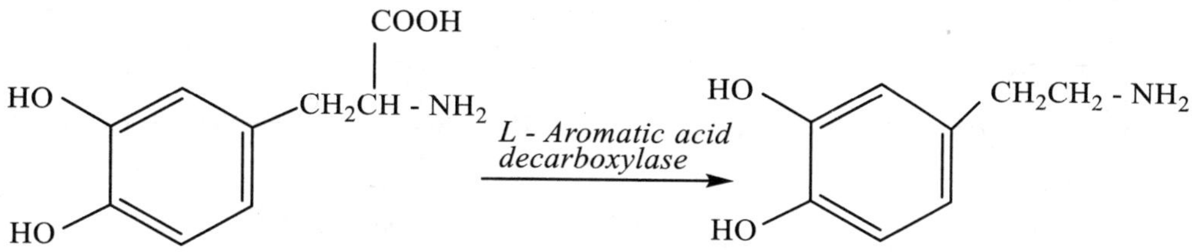


L - Dihydroxy phenyl alanine Dopamine

### e) Prodrug for Prolonged Duration of Action

Frequent dosing is required for drugs having short biological half life; this can also be overcome by prodrug approach. This can be achieved by either controlling the release rate of drug from the site of application or the conversion of prodrug into active drug. For example, the diester of Pilocarpine has prolonged therapeutic effect than the Pilocarpine. The diester of the drug when applied as ophthalmic solution showed better intraocular penetration due to improved lipophilicity and slow conversion of ester prodrug to active Pilocarpine prolong the activity.

The prodrug by its improved characteristics get closer to the receptor site for longer period of time and the conversion to the active drug takes place at the site of action.

Nordazepam, a sedative drug loses activity quickly due to metabolism and excretion. A prodrug Diazepam improves the retention characteristics, due to the presence of N-methyl group. Slow release of the Nordazepam in the liver by demethylation prolongs the activity.

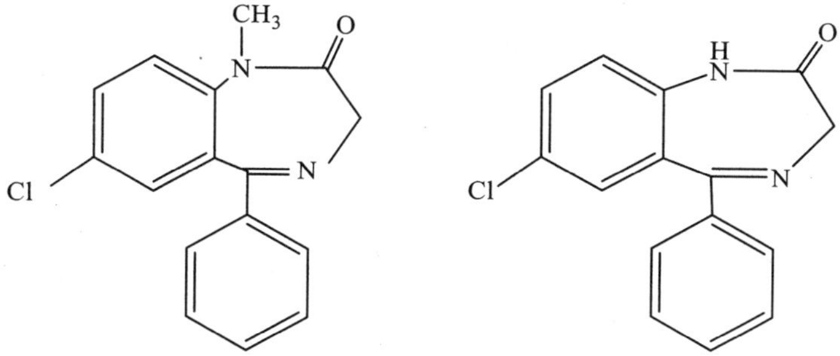


Diazepam Nordazepam

Replacement of less oxidizable chlorine group by vulnerable moiety-a methyl in Tolbutamide results in long acting prodrug Chlorpropamide, with half-life six-fold greater than its parent.

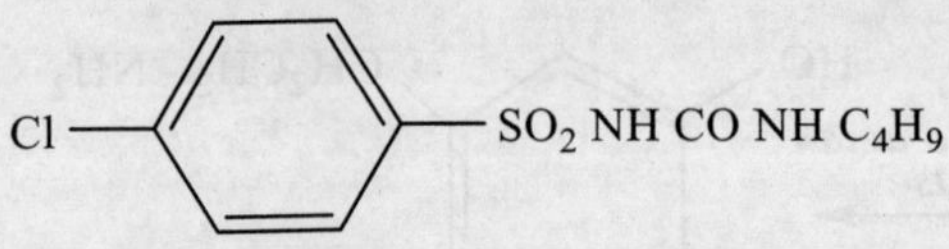

Tolbutamide

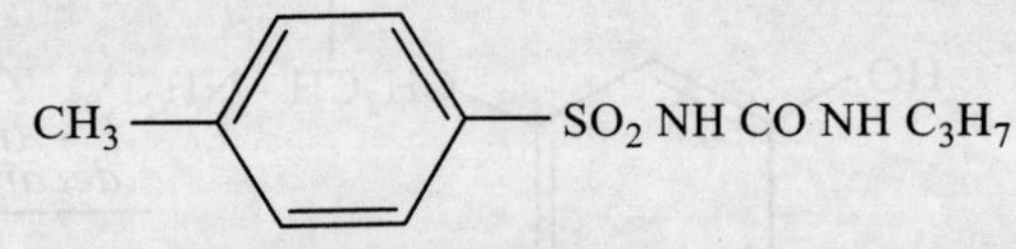

Chloropropamide

The utility of slow and prolonged release of prodrug is

i. It reduces the number and frequency of dose required
ii. It eliminates night-time administration of drugs.
iii. Because the drug is taken frequently, it minimizes patient non-compliance.
iv. When fast release drug is taken, due to metabolism the concentration of the drug diminished. A slow release drug would eliminate these peaks and valleys of fast-release drugs, which place a strain on cells.
v. Because a constant lower concentration of the drug is being released, the toxic level of drug in reduced.
vi. It reduces the gastro intestinal side effects.

Chapter

3

# ANTIMALARIAL DRUGS

## 1. INTRODUCTION

Malaria is one of the most widespread diseases caused by the protozoan parasite of the genus, *Plasmodium*. These parasites spend an asexual phase in the man and sexual phase in female anopheles mosquito. Malaria is caused by five species of one-cell protozoan of the *Plasmodium* genus: *P. falciparum*, *P. vivax*. *P. malariae*, *P. ovale* and *P. knowlesi*. No single antimalarial drug is effective against all five species. The majority of infections are caused by *P. falciparum* and *P. vivax.*

### 1.1 Etiology of Malaria

Malaria is a mosquito-borne parasitic infection spread by a female anopheles mosquito infected by the Plasmodium parasite. It is a single-celled parasite that multiplies amongst the red blood cells of humans as well as in the mosquito's intestine. When the female mosquito feeds on an infected person, the parasites are ingested along with the human blood. The parasites multiply in the mosquito's gut and these infectious forms are passed onto another human when the mosquito feeds again. Malaria can be obtained:

- If bitten by an infected female anopheles mosquito
- If receive infected blood from a malaria patient during a blood transfusion

Malaria can also be transmitted from an infected mother to the child during pregnancy through the placenta, or be transferred to the baby through blood during childbirth, resulting in 'congenital malaria' (malaria which has been passed from mother to infant). The symptoms of the disease may occur within 1 to 3 weeks after being infected.

A malaria patient is likely to suffer from the symptoms like abdominal pain, chills and sweats, diarrhea, nausea and vomiting, headache, high fever, low blood pressure, feeling dizzy when shifting from a lying or a sitting position to a standing position, muscle aches, Poor appetite.

In patients infected with the *P. falciparum* parasite, the symptoms like anaemia caused by the destruction of infected red blood cells, extreme tiredness, delirium, unconsciousness, convulsions and coma, kidney failure, pulmonary edema may also occur. The parasites, *P. vivax and P. ovale* can lie dormant in the liver for up to a year before causing any symptoms. They can even remain dormant in the liver again and cause relapses later.

## 1.2 Life Cycle of Malaria Parasite

The malaria parasite has a multistage life cycle occurring within two living beings, the vector mosquitoes and the vertebrate hosts.

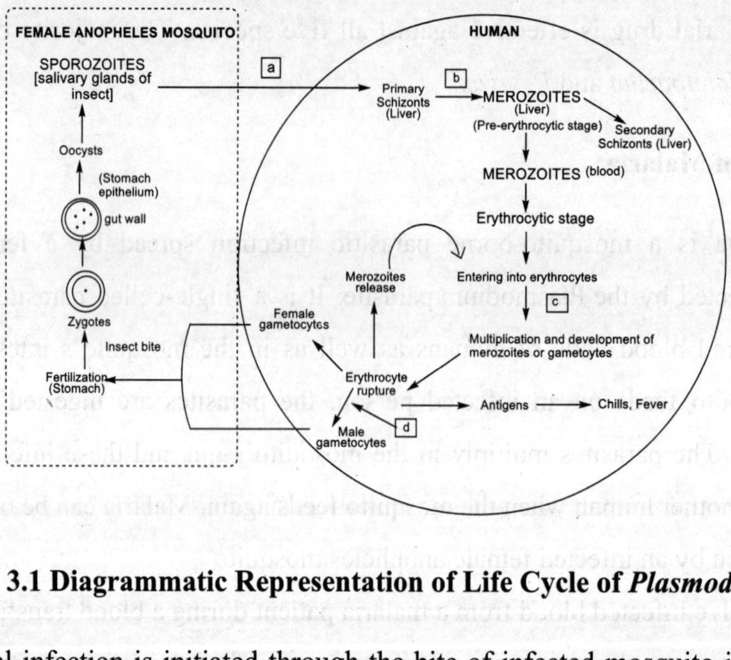


**Fig. 3.1 Diagrammatic Representation of Life Cycle of *Plasmodium***

- Malarial infection is initiated through the bite of infected mosquito into the human blood stream. The mosquito stores the sporozoites form of the protozoan in its salivary glands.
- The sporozoites in the blood stream enter into the parenchyma cell of host liver, where they become primary schizonts and then merozoites. Depending upon the plasmodium the merozoite either ruptures the infected hepatocytes and enters the systemic circulation or infects other liver cells.

- Merozoites now enter into the circulation and invade erythrocytes, where they reside for 3 to 4 days and reproduce. The reproduction stage in the erythrocyte can produce either more merozoites or another form called gametocytes. Due to this repeated multiplication erythrocyte may rupture and release merozoites into the circulation. Each merozoites again invades fresh erythrocytes and the cycle of asexual multiplication is repeated again. This stage is known as schizogony phase of infection which causes severe fever and chills.
- When such infected blood was ingested by female anopheles mosquito, the gametocytes (male and female) undergo sexual reproduction within the gut of the insect. The resulting zygotes through various stages of development migrate as sporozoites to the mosquito salivary gland. The cycle begins when a mosquito bites a human.

**1.3 Site of Antimalarial Agents: (Fig. 3.1)**

a) Kills the sporozoites injected by the mosquito and / or prevail the entering of sporozoites entering the liver. The drugs used in this stage in known as prophylactic agent. Since no drug is effective in this stage, true prophylaxis does not exist for malarial parasites.

b) Drug active against erythrocytic phase. These drugs are known as schizonticidal agents eg. Amodiaquine, Chloroquine, Quinine, Pyrimethamine.

c) Kills the merozoites in the blood and/or prevent their multiplication known as suppressive agent eg. Chloroquine, Amodiaquine.

d) Kill the gametocytes before they enter the mosquito and reproduce into zygotes. eg. Primaquine.

## 2. CLASSIFICATION

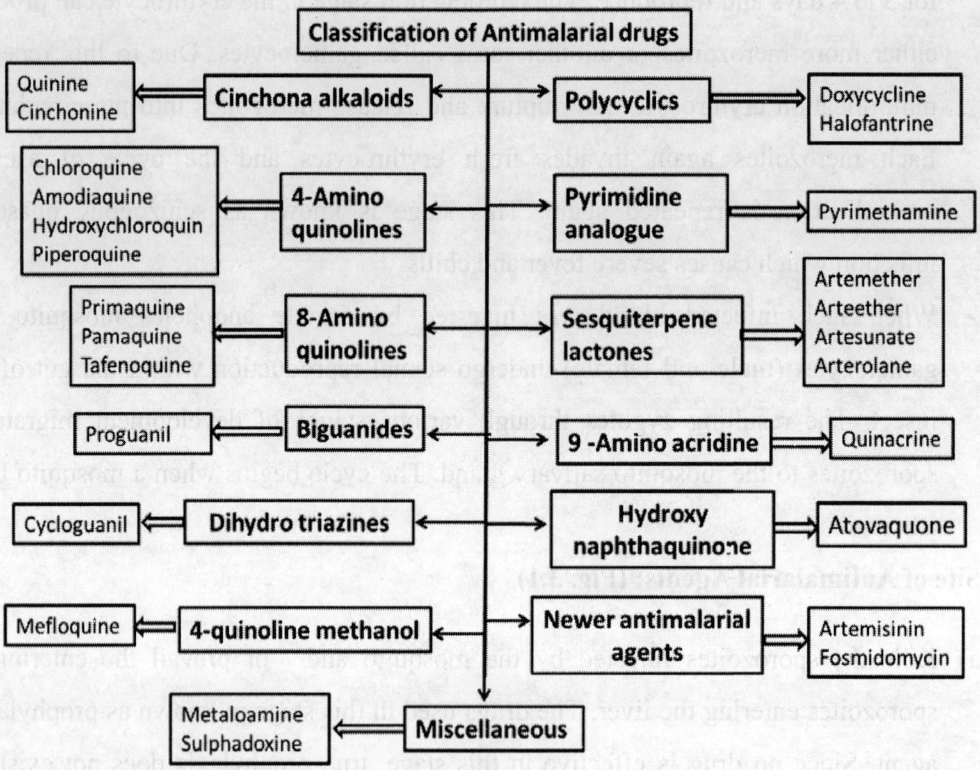


### 2.1 Cinchona Alkaloids

Quinine was the first known antimalarial. It is an alkaloid obtained from the bark of cinchona tree used to treat malaria from as early as 1600s, when it was referred as "Jesuits' bark" "cardinal's bark" or "sacred bark". Cinchona bark contains about 30 alkaloids, of which the most important are Quinine, Quinidine, Cinchonine and Cinchonidine. It is a 4-quinoline methanol derivative bearing a substituted quinuclidine ring. Quinine, Quinidine, Cinchonidine and Cinchonine contains a quinoline moiety attached through a secondary alcohol linkage to a quinuclidine ring having a vinyl group. Quinine and Quinidine each contains a methoxy group, that is absent in Cinchonidine and Cinchonine. Four stereo isomeric chemical centers exist in the molecule at $C_3$, $C_4$, $C_8$ and $C_9$. Quinine has absolute configuration of 3R: 4S: 8S: 9R. The *dextro* isomer of Quinine is Quinidine which is used as antiarrhythmic agent. Quinine has rapid schizonticidal action against intra-erythrocytic malaria parasites. It is also gametocytocidal for *Plasmodium vivax* and *Plasmodium malariae*, but not for *Plasmodium falciparum.* Quinine has been the lead compound for the development of a large number of antimalarial drugs.

### 2.1.1 Structure Activity Relationship

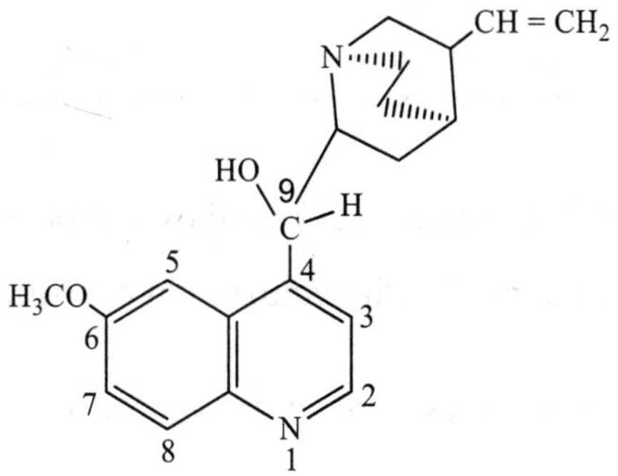


- Any alteration in the structure of quinine has not improved its antimalarial action.
- The methoxy group of the quinoline ring and the vinyl group of quinuclidine are not required for antimalarial activity.
- Saturation of vinyl group, results in formation of Dihydroquinidine which is slightly more potent than Quinine.
- The secondary alcohol group is essential for activity. Reduction of the alcohol group increases toxicity as well as moderating antimalarial activity.
- Quinuclidine portion is not required, but the presence of an alkyl tertiary amino group is essential for activity.
- Replacement of trifluoro methyl group in $C_2$ position decreases the phototoxicity. eg. Mefloquine
- Since the development of potent synthetic agents, Quinine had fallen into abandon as a first-line antimalarial.

### A. Quinine sulphate (Qualaquin)

It is a di-acidic tertiary base and its forms salts with two equivalents of an acid.

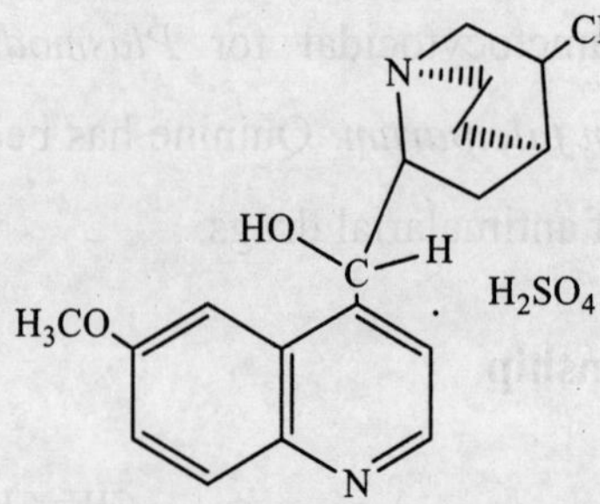


[(1S,2S,4S,5R) - 5 - ethenyl - 1 - azabicyclo[2.2.2]octan - 2 - yl](6 - methoxyquinolin - 4 - yl)methanol) sulfuric acid

**Mechanism of action:** It inhibits nucleic acid synthesis, protein synthesis and glycolysis in *Plasmodium falciparum* and can bind with hemozoin in parasitized erythrocytes.

**Use:** It is used to treat Chloroquine-resistant strains of *Plasmodium falciparum*.

## 2.2 4 – Amino Quinolines

### 2.2.1 Structure Activity Relationship

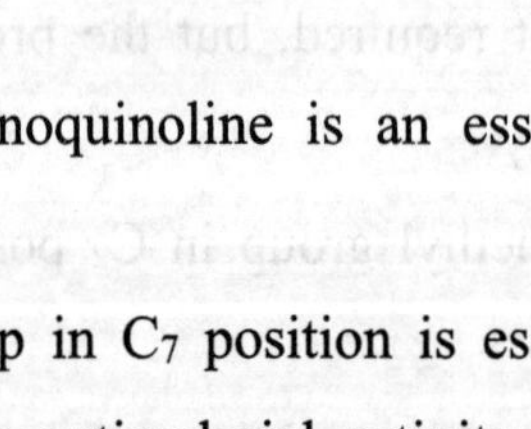


- The basic nucleus 4-aminoquinoline is an essential component for antimalarial activity.
- Introduction of halo group in $C_7$ position is essential for inhibition of β-hematin formation and optimal for antimalarial activity. Other electron donor groups like $-NH_2$ or $-OCH_3$ and electron withdrawing groups like $-NO_2$ in the place of $C_7$ position reduces the antimalarial activity.
- Modification of diaminoalkyl side chain provides the required pharmacokinetic properties for drug transport.
- 2 to 5 carbon between nitrogen atom is optimum for activity.

- 3° amine is important for activity and ethyl group is best for activity. Substitution of –OH group on one of the ethyl group on 3° amine reduces the activity and increases the plasma concentration. eg. Hydroxy chloroquine.
- Incorporation of an aromatic ring in the side chain reduces the activity and toxicity. eg. Amodiaquine.
- Introduction of methyl group at $C_3$ position reduces the antimalarial activity.

**A. Chloroquine (Lariago)**

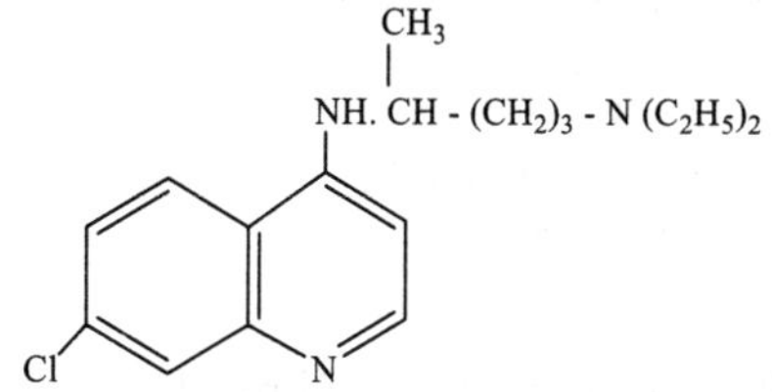


7 - Chloro - 4 - {[4 - (diethylamino) -1- methyl butyl] amino} quinoline

Synthesis

Step - I: Preparation of 4, 7 - Dichloro quinoline

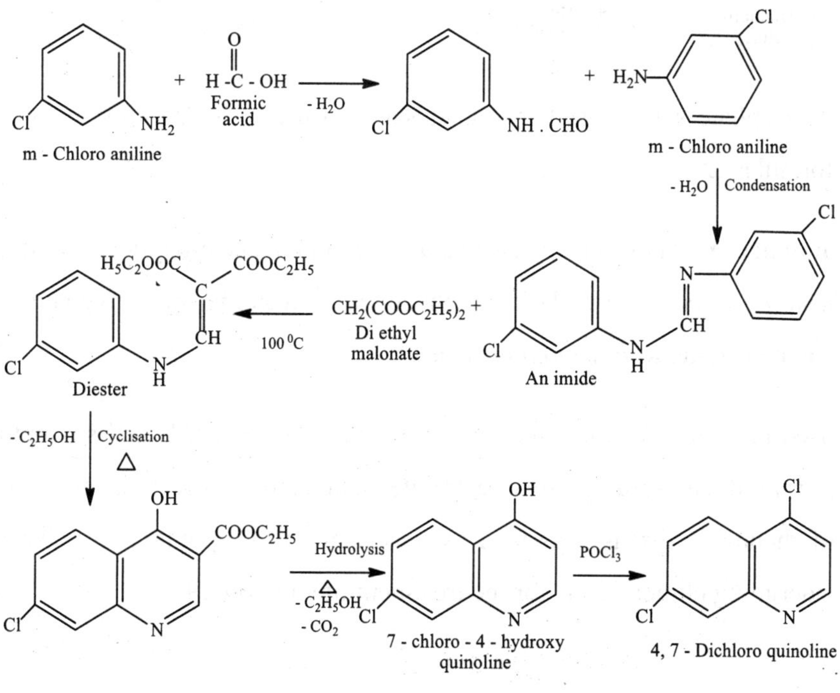

Step II: Preparation of 4- Amino -1- diethylamino pentane

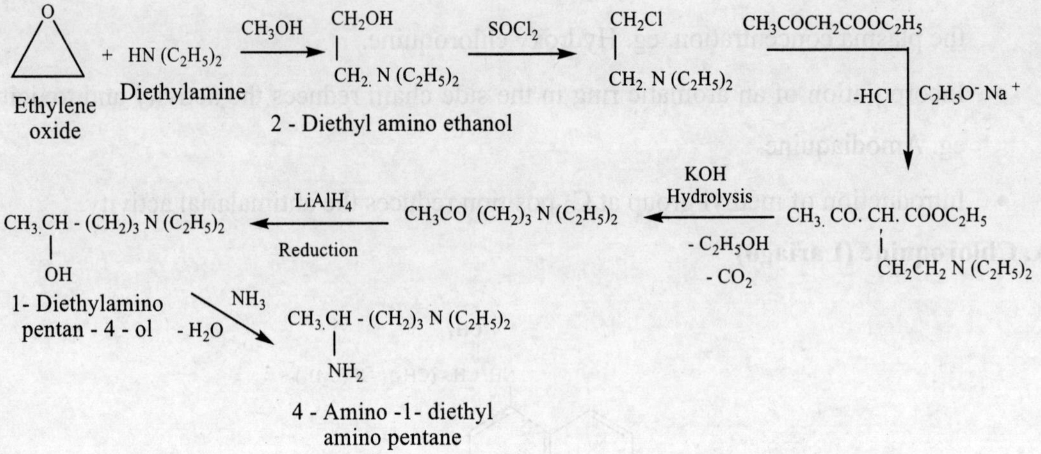


Step - III: Condensation of step - I and step - II products

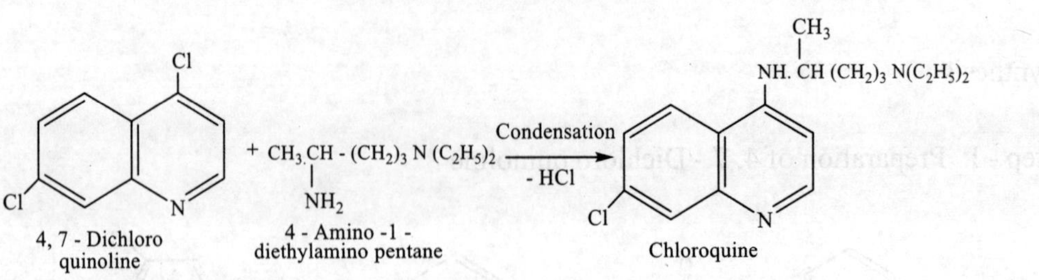


The phosphate salt is used in oral dosage form and hydrochloride salt is used in parenteral formulation.

**Mechanism of action:** They act against *Plasmodium* in the erythrocytic stage. It inhibits the action of *heme polymerase* in malarial trophozoites, preventing the conversion of heme to hemozoin. Heme is toxic to *Plasmodium* species.

**Use:** It is used to treat infections of *P. vivax*, *P. malariae*, *P. ovale* and susceptible strains of *P. falciparum*. It is useful to treat extraintestinal amoebiasis. It is also used for the treatment of rheumatic diseases, as well as treatment and prophylaxis of Zika virus. It is currently undergoing clinical trials for the treatment of COVID-19.

**B. Amodiaquine (Camoquin)**

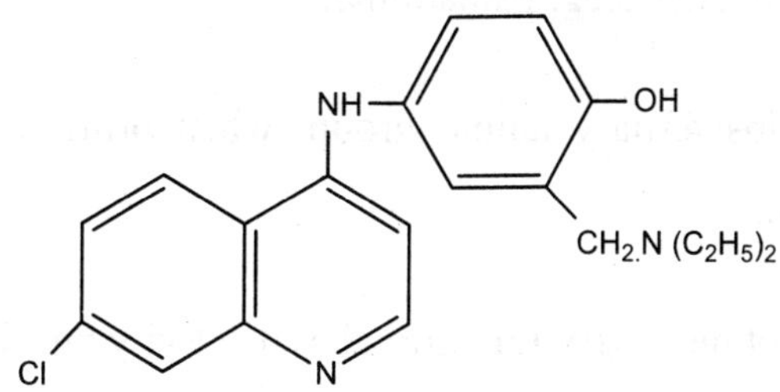


7 - Chloro - 4 - (3 - diethylamino methyl - 4 - hydroxyanilino) quinoline

**Mechanism of action:** It inhibits heme *polymerase* activity results in accumulation of free heme, which is toxic to the parasites. The drug-heme complex is toxic and disrupts membrane function.

**Use:** It is used as a suppressive agent in malaria. It also possesses anti-inflammatory property.

**2.3 8 - Amino Quinolines**

**2.3.1 Structure Activity Relationship**

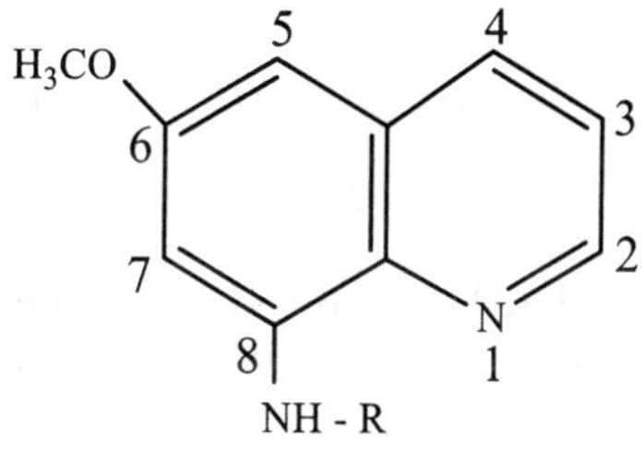


- Drug in this group have amino substitution at $8^{th}$ position at quinoline ring. Such ring has $-OCH_3$ group at $6^{th}$ position.
- Pamaquine, Primaquine and Tafenoquine are antimalarial drug that belongs to 8-aminoquinoline family. Pamaquine is closely related to Primaquine. Compared to Primaquine, Pamaquine is more toxic and less efficacious.

- When side chain is introduced at amino group, antimalarial activity is intensified. It causes hemolysis of RBCs.eg. Pamaquine.

- Pamaquine contains tertiary amino group, when primary amino group is placed, toxicity is reduced.

- -$OCH_3$ group is not necessary for antimalarial activity but when replaced by –$OC_2H_5$ the compound become less active and more toxic. eg. Primaquine.

- When -$OCH_3$ group is replaced with –$CH_3$ group, the compound becomes inactive.

- Introduction of halogen increases toxicity.

- Presence of quinoline ring is essential for antimalarial activity. When pyridine ring is converted to piperidine the compound become inactive.

**A. Pamaquine (PMQ, Malquine)**

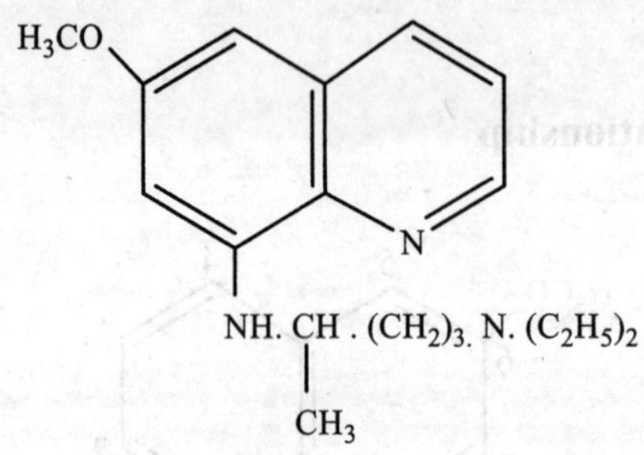


8 - [(4 - Diethyl amino -1- methyl butyl) amino] - 6 - methoxy quinoline

Synthesis

Step - I: Preparation of 8 - Amino - 6 - methoxy quinoline

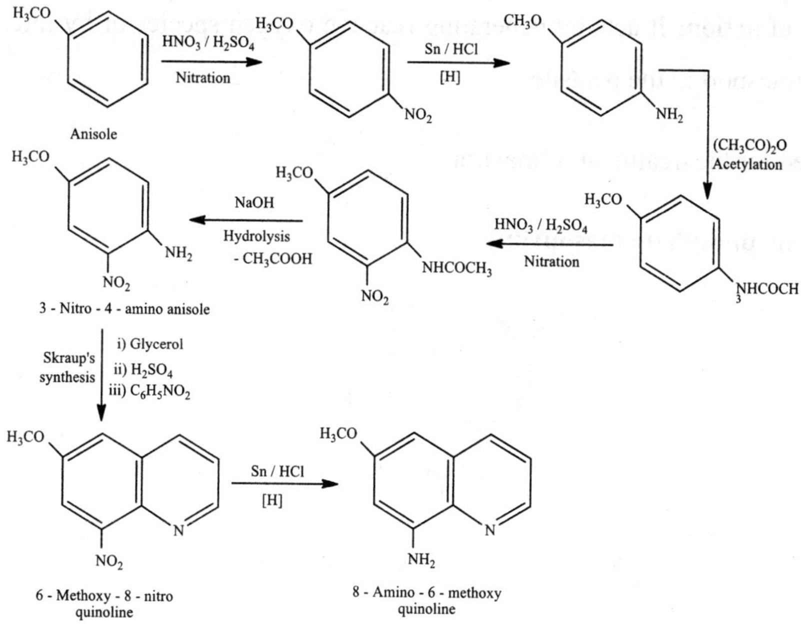


## Step - II: Preparation of 4 - Bromo -1- diethyl amino pentane

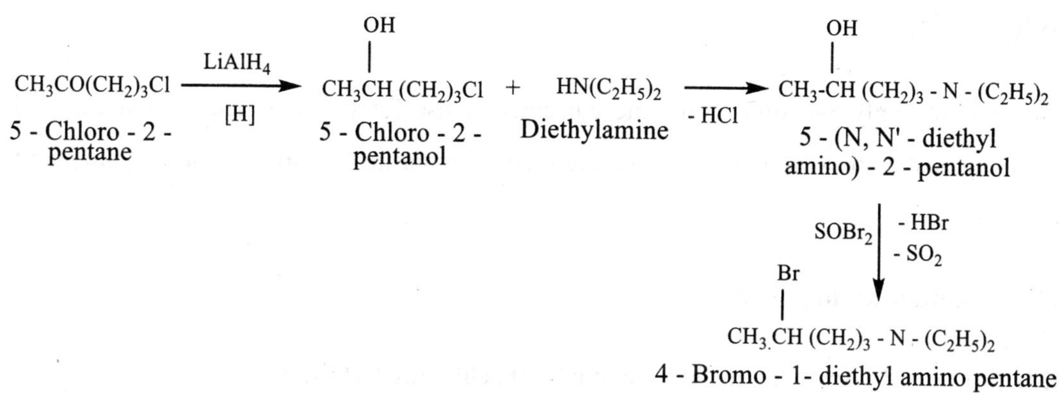


## Step - III: Condensation of step - I and II product

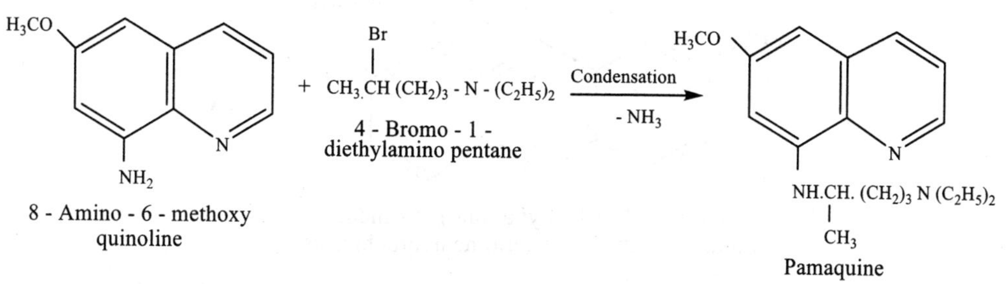

**Mechanism of action:** It acts by generating reactive oxygen species or by interfering with the electron transport in the parasite.

**Use:** It is used for the treatment of malaria.

**B. Primaquine phosphate (Jasoprim)**

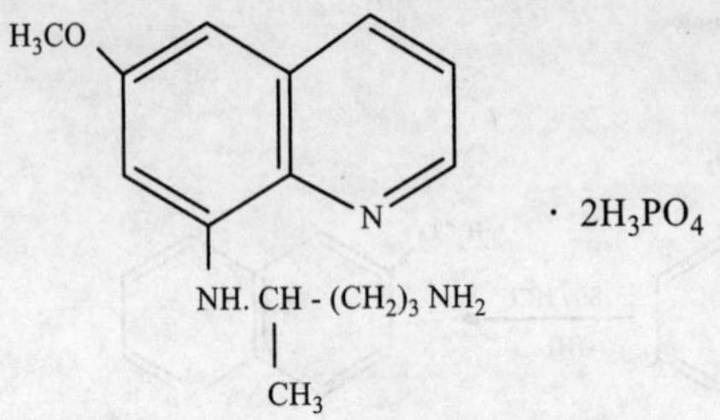

8 - [(4 - Amino - 1- methyl butyl) amino] - 6 - methoxy quinoline

**Mechanism of action:** It acts by generating reactive oxygen species or by interfering with the electron transport in the parasite. It may bind to and alter the properties of protozoal DNA.

**Use:** It is the only 8-Amino quinoline currently in use for the treatment of malaria. It is active against exoerythrocytic *Plasmodium vivax* malaria and also inhibits gametocyte stage.

**2.4 9 - Amino Acridines**

**A. Quinacrine hydrochloride/Mepacrine hydrochloride (Atabrine)**

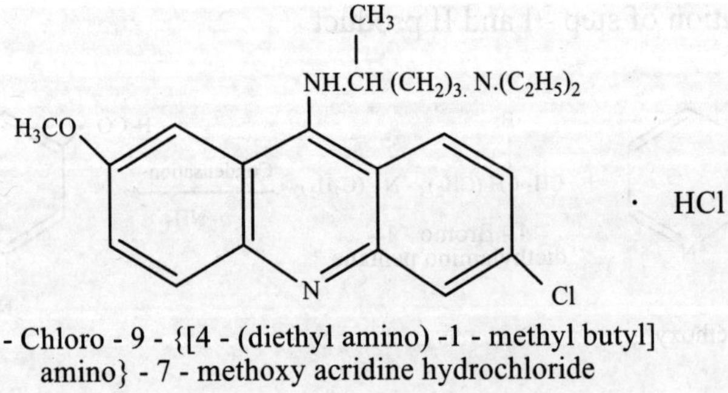

3 - Chloro - 9 - {[4 - (diethyl amino) -1 - methyl butyl] amino} - 7 - methoxy acridine hydrochloride

**Mechanism of action:** It binds to deoxyribonucleic acid (DNA) *in vitro* by intercalation between adjacent base pairs, inhibiting transcription and translation to ribonucleic acid (RNA).

**Use:** It is used as antimalarial agent. It has also been used as an anthelmintic and in the treatment of giardiasis and malignant effusions.

## 2.5 Biguanides

### A. Proguanil (Malarone)

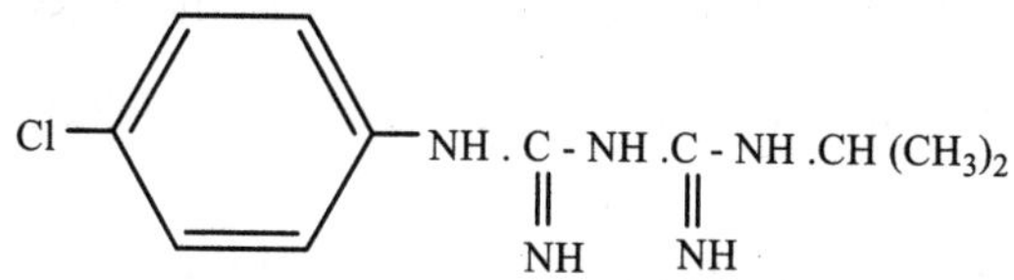

1- (p - Chloro phenyl) - 5 - isopropyl biguanide

**Mechanism of action:** It is a prodrug metabolized by CYP2C19 to bioactive Cycloguanil. It interferes with deoxy thymidylate synthesis by inhibiting *dihydrofolate reductase*.

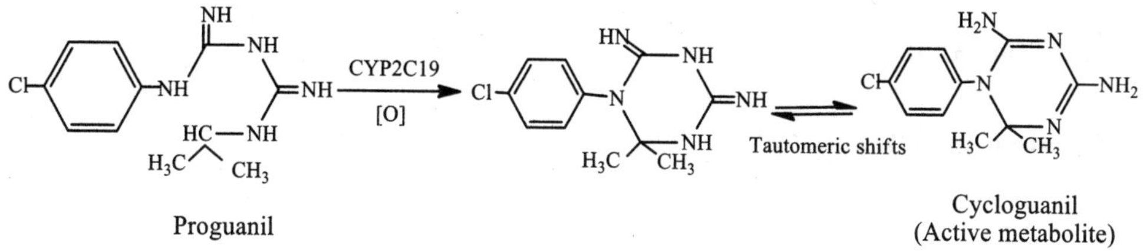

Proguanil and Atovaquone are administered in combination for synergistic effect. Atovaquone is a selective inhibitor of plasmodium's mitochondrial electron transport system and Cycloguanil is a *dihydrofolate reductase* inhibitor.

**Use:** It is used in prophylactic treatment of malaria. It is active against pre-erythrocytic form of malaria.

## 2.6 Dihydro triazine

### A. Cycloguanil pamoate

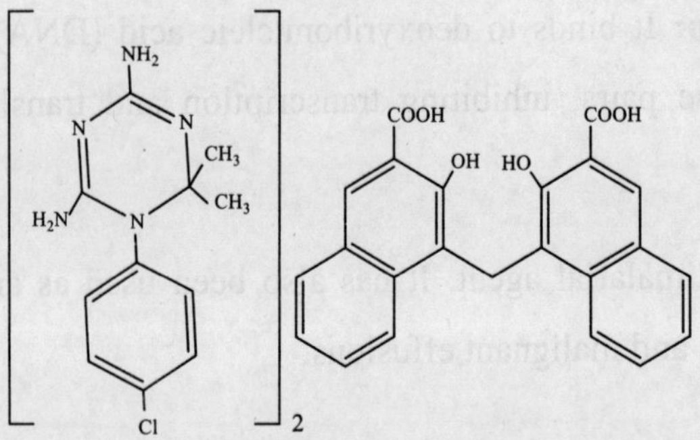

Bis(1 - (4 - chlorophenyl) - 6,6 - dimethyl - 1,6 - dihydro - 1,3,5 - triazine - 2,4 - diamine); 4 - [(3 - carboxy - 2 - hydroxynaphthalen -1 - yl)methyl] -3 - hydroxynaphthalene - 2 - carboxylic acid

It is an active metabolite of Proguanil. It belongs to the class of organic compounds known as amino triazines in which amino group attached to a triazine ring.

**Mechanism of action:** It is a *dihydrofolate reductase* inhibitor and is a metabolite of the antimalarial drug Proguanil. It is one of the few antimalarial drugs that act on both erythrocytic and on the pre-erythrocytic (hepatic) forms of the malarial parasites.

**Use:** It is employed for the suppression of malaria.

## 2.7 Pyrimidine Analogues

### A. Pyrimethamine (Daraprim)

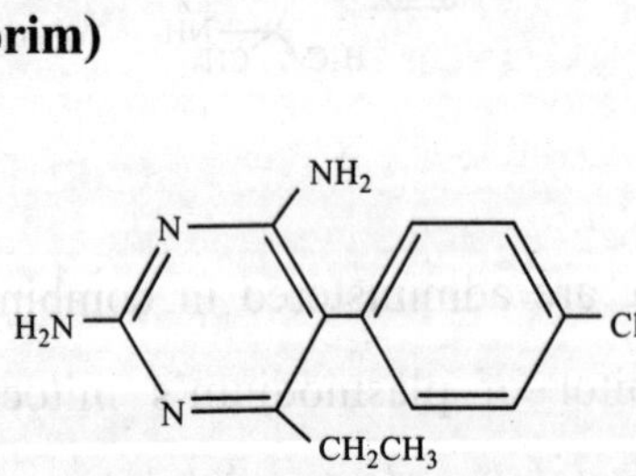

2,4 - Diamino - 5 - (p - chloro phenyl) - 6 - ethyl pyrimidine

**Mechanism of action:** It inhibits the *dihydrofolate reductase* of plasmodia and thereby blocks the biosynthesis of purines and pyrimidines, which are essential for DNA synthesis and cell multiplication. This leads to failure of nuclear division at the time of schizont formation in erythrocytes and liver.

**Use:** It is active against *Plasmodium falciparum* and *Plasmodium vivax* in combination with Sulfadiazine.

## 2.8 Sesquiterpene Lactones

### 2.8.1 Structure Activity Relationship

- Artemisinin is a natural product that can be extracted from the leaves of *Artemisia annua*.
- Artemisinin serves as a lead compound for the development of newer antimalarials with improved properties.
- The lactone group can be reduced and form Dihydro artemisinin, which is used to produce semi-synthetic prodrugs that are more water and oil soluble.
- Compared to Artemisinin, Artemether, Artesunate and Dihydro artemisinin are more active.
- The hydroxyl group can be alkylated to give oil soluble ether derivatives such as Artemether and Arteether.
- Esterification of the hydroxyl group with succinic acid gives the water soluble derivative Artesunate.

### A. Artemether (Larither, Paluther)

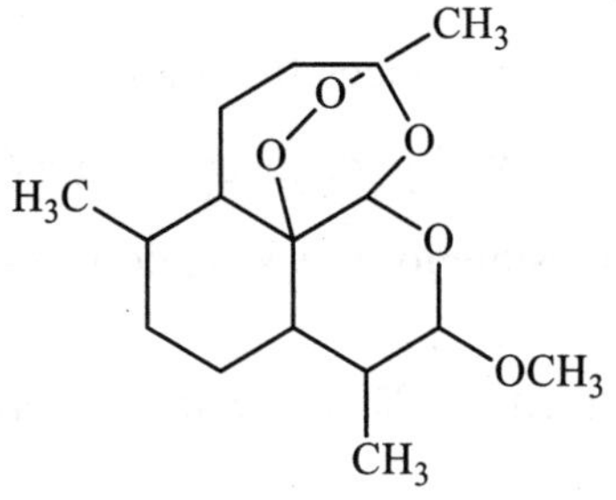


Decahydro - 10 - methoxy - 3,6,9 - trimethyl - 3,12 - epoxy - 12H - pyrano [4,3 - j] - 1,2 - benzodioxepine

Artemether is a methyl ether derivative of Artemisinin, which is a peroxide-containing lactone, isolated from the antimalarial plant *Artemisia annua*.

**Mechanism of action:** It acts against the erythrocytic stages of *Plasmodium falciparum* by inhibiting nucleic acid and protein synthesis.

**Use:** It is used for the treatment of malaria in injectable formulation. It is available in combination with Lumefantrine as oral tablet.

**B. Artesunate (Asunate, Ulteria)**

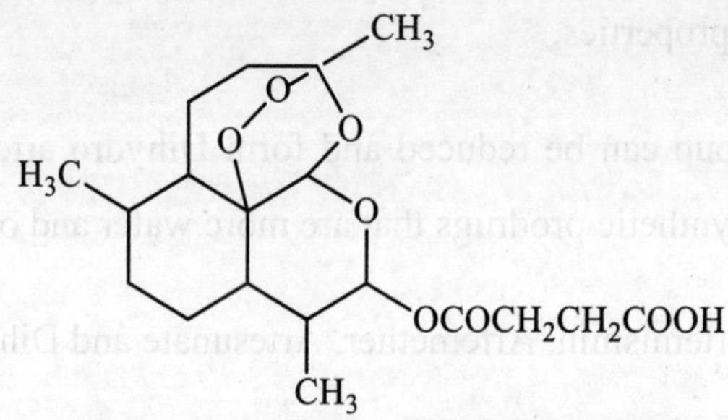


Decahydro - 3,6,9 - trimethyl - 3,12 - epoxy - 12H - pyrano[4,3-j]1,2 - benzodioxepin - 10 - ol - hydrogen succinate

Artesunate is a water-soluble hemi-succinate derivative of Artemisinin. It is an Artemisinin drug capable of killing all erythrocytic stages of the malaria parasite including the ring stage, late schizonts and the gametocytes responsible for transmission of malaria.

**Mechanism of action:** The mechanism involves the cleavage of the endoperoxide bond through reaction with heme. This produces free radicals which alkylate parasitic proteins. It has been shown to inhibit an essential parasite calcium *adenosine triphosphatase* enzyme. It inhibits malaria proteins, responsible for breaking down cytotoxic hematin.

**Use:** It is effective in the treatment of *Plasmodium falciparum* gametes.

## 2.9 Hydroxy Naphthoquinone

### A. Atovaquone (Mepron)

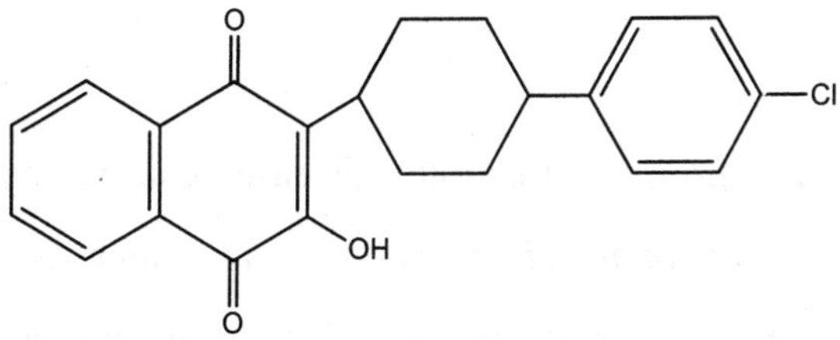


2 - (4 - (p - Chlorophenyl) cyclohexyl) - 3 - hydroxy -1, 4 - naphthoquinone

**Mechanism of action:** It acts by selectively affecting mitochondrial electron transport and parallel processes such as ATP and pyrimidine biosynthesis in Atovaquone-responsive parasites.

**Use:** It is used as antimalarial agent. It also possesses antimicrobial and anti-pneumocystis activities.

## 2.10 Quinoline

### A. Mefloquine (Lariam)

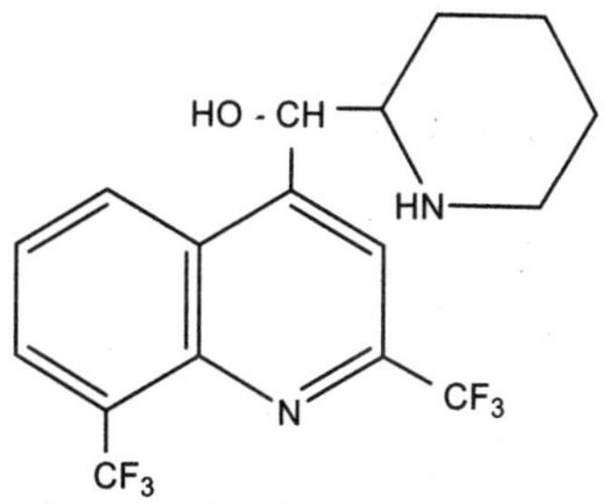


*DL - Erythro* - α - 2 - piperidyl - 2, 8 - bis - (trifluromethyl) - 4 - quinoline methanol

**Mechanism of action:** It acts by forming toxic complexes with free heme that damage membranes and interact with other plasmodial compounds.

**Use:** It is used for the treatment of mild to moderate acute malaria caused by strains of *Plasmodium falciparum* and *Plasmodium vivax*.

Chapter 4

# ANTITUBERCULAR AGENTS

## 1. INTRODUCTION

Tuberculosis is a chronic infectious disease caused by various strains of *Mycobacterium* especially *Mycobacterium tuberculosis* which is an acid fast aerobic bacillus. It is transmitted via the respiratory route. The organism appears in water droplets expelled during coughing, sneezing or talking. Either in droplet form or through the air, the organism enters the respiratory tract. It mainly affects the lungs but can spread through blood stream and lymphatic system to the brain, bones, eyes and skin. In pulmonary tuberculosis the bacilli reach the alveoli and are ingested by pulmonary macrophages. Substance secreted by the macrophages stimulates surrounding fibroblast to enclose the infection site leading to formation of granuloma or tubercles. Extra pulmonary tuberculosis is much more common in HIV infected patients. The drugs used in the treatment of tuberculosis are called antitubercular agents, which can be divided into two major categories like first line agents and second line agents.

All first line agents have a standard three letter and a single letter abbreviation as follows,

- Ethambutol is EMB or E,
- Isoniazid is INH or H,
- Pyrazinamide is PZA or Z,
- Rifampicin is RMP or R,
- Streptomycin is STM or S.

Drug regimens are similarly abbreviated in a standardized manner. The drugs are listed using their single letter abbreviations. A prefix denotes the number of months the treatment should be given for and a subscript denotes intermittent dosing and no subscript means daily dosing. Most regimens have an initial high intensity phase, followed by a continuation phase (also called a consolidation phase or eradication phase) and the two phases divided by a slash. So, $2HREZ/4HR_3$: means Isoniazid, Rifampicin, Ethambutol, Pyrazinamide daily for two months, followed by four months of Isoniazid and Rifampicin given three times a week.

## 2. CLASSIFICATION

**Classification of Antitubercular Drugs**

| First line oral drugs | Antibiotics | Second line oral drugs | Fluoroquinolones |
|---|---|---|---|
| Isoniazid | Streptomycin | Ethionamide | Ciprofloxacin |
| Ethambutol | Kanamycin | Prothionamide | Ofloxacin |
| Pyrazinamide | Amikacin | Para amino salicylic acid | Levofloxacin |
| Rifampicin | Capreomycin | Cycloserine | Gatifloxacin |
| Rifabutin | Vincomycin | | |
| | Rifampicin | | |
| | Rifabutin | | |
| | Cycloserine | | |

### 2.1. First-line Oral Drugs

### A. Isoniazid (INH) (Isonex, Nydrazid)

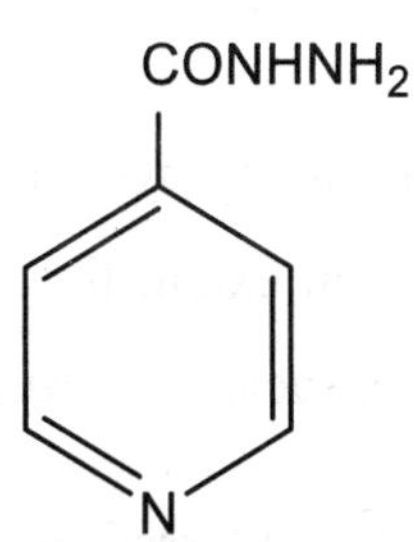


4 - Pyridine carboxylic acid hydrazide

Synthesis

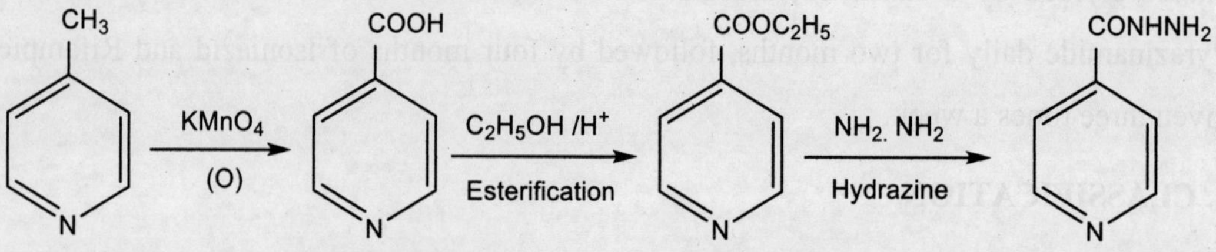


γ- Picoline Isonicotinic acid Ethyl isonicotinate Isoniazid

**Mechanism of action:** It is a prodrug that is activated through an oxidation reaction by bacterial *catalase-peroxidase* enzyme in *Mycobacterium tuberculosis.* The activated INH acylates the enzyme system found exclusively in *Mycobacterium tuberculosis* which is essential for the synthesis of mycolic acid, a fatty acid stabilizes the bacterial cell wall.

**Use:** It is a most potent and selective of the known primary drug for tuberculosis.

**B. Pyrazinamide (Pyzid, Zypyra)**

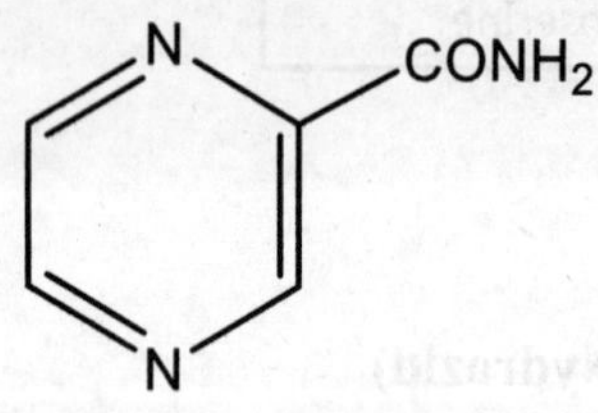


Pyrazine - 2 - carboxamide

**Mechanism of action:** It acts by producing pyrazinoic acid, which lowers the pH of the surrounding *M. tuberculosis*, to such an extent that the organism is unable to grow. The Pyrazinamide is converted to Pyrazinoic acid by *pyrazine amidase* produced by organism.

**Use:** It is a secondary tuberculostatic agent used in combination with other antitubercular drugs (INH and Rifampin). It is used to treat intracellular tubercle bacilli that are not affected by other drugs.

**C. Ethambutol (Mycoback, Mycobutol)**

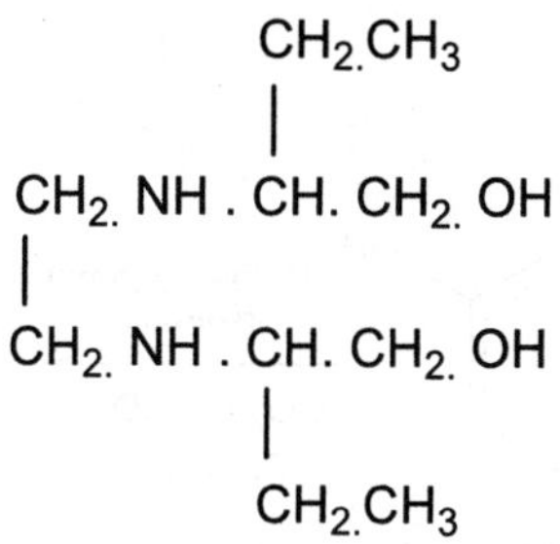

2, 2' - (1, 2 - Ethane diyldiamino) bis - 1 - butanol

(+) Ethambutol is 200 to 500-fold more active than its (-) enantiomer.

**Mechanism of action:** It inhibits the formation of mycobacterial cell wall by affecting the synthesis of mycobacterial arabinogalactan. The enzyme polymerizes D-arabino furanose to arabinoglycan, an essential cell wall component.

**Use:** It is a tuberculostatic drug that is effective against tubercle bacilli resistant to Isoniazid or Streptomycin.

### 2.2 Second-line Oral Drugs

**A. Para-aminosalicylic Acid (Paser)**

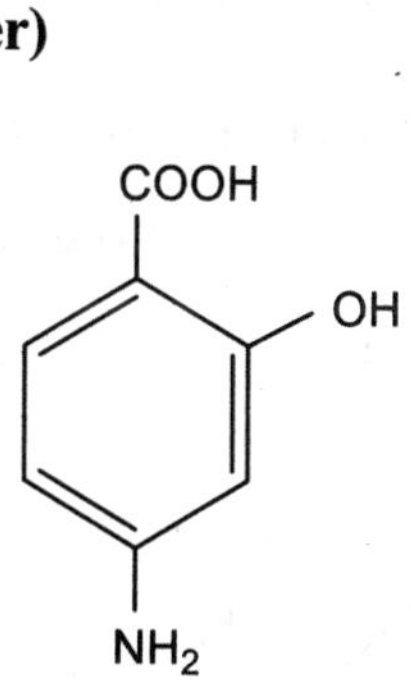

4 - Amino - 2 - hydroxy benzoic acid

Synthesis

Method - I

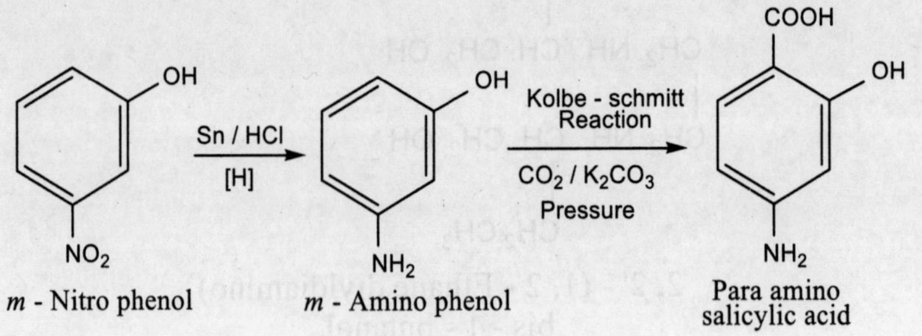


Method - II

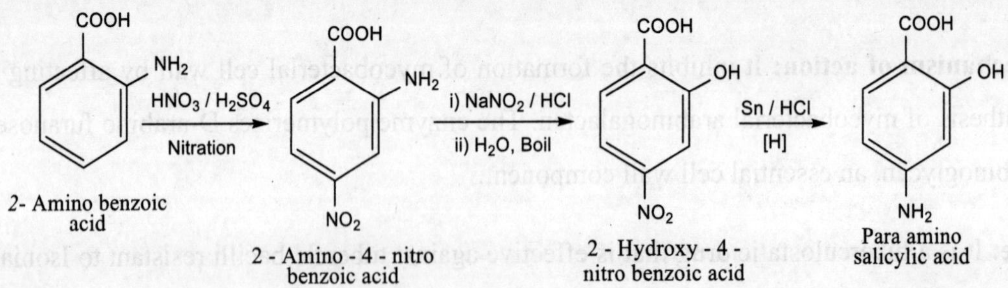


**Mechanism of action:** It inhibits folic acid synthesis which is needed for bacterial growth. It may inhibit the synthesis of the cell wall component, mycobactin, thus reducing iron uptake by *M. tuberculosis* and it delay bacterial resistance to Streptomycin and Isoniazid.

**Use:** It is used in the treatment of tuberculosis. PAS is bacteriostatic, so that it only arrest but does not eradicate the *tubercle bacilli*. Therefore, PAS is always used in combination with one or two other antitubercular drugs.

**B. Ethionamide (Ethide, Mycotuf)**

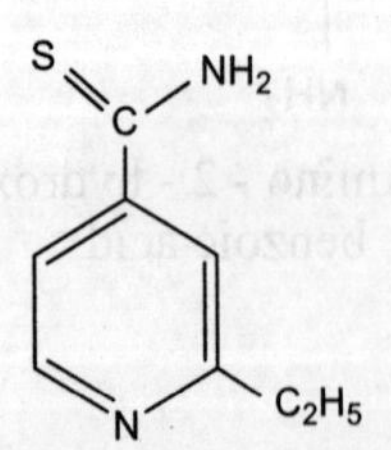


2 - Ethyl - 4 - pyridine carbothioamide

**Mechanism of action:** It is a prodrug that is activated through an oxidation reaction catalyzed by an endogenous enzyme *catalase peroxidase*. The activated acetylated Ethionamide deactivates *enoyl reductase* enzyme found exclusively in *M. tuberculosis* which is essential for the synthesis of mycolic acid.

**Use:** It is less potent and more toxic than INH, so its general use should be avoided. It should be used only when the usual combination of Streptomycin, PAS and INH are ineffective or cannot be tolerated.

### 2.3 Antibiotics

**A. Streptomycin (Refer to Chapter 1 Antibiotics; Page No.45)**

**B. Capreomycin sulphate (Capastat)**

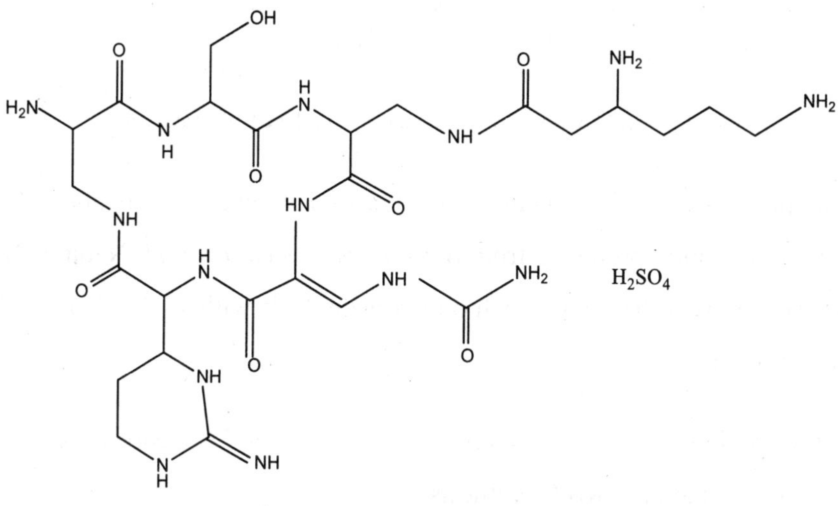


It is an antibiotic isolated from *Streptomyces capreolus*, is a mixture of polypeptide. It consists of four active components- Capreomycin IA, IB, IIA and IIB. The agent clinically used contains primarily IA and IB. It should be administered only in combination with other antitubercular drug such as INH or Ethambutol. Capreomycin is a fourth or fifth choice of drug in tuberculosis therapy.

**Mechanism of action:** It inhibits protein synthesis by binding to the 70S ribosomal unit and also interferes with lipid and nucleic acid biosynthesis ultimately fatal to the bacteria.

**Use:** It is active against *Mycobacterium tuberculosis* and some atypical mycobacterium, particularly *Mycobacterium kansasii.*

**C. Rifampicin (Rifampin, Rimpacin)**

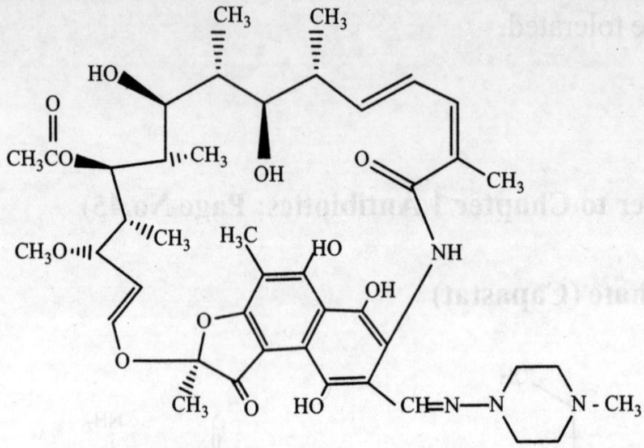

3 - [[(4 - Methyl - 1 - piperazinyl) imino] methyl] rifamycin

Rifampicin is a semi-synthetic derivative of Rifamycin, a member of ansamycin class of natural antibiotic produced from *Streptomyces mediterranei*. Natural Rifamycin is converted to 3- Formyl rifamycin, which on hydrazinolysis with 4 - Methyl - 1 - piperazine amine gives Rifampicin.

**Mechanism of action:** It inhibits bacterial *DNA-dependent RNA polymerase* (DDRP) and blocks the chain formation of RNA synthesis.

**Use:** It is a broad spectrum antibiotic effective against most of the Gram-positive bacteria and variably active against Gram-negative organisms. Both *Mycobacterium tuberculosis* and *Mycobacterium leprae* are very susceptible to the drug. Its clinical use is mainly for the treatment of tuberculosis.

## D. Rifabutin (Mycobutin)

Rifabutin is the spiro imidazole-piperidyl derivative of Rifamycin B. It is a very lipophilic compound with high affinity for tissues.

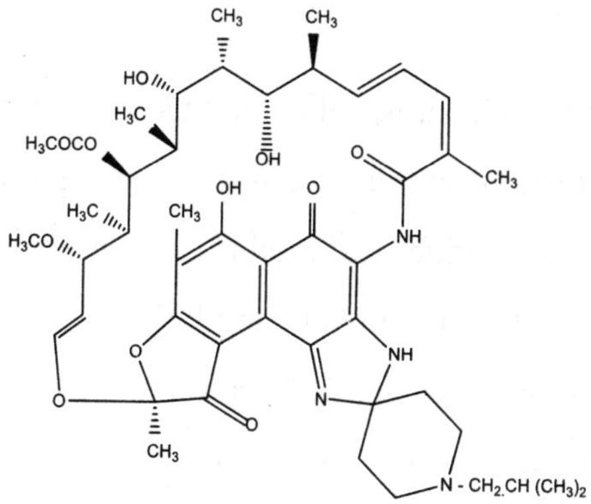

**Mechanism of action:** It inhibits *DNA-dependent RNA polymerase* in gram-positive and some gram-negative bacteria, leading to a suppression of RNA synthesis and cell death.

**Use:** It is a broad-spectrum antibiotic used as prophylaxis against disseminated *Mycobacterium avium* complex (MAC) disease in patients with advanced HIV infection.

## E. Cycloserine (Cyclokox, Seromycin)

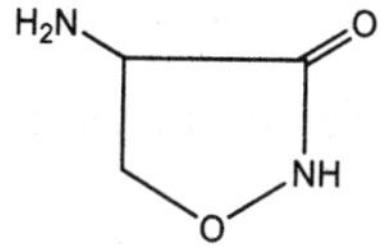

4 - Amino - 3 - isoxazolidinone

It is an antibiotic, produced by *Streptomyces garyphalus*. It slowly dimerizes on standing or in solution.

**Mechanism of action:** It acts by blocking the formation D-alanine and D-alanine peptidoglycans, then the bacteria become weak and results in death of the bacteria.

**Use:** It is useful in the therapy of tuberculosis resistant to other drugs. It is always combined with other antitubercular drug.

Chapter

5

# URINARY TRACT ANTI-INFECTIVE AGENTS

## 1. INTRODUCTION

Urinary anti-infective are drugs that are used to prevent or treat urinary tract infections. Urinary tract infections are divided into two categories: infections involving only the lower urinary tract (i.e. the bladder and urethra) and infections involving both upper and lower tracts. "Upper UTI involves the ureters and kidneys. When the kidneys are involved, the term "acute pyelonephritis" is applied. "Cystitis" is the term applied to bladder inflammation, the commonest cause of which is infection of urine in the bladder. The organism causing UTI infections *are Escherichia coli, Pseudomonas aeruginosa, Streptococcus faecalis, Staphylococcus epidermidis* and *Proteus mirabilis.* Symptoms of lower urinary tract infection are pain with urination, frequent urination and feeling the need to urinate despite having an empty bladder. Symptoms of a kidney infection include fever and flank pain usually in addition to the symptoms of a lower UTI.

### 1.1 The Bacterial Cell

The success of antibacterial agents is due to the fact that, they can act selectively against bacterial cells rather than animal cells. This is largely due to the fact that, bacterial cells and animal cells differ both in their structure and in the biosynthetic pathways. The differences between bacterial and animal cells are

- The bacterial cell has a cell wall, as well as a cell membrane, whereas the animal cell has only a cell membrane. The cell wall is crucial to the bacterial cell's survival. Bacteria have to survive a wide range of environments and osmotic pressures, whereas animal cells do not. The cell wall does not stop water flowing into the cell directly, but it does prevent the cell from swelling and so indirectly prevents water entering into the cell.
- The bacterial cell does not have a defined nucleus, whereas the animal cell does.

- Animal cells contain a variety of structures called organelles (e.g. mitochondria, etc.,) whereas the bacterial cell is relatively simple.
- The biochemistry of a bacterial cell differs significantly from that of an animal cell. For example, bacteria may have to synthesize essential vitamins where as animal cells can acquire intact from food. The bacterial cells must have the enzymes to catalyze these reactions. Animal cells do not, since the reactions are not required.

### 1.2 General Mechanisms of Antibacterial Agents

**Inhibition of nucleic acid transcription and replication**: Inhibition of nucleic acid function prevents cell division and/or the synthesis of essential enzymes. eg. Quinolones.

## 2. CLASSIFICATION

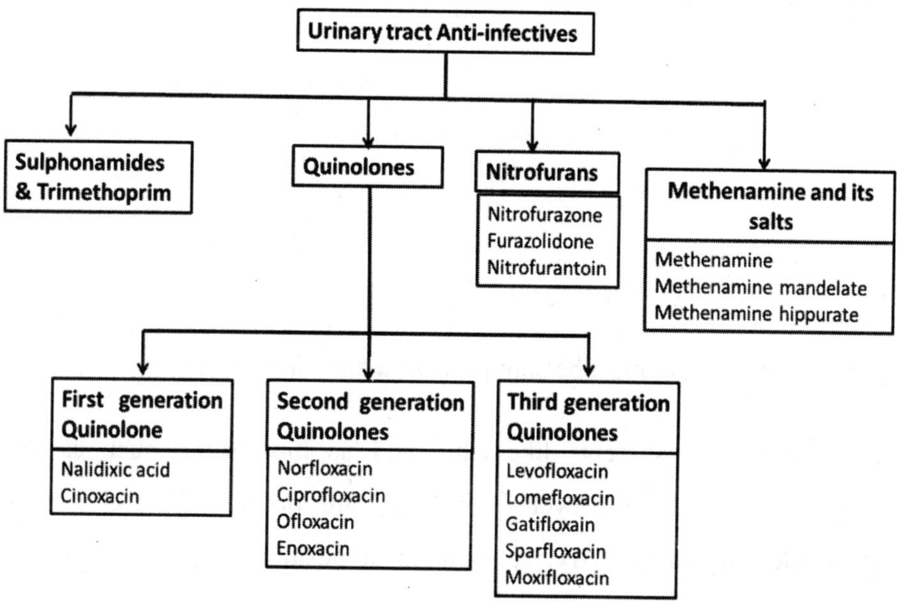


### 2.1 Quinolones

Quinolone antibacterial drugs have been in use since 1964 when Nalidixic acid was released. A second generation of this class of drugs was introduced in 1987 with Ciprofloxacin. Quinolones binds to the bacterial enzymes *DNA gyrase* (*topoisomerase II*) and *topoisomerase IV* and prevent supercoiling of DNA (required for normal transcription) thereby inhibit DNA synthesis. The majority of quinolones in clinical use belong to the subclass fluoroquinolones, which have a fluorine atom attached to the central ring system, typically at the $C_6$ position or $C_7$ position. It is a broad-spectrum antibacterial agent, effective for both Gram-negative and Gram-positive bacteria. It is used in the treatment of urinary tract infections. It can be chemically classified as

a) 1, 8-Naphthyridine-4-one-3-carboxylic acid: eg. Nalidixic acid, Enoxacin.

b) Cinnoline-4-one-3-carboxylic acid: eg. Cinoxacin.

c) 4-Quinolinone-3-carboxylic acid: eg. Norfloxacin, Lomefloxacin, Ciprofloxacin.

### 2.1.1 Structure Activity Relationship

- The minimum pharmacophore essential for antibacterial activity is 1, 4-Dihydro-4-oxopyridine-3-carboxylic acid moiety.

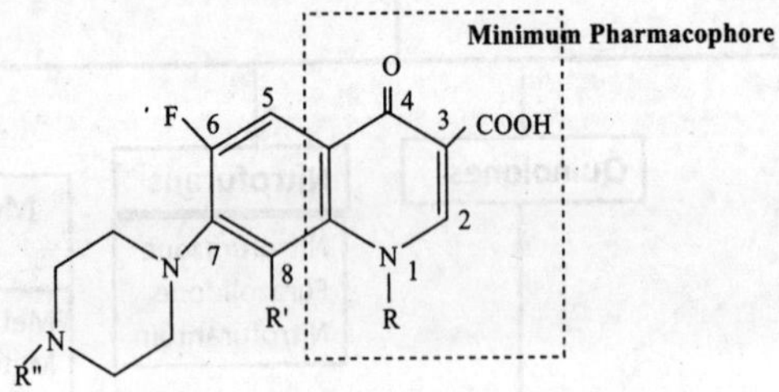


- The pyridone system must be annulated with an aromatic ring.

- At position 1 substituents like ethyl and its bioisosteres such as fluoroethyl, methylamino, methoxy, cyclopropyl etc., are optimal for the activity of the quinolone compounds. Aryl substitution at position 1 is also having consistent activity.

- Introduction of substituent at position 2 greatly reduces the activity. Replacement of nitrogen for $C_2$ gives Cinoxacin, has a good antibacterial activity and pharmacokinetic properties. Reduction of 2, 3 double bonds eliminate the activity.

- Positions 3 and 4, having a carboxylic acid group and the keto group, are generally considered necessary for the binding of quinolones to *DNA gyrase*.

- The replacement of the 3-carboxylic acid function by acidic groups such as sulfonic acid, acetic acid, hydroxamic acid, sulfonamide and phosphoric acid resulted in a substantial decrease in antibacterial activity.

- Presence of 4-oxo group is must for activity.

- Amino and chloro groups are found to be beneficial for positions 5 and 8 respectively. The $C_5$ amino substitution enhances absorption or tissue distribution and reduces phototoxicity.

- Of the various $C_6$ substituent's (H, F, Cl, Br, $CH_3$, $SCH_3$, $COCH_3$, CN and $NO_2$), the addition of a fluorine atom resulted in a dramatic increase in antibacterial potency. The fluoro group at position $C_6$ seems to improve both the *DNA gyrase* complex binding (2 to 17-fold) and cell penetration. Because of such an enhancement of antibacterial potency, nearly all of the recently synthesized quinolones carry a $C_6$ fluorine substituent.

- Piperazine, N-methyl piperazine and pyrrolidine ring substitution at position 7 gives active compounds. Piperazine group at position 7 broadens the spectrum to include Gram-negative bacteria. But it also increases the affinity to GABA receptors which results in CNS side effects. This is overcome by adding a methyl or ethyl group to the piperazine ring (Sparfloxacin, Ofloxacin) or by placing bulky substituents (cyclopropyl) at N-1 position (Ciprofloxacin).

- Replacement of $C_8$ by nitrogen gives naphthyridine ring (Enoxacin) increases bioavailability. Whereas a methoxy group (Gatifloxacin) on $C_8$ position in place of hydrogen provides less phototoxicity. Second fluorine at $C_8$ resulted in increased activity and also increased phototoxicity.

- Compounds with ring fusion at 1, 8 (Ofloxacin) at 5, 6, 7 and 7, 8 are active.

### 2.1.1.1 First Generation Quinolones

#### A. Nalidixic acid (Gramoneg)

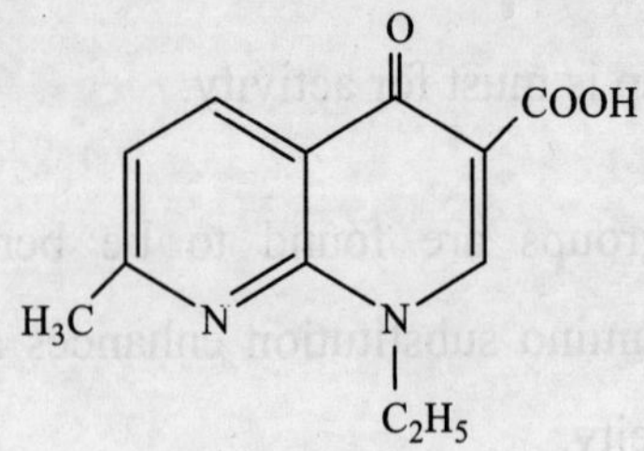

1 - Ethyl - 1, 4 - dihydro - 7 - methyl - 4 - oxo - 1, 8 - naphthyridin - 3 - carboxylic acid

**Mechanism of action:** It inhibits the enzyme *DNA gyrase,* which is responsible for unwinding and supercoiling of bacterial DNA before it replicates causes bacterial cells to die.

**Use:** It is particularly effective against Gram-negative bacteria that cause urinary tract infection.

### 2.1.1.2 Second Generation Quinolones

#### A. Norfloxacin (Normax)

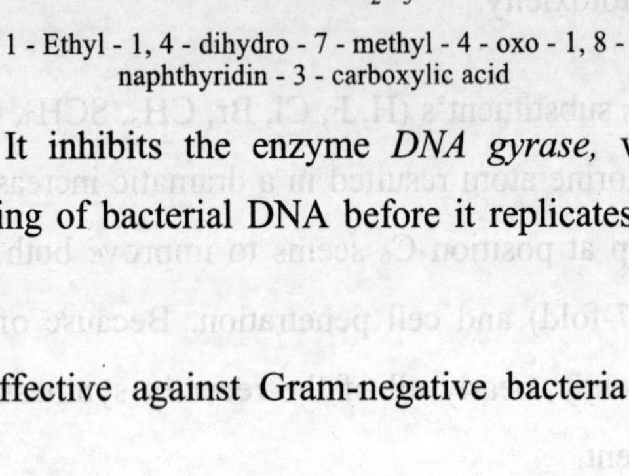

1 - Ethyl - 6 - fluoro - 1, 4 - dihydro - 4 - oxo - 7 - (1- piperazinyl) - 3 - quinoline carboxylic acid

**Mechanism of action:** It inhibits the enzyme *DNA gyrase,* which unwinds and supercoils bacterial DNA before it replicates leads to interferes with bacterial cell replication and causes cell death.

**Use:** It is used for the treatment of urinary tract infections caused by *E. coli, K. pneumoniae and P. mirabilis,* indole-positive *Proteus spp. including P. vulgaris, P. aeruginosa, S. aureus, S. epidermidis* and group *D Streptococci*.

**B. Enoxacin (Penetrex)**

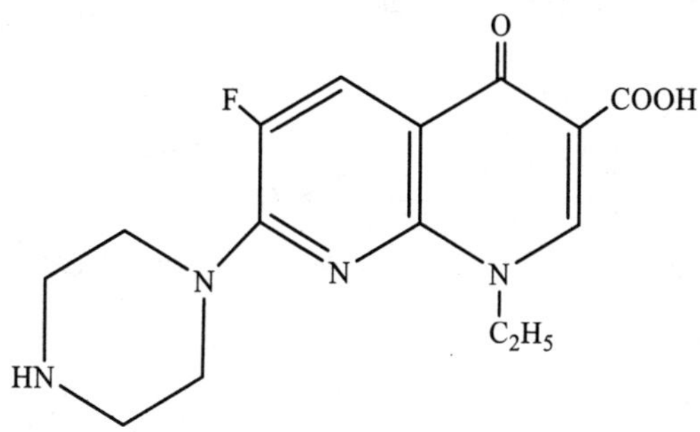


1 - Ethyl - 6 - fluoro - 1, 4 - dihydro - 4 - oxo - 7 - (1 - piperazinyl) - 1, 8 - naphthyridine - 3 - carboxylic acid

**Mechanism of action:** It inhibits the enzyme *DNA gyrase*, which unwinds and supercoils bacterial DNA before it replicates leads to interferes with bacterial cell replication and causes cell death.

**Use:** It is a broad-spectrum antibacterial agent used primarily for the treatment of urinary tract infection and sexually transmitted diseases.

**C. Ciprofloxacin (Cipro)**

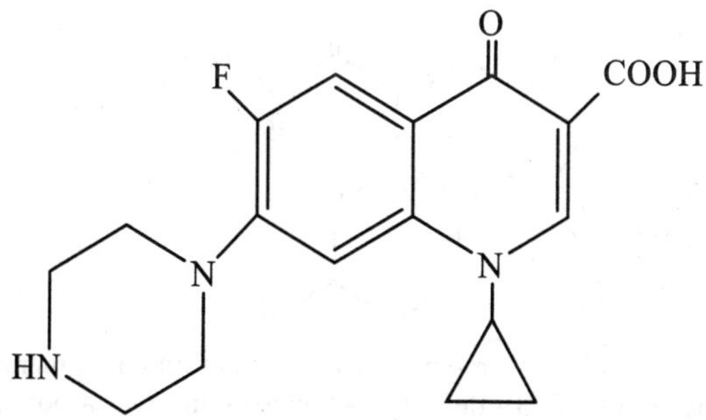


1- Cyclopropyl - 6 - fluoro - 1, 4 - dihydro - 4 - oxo - 7 - (1-piperazinyl) - 3 - quinolin carboxylic acid

Synthesis

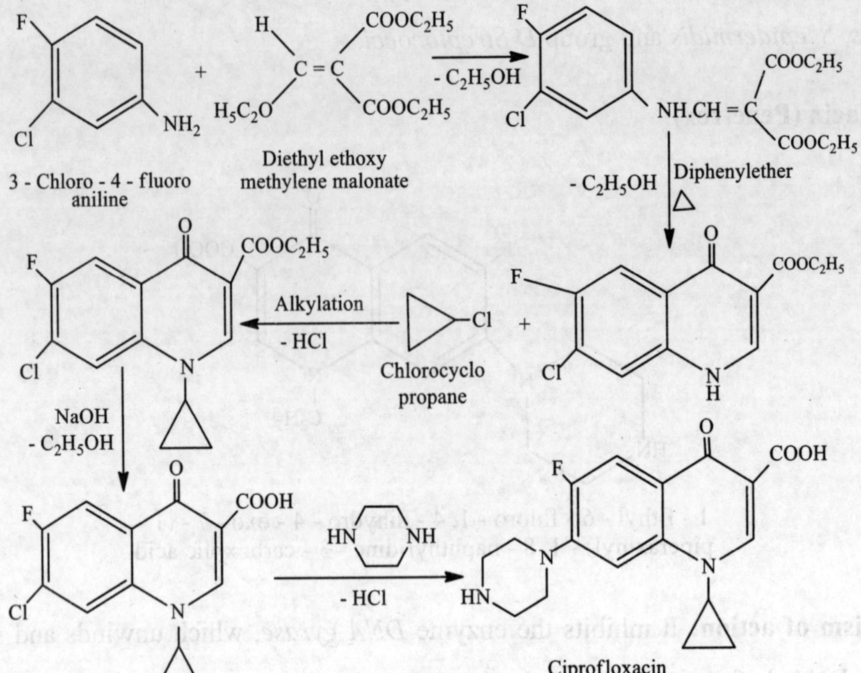


**Mechanism of action:** It acts by inhibiting *DNA gyrase* and a type II *topoisomerase, topoisomerase IV*, necessary to separate bacterial DNA, thereby inhibiting cell division.

**Use:** It is an effective drug for the treatment of urinary tract infection.

**D. Ofloxacin (Alproxen)**

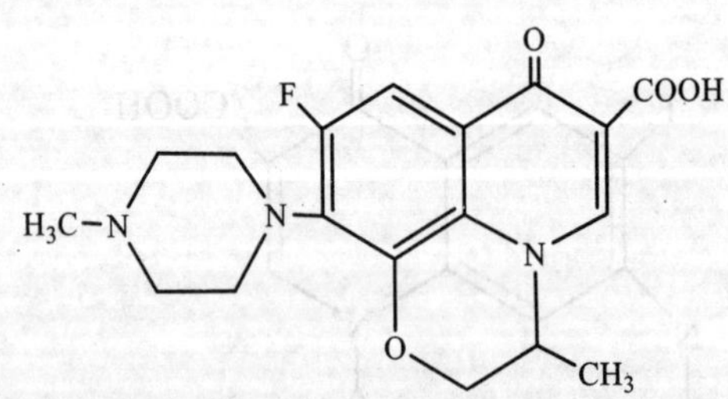

9 - Fluoro - 2, 3 - dihydro - 3 - methyl - 10 - (4 - methyl - 1 - piperazinyl) - 7 - oxo - 7H - pyridol [1, 2, 3 - de] - 1, 4 - benzoxacin - 6 - carboxylic acid

S- Enantiomer called Levofloxacin is 10 folds more potent than R- isomer

**Mechanism of action:** It inhibits the synthesis of the bacterial enzyme *DNA gyrase* by counteracting excessive supercoiling of DNA during replication or transcription. Inhibition of *DNA gyrase* causes rapid- and slow-growing bacterial cells to die.

**Use:** It is used in the treatment of infections of lower respiratory tract, including chronic bronchitis and pneumonia caused by Gram-negative bacilli and pelvic inflammatory disease and is highly active against both *Gonococci* and *Chlamydia.*

### 2.1.1.3 Third Generation Quinolones

#### A. Lomefloxacin (Lomitas)

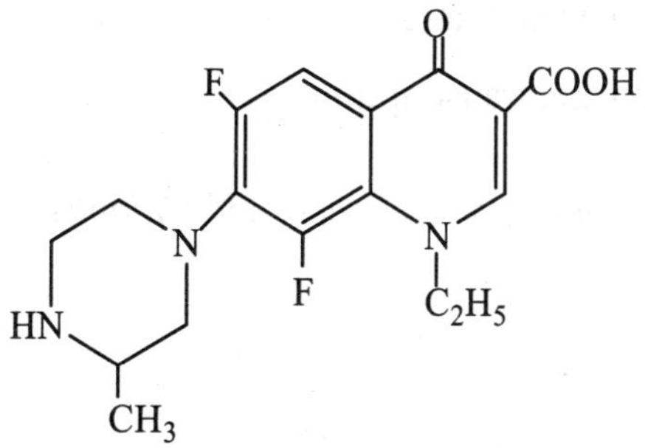


1 - Ethyl - 6, 8 - difluoro - 1, 4 - dihydro - 7 - (3 - methyl - 1 - piperazinyl) - 4 - oxo - 3 - quinoline carboxylic acid

It is a difluorinated quinolone with a longer elimination half-life (7 to 8 hours) than any other member of this class.

**Mechanism of action:** It acts by inhibiting enzymes *DNA gyrase* and *topoisomerase IV*, which are needed for the transcription and replication of bacterial DNA. As a result, DNA replication and transcription are inhibited.

**Use:** It is used to treat bacterial infections including bronchitis and urinary tract infections.

**B. Sparfloxacin (Zespar)**

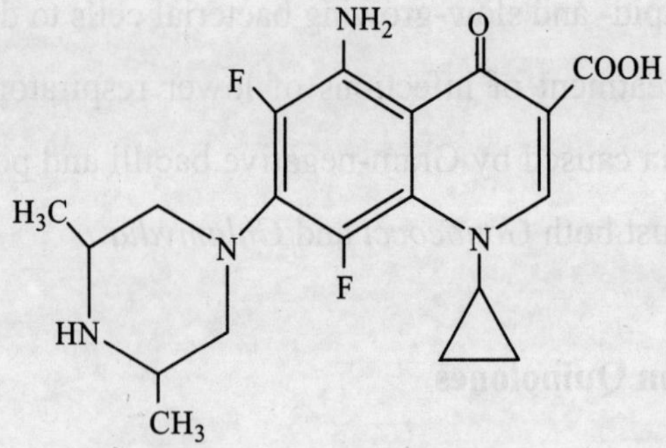

Cis - 5 - amino - 1 - cyclopropyl - 7 - (3, 5 - dimethyl) - 1 - piperazinyl) - 6, 8 - difluoro - 1, 4 - dihydro - 4 - oxoquinoline - 3 - carboxylic acid

**Mechanism of action:** It inhibits the bacterial *DNA gyrase* or the *topoisomerase IV* enzyme, thereby inhibiting DNA replication and transcription.

**Use:** It is effective against *Staphylococci, Streptococci* and *Chlamydia.*

**C. Gatifloxacin (Zymar)**

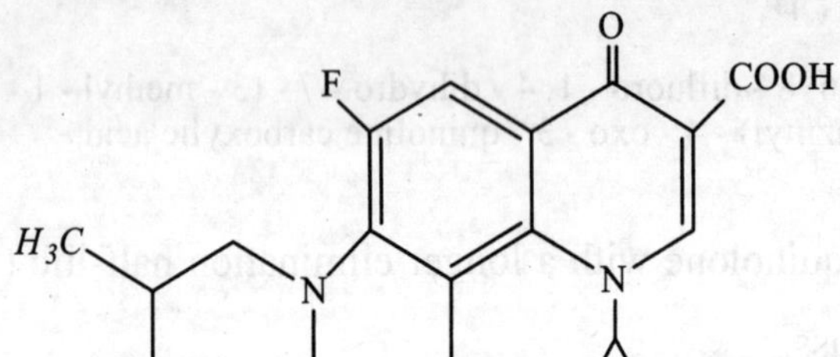

1- Cyclopropyl -1, 4 - dihydro - 6 - fluoro - 8 - methoxy - 7 - (3 - methyl - 1 - piperazinyl) - 4 - oxo - 3 - quinoline carboxylic acid

**Mechanism of action:** It acts by inhibiting the enzymes *topoisomerase* II (*DNA gyrase*) and *topoisomerase* IV, which are required for bacterial DNA replication, transcription, repair and recombination.

**Use:** It is used for the treatment of bronchitis, sinusitis, community-acquired pneumonia and skin infections caused by *Streptococcus pneumoniae, Haemophilus influenza, Staphylococcus aureus, Mycoplasma pneumonia* and *Streptococcus pyogenes*.

### D. Moxifloxacin (Avelox)

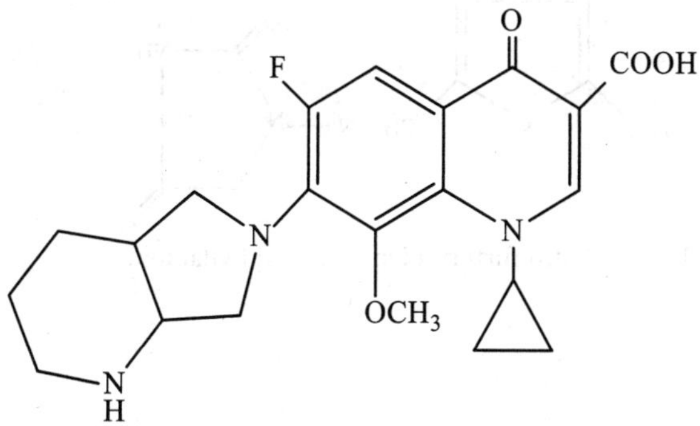

1- Cyclopropyl - 1, 4 - dihydro - 6 - fluoro - 8 - methoxy - 7 - (octahydro - 6H - pyrrolo (3, 4 - b) pyridin - 6 - yl) - 4 - oxo - 3 - quinoline carboxylic acid

**Mechanism of action:** Same as Gatifloxacin.

**Use:** It is a broad-spectrum antibiotic active against both Gram-positive and Gram-negative bacteria. It is used to treat infections caused by *Corynebacterium* species, *Micrococcus luteus*, *S. aureus*, *S. epidermidis*, *S. haemolyticus*, *S. hominis*, *S. warneri*, *Streptococcus pneumoniae* and *Streptococcus viridans* group.

## 2.2 Nitrofurans

The first heterocyclic compounds to be introduced into chemotherapy were the nitrofurans. They are used for the treatment of various kinds of bacterial infections. Nifurtimox is used as an antiprotozoal agent to treat trypanosomiasis and leishmaniasis. Another important nitro heterocyclic compound is Metronidazole, which is used in the treatment of systemic infections caused by anaerobic bacteria.

The nitrofurans are derivatives of 5-Nitro-2-furaldehyde. Antimicrobial activity is present only when the nitro group is in the 5$^{th}$ position.

**A. Nitrofurantoin (Macrobid)**

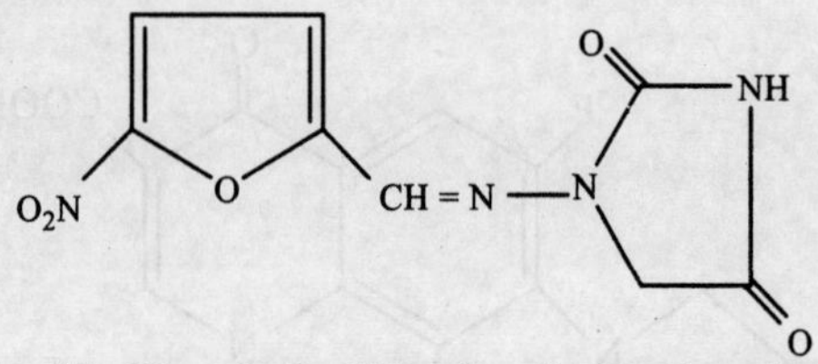

1 - [(5 - Nitro furfurylidene) amino] hydantoin

Synthesis

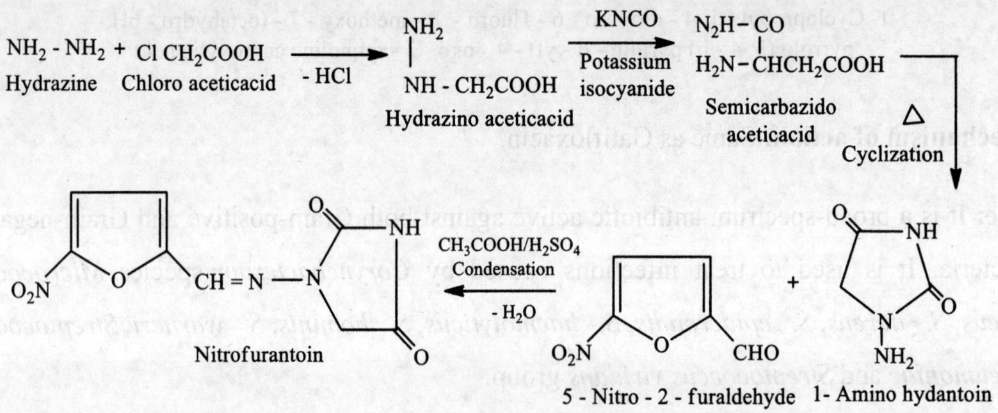

**Mechanism of action:** It acts by inhibiting bacterial protein synthesis, aerobic energy metabolism, DNA synthesis, RNA synthesis and cell wall synthesis.

**Use:** It is effective against a majority of urinary tract pathogens, including certain strains of *E. coli, Klebsiella, Proteus spp.*, *Pseudomonas* and *Aerobacter spp*. It is also effective against *Staphylococci*, *Clostridia* and *Bacillus subtilis*.

**B. Furazolidone (Furoxone)**

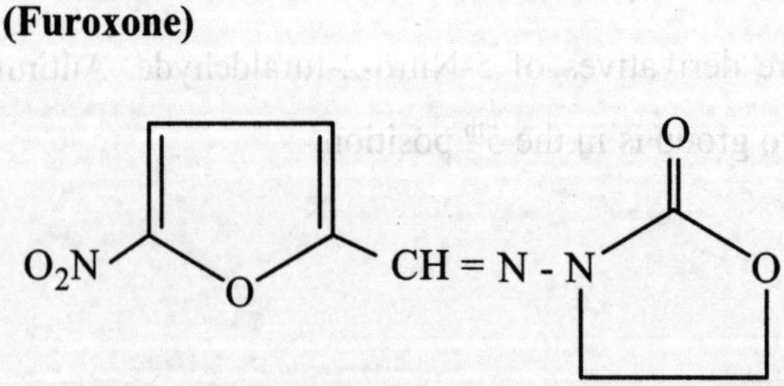

3 - [(5- Nitro furylidene) amino] - 2 - oxazolidinone

**Mechanism of action:** It interferes with several bacterial enzyme systems through DNA strand damage. It also prevents the inactivation of tyramine by GI and hepatic MAO because it is similar in structure and actions to MAO inhibitors.

**Use:** It is effective against *S. aureus, E. coli, Salmonella, Shigella, Proteus spp., Enterobacter and Vibrio cholerae.* It is recommended for the oral treatment of bacterial or protozoal diarrhea caused by susceptible organisms.

### 2.3 Methenamine and its Salts

### A. Methenamine (Hiprex)

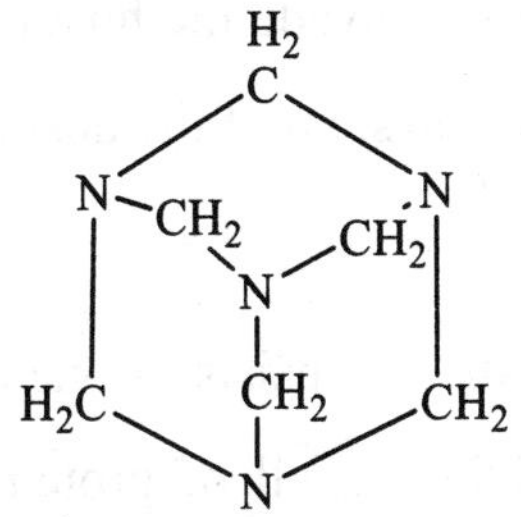

Hexamethylene tetramine

**Mechanism of action:** It is an inactive weak base hydrolyzed to formaldehyde and ammonia in an acidic environment, such as urine, producing greater amounts of formaldehyde as pH decreases. Formaldehyde has bactericidal action, possibly by denaturing proteins. To facilitate hydrolysis, Methenamine is formulated with weak organic acid, such as hippuric acid or mandelic acid.

**Use:** It is used internally as urinary antiseptic for the treatment of chronic urinary tract infections.

Chapter 6

# ANTIVIRAL AGENTS

## 1. INTRODUCTION

Antiviral drugs are a class of medication used specifically for treating viral infections. Viruses are obligate intracellular parasite, smallest of all self-replicating organisms able to pass through filter that retain the smallest bacteria. Virus conducts no metabolic process on their own. They invade the host cell, which may be bacteria, animal or plant cell. It turns the biochemical system of the host cell to its own purposes completely subverting the infected cell.

Virus does not possess cell wall. It consists of one or more of linear or helical strands of either DNA or RNA enclosed in a shell of protein known as capsid. The capsid is composed of several sub-units known as capsomers. In certain cases, capsid may be surrounded by an outer protein or lipoprotein envelope. Viral life cycle varies with species, but they all share a general pattern (Fig. 6.1) can be sequenced as follows:

a) **Adsorption:** Attachment of virus to the host cell.

b) **Penetration:** Penetration of virus into the cell.

c) **Uncoating:** The genetic material or viral genome (DNA or RNA) passes into the host cell, leaving the capsid covering outside of the host cell.

d) **Transcription:** Production of viral mRNA from the viral genome.

e) **Translation:** Viral genome enters the cytoplasm or nucleoplasm and direct or utilizes the host nucleic acid machinery for the synthesis of new viral protein and also for the production of more viral genome. The viral protein modifies the host cell and allows the viral genome to replicate by using host and viral enzyme. This is often the stage at which the cell is irreversibly modified and eventually killed.

f) **Assembly of viral particle:** New viral coat protein assembles into capsid and viral genomes.

g) Release of the mature virus from the cells by budding process or rupture of the cell and repeat of the process, in fresh host cell. Since the host cell machinery is totally utilized for production of new virions, the normal cell function ceases at the time of replication.

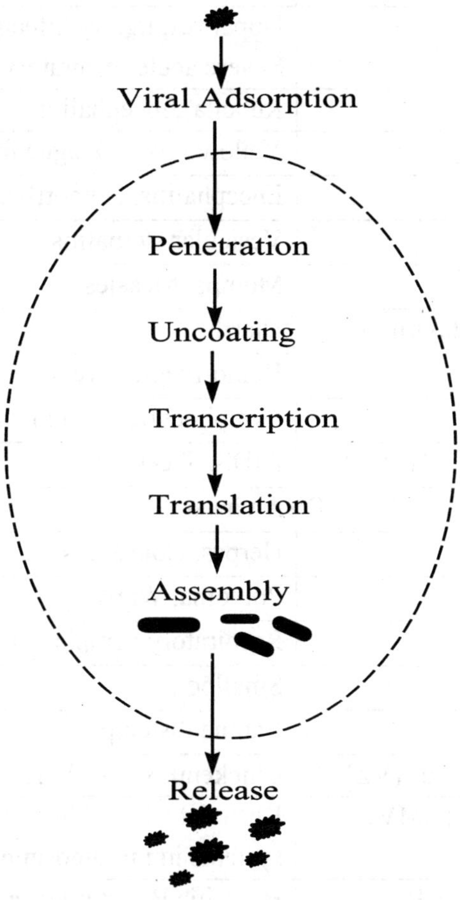


**Fig. 6.1 Virus Life Cycle**

Viral diseases include influenza, rabies, poliomyelitis, yellow fever, ornithosis, mumps, measles, Ebola human immunodeficiency syndrome, herpes, warts small pox etc., (Table 6.1)

**Table 6.1 List of Some Virus and Diseases**

| Virus | Diseases |
|---|---|
| **RNA Viruses** | |
| Picornaviruses | Polio, Hepatitis A |
| Rhinovirus | Common cold, Pneumonia |
| Coronovirus | Upper respiratory infections and common cold; Severe acute respiratory syndrome (SARS) |
| Togavirus | Rubella, Encephalitis |
| Flavivirus | Yellow fever, Dengue fever, St.Louis encephalitis |
| Bunyaviruses | Encephalitis, Hemorrhagic fever |
| Rhabdoviruses | Vesicular stomatitis |
| Myxoviruses | Mumps, Measles |
| Reoviruses or Rotaviruses | Diarrhea |
| Ebola, Marburg | Hemorrhagic fevers |
| Arenaviruses | Lymphocytic choriomeningitis |
| Retroviruses (HIV; HTLV) | AIDS; T-cell leukemia |
| **DNA viruses** | |
| Herpesviruses | Herpes, Cold sores |
| Papovaviruses | Polyoma, Warts |
| Adenoviruses | Respiratory complaints |
| Poxvirus | Smallpox |
| Parvovirus | Canine distemper |
| Varicella-zoster virus (VZV) | Chickenpox and shingles |
| Cytomegalovirus (CMV) | Birth defects and infections of a variety of body systems in immunosuppressed individuals |
| Hepatitis B virus (HBV) | Hepatitis B and liver cancer |
| Influenza viruses A, B, and C | Influenza |

The best time to attack virus is as early as possible in its life cycle that is exactly what vaccines do. Vaccines consists of a weakened or killed version of pathogen, though more recently subunit vaccine have been devised that consists strictly of protein targets from the pathogens. They stimulate the immune system without doing serious harm to the host and so when the real pathogens attack the subject, the immune system responds to it quickly and blocks it. Vaccines have an excellent effectiveness, but they are of limited use in treating a patient who has already been infected. That's where antiviral drug come in because of unique properties of virus and the need for host cell metabolic activities. Antiviral agents have been developed to act at various stages in the viral replication cycle, such as attachment, replication and release of the virus.

## 2. CLASSIFICATION

### I. Based on Enzyme Inhibition

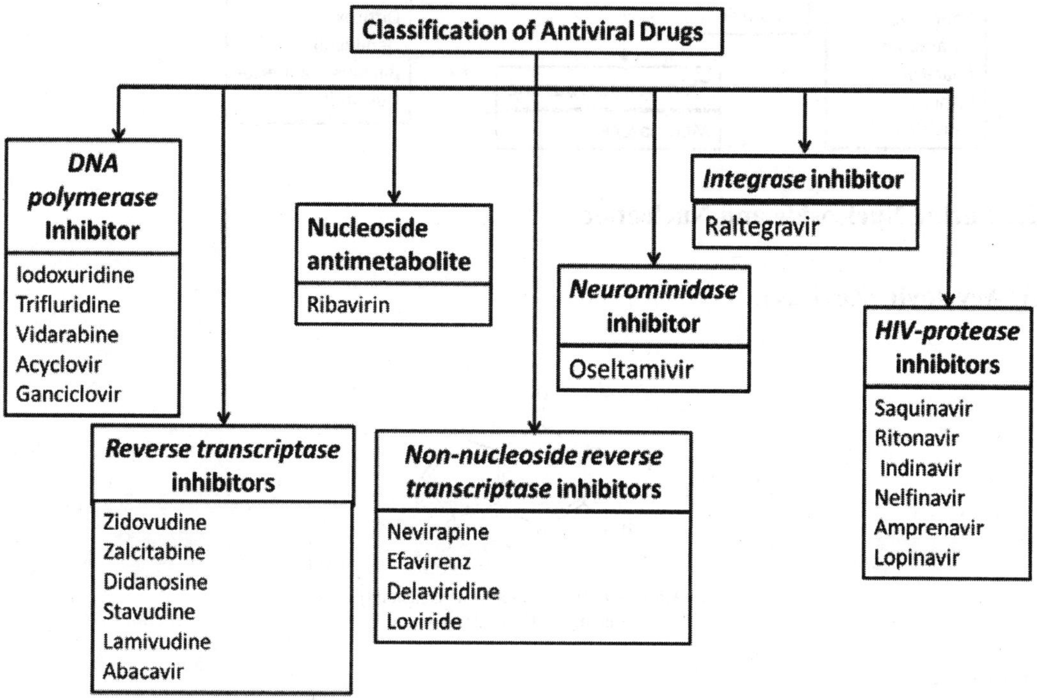


### II. Based on Treatment Protocol

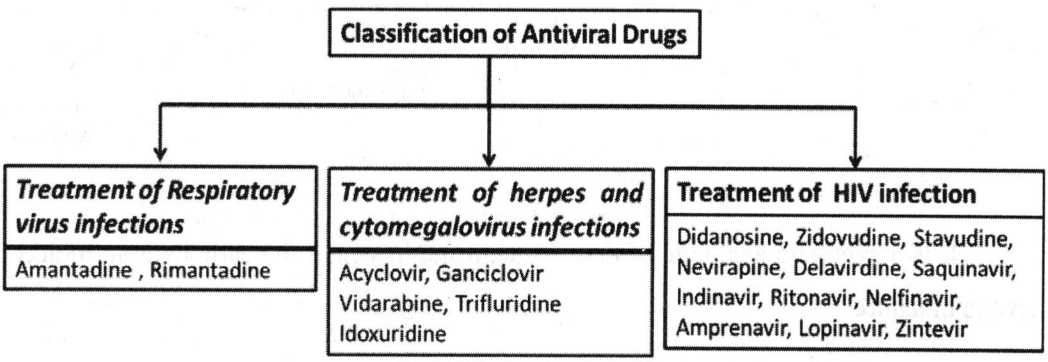

### III. Based on Chemical Structure

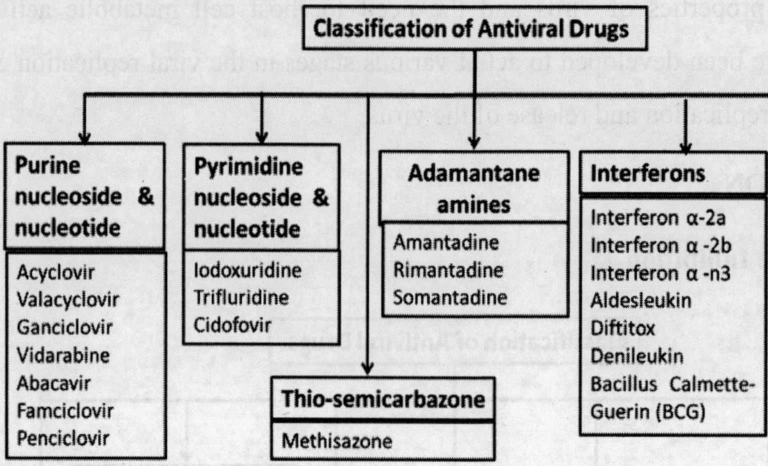


## 2.1 Purine Nucleoside and Nucleotide

### A. Acyclovir (Zovirax)

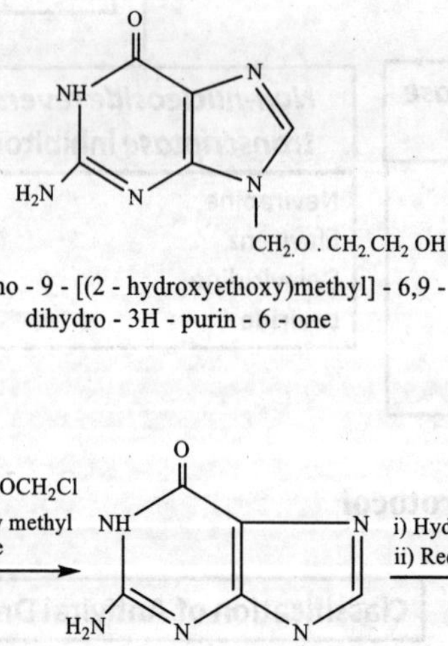

2 - Amino - 9 - [(2 - hydroxyethoxy)methyl] - 6,9 - dihydro - 3H - purin - 6 - one

Synthesis

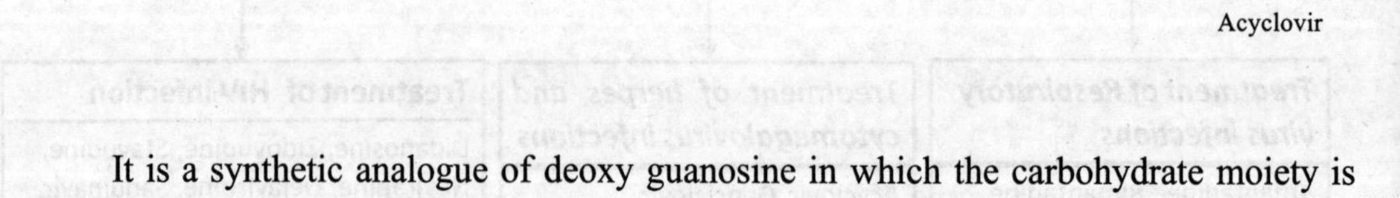


It is a synthetic analogue of deoxy guanosine in which the carbohydrate moiety is acyclic in nature.

**Mechanism of action:** The mode of action of Acyclovir consists of the following consecutive mechanism. (Fig. 6.2)

i) Acyclovir itself is inactive, but it is selectively phosphorylated by a viral *thymidine kinase* to the corresponding monophosphate. This phosphorylation reaction occurs faster in infected cell than normal cell, because Acyclovir is a poor substrate for the normal cell *thymidine kinase.* Acyclovir monophosphate is further converted into di and triphosphate by a normal cellular enzyme *guanosine monophosphate kinase.*

ii) Acyclovir triphosphate inhibits viral *DNA polymerase* by competing deoxy guanosine triphosphate. The triphosphate drug is also incorporated into viral DNA where it acts as a chain terminator; because it has 3'- hydroxy group, like cyclic sugar, 3' 5'- phosphodiester bond can be formed. It acts as suicide inhibitor because the terminated DNA template containing Acyclovir as ligand binds irreversibly with *DNA polymerase* and inactivates. It is a drug of choice in both prophylaxis and treatment of herpes simplex virus.

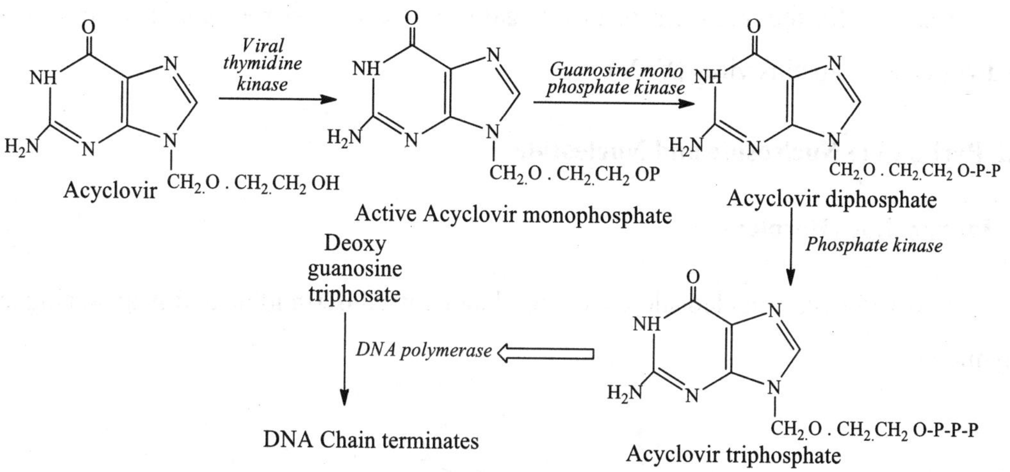


**Fig. 6.2 Mechanism of Action of Acyclovir**

**Use:** It is effective against several DNA viruses including herpes simplex virus (HSV-1 and HSV- 2) and against Varicella Zoster Virus (VZV). It is used for short term treatment of shingles and chicken pox caused by VZV.

**B. Ganciclovir (Cytovene)**

It is an analogue of Acyclovir, with an additional hydroxy methyl group on the acylic side chain.

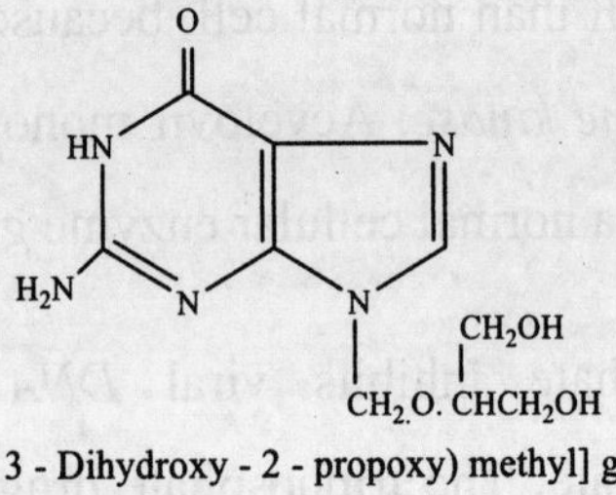

9 - [(1, 3 - Dihydroxy - 2 - propoxy) methyl] guanine

**Mechanism of action:** It is phosphorylated to monophosphates by viral and *cellular kinase* and then to di and triphosphate by cellular enzymes. The triphosphate is a competitive inhibitor by incorporating deoxyguanosine triphosphate into DNA and it inhibits *DNA polymerase* selectively.

**Use:** It is used for the treatment of cytomegalovirus (CMV), herpes simplex virus (HSV) and vesicular stomatitis virus (VSV).

**2.2 Pyrimidine Nucleoside and Nucleotide**

**A. Idoxuridine (Herplex)**

Idoxuridine is a nucleoside containing halogenated pyrimidine and is an analogue of thymidine.

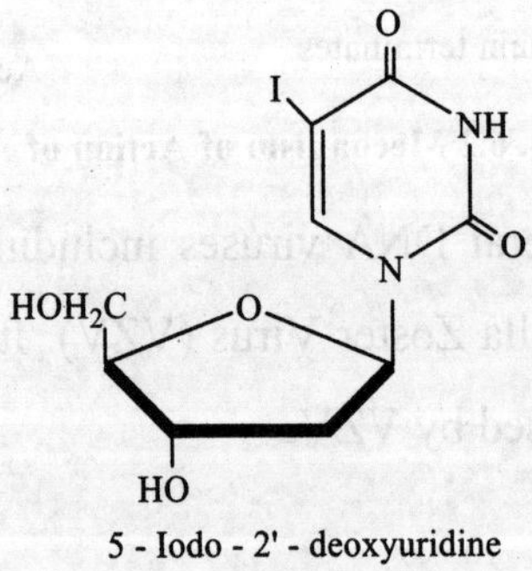

5 - Iodo - 2' - deoxyuridine

**Mechanism of action:** It acts as antiviral agent against DNA virus. Idoxuridine is phosphorylated by *thymidine kinase* to active triphosphate. This phosphorylated drug inhibits HSV *DNA polymerase* which is necessary for the synthesis of viral DNA. The ability of idoxuridylic acid substitute for deoxythymidic acid in the synthesis of DNA may be due to the similar Vander-Waal's radii of iodine (2.15A°) and the thymidine methyl group (2.0A°).

**Use:** It is used for the topical treatment of herpes simplex virus (HSV) keratitis, which causes blindness. Idoxuridine in dimethyl sulfoxide is used in mucocutaneous HSV infection.

**B.Trifluridine (Viroptic)**

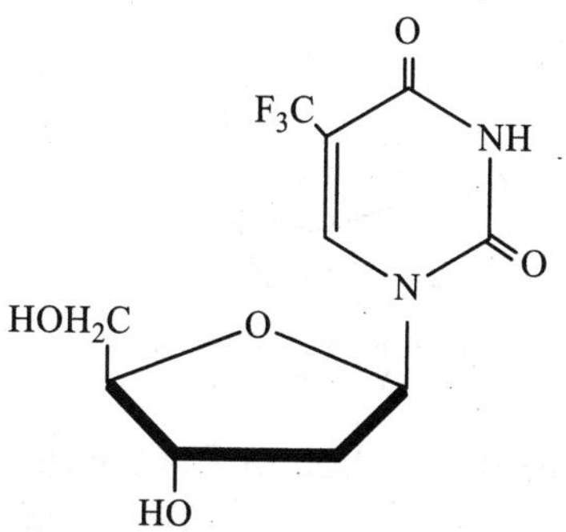


5 - Trifluoromethyl - 2 - deoxyuridine

It is a fluorinated pyrimidine nucleoside that is structurally related to Idoxuridine

**Mechanism of action:** Trifluridine monophosphate irreversibly inhibits *thymidylate synthetase* and the triphosphate competitively inhibits *DNA polymerases* with respect to thymidine triphosphate. It involves the inhibition of viral replication.

**Use:** It is an active antiviral agent in ophthalmic solutions used mainly in the treatment of primary keratoconjunctivitis and recurrent epithelial keratitis due to herpes simplex virus. It is effective against Herpes simplex virus type 1 and 2.

## 2.3 Adamantane Amines

Adamantane inhibits influence type A infection. These agents interfere with influenza type A replication by preventing the early stage of viral uncoating and disturbing the late stage of viral assembly.

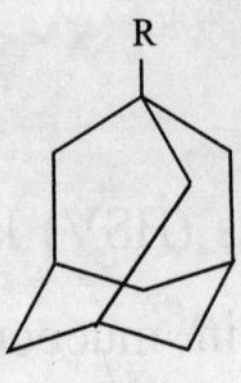

| S. No | Name | R |
|---|---|---|
| 1. | Amantadine | $-NH_2$ |
| 2 | Rimantadine | $H_2N-CH\ CH_3$ |

### A. Amantadine hydrochloride (Symmetral)

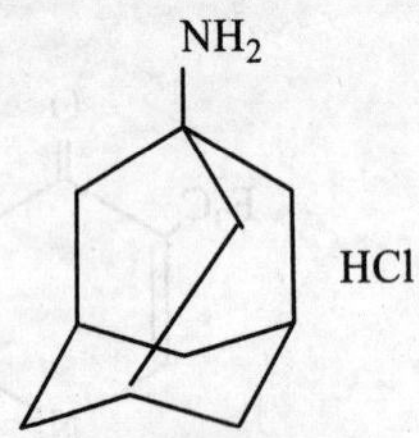

1 - Amino adamantane hydrochloride

**Mechanism of action:** It inhibits penetration of RNA virus particle. It interferes with the release of infectious viral nucleic acid into the host cell through interaction with the transmembrane domain of the viral protein, M2 (an ion channel), which is needed for the viral particle to become "uncoated" once it is taken inside the cell by endocytosis.

**Use:** It is used in the treatment of Parkinson's disease. It is effective against influenza type A virus, para influenza and some RNA virus.

### B. Rimantadine hydrochloride (Flumadine)

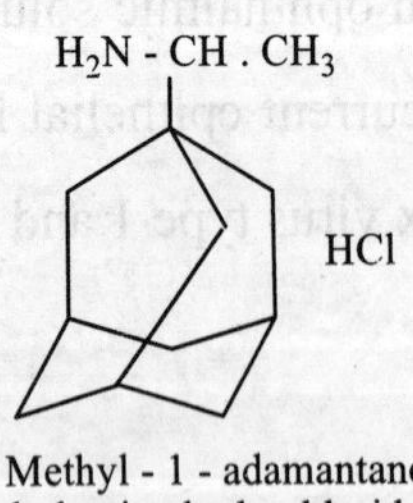

α - Methyl - 1 - adamantane methylamine hydrochloride

Rimantadine is 4 to 10fold more active than Amantadine. It is more effective against influenza A virus.

**Mechanism of action:** It interferes with the release of infectious viral nucleic acid into the host cell through interaction with the transmembrane domain of the viral protein, M2 (an ion channel), which is needed for the viral particle to become "uncoated" once it is taken inside the cell by endocytosis. It also appears to prevent virus assembly during replication in some cases.

**Use:** It is used for prevention of infection caused by various strains of influenza virus A.

### 2.4 Miscellaneous Agents

#### A. Ribavirin (Rebetol, Ribamac)

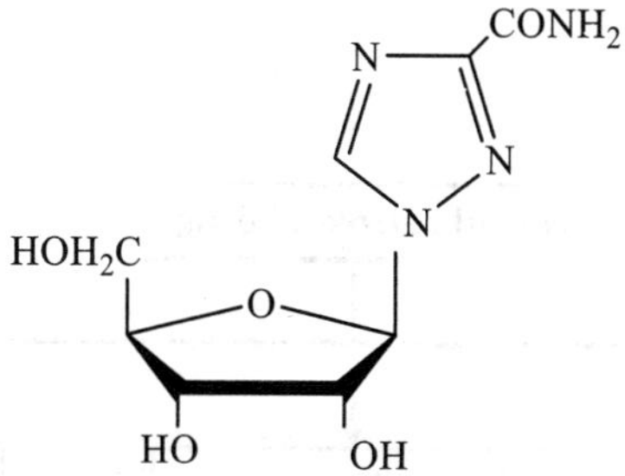


1β - D - Ribofuranosyl - 1H - 1, 2, 4 - triazole - 3 - carboxamide

Ribavirin is also known as Tribavirin and it is a purine nucleoside analogue with a modified base and a D- ribose sugar moiety.

**Mechanism of action:** The nucleotide is bio-activated by viral and host *cellular kinase* to give the Ribavirin monophosphate (RMP) and Ribavirin triphosphate (RTP). RMP inhibits *inosine monophosphate dehydrogenase,* thereby preventing the conversion of inosine monophosphate to xanthine monophosphate, which is required for the synthesis of guanosine triphosphate. RTP inhibits viral RNA.

**Use:** It is used in the treatment of influenza types A and B, hepatitis, general herpes and lassa fever.

## 3. ANTI-HIV AGENTS

### 3.1 Introduction

Human immuno deficiency virus (HIV) is the cause of acquired immunodeficiency syndrome (AIDS). Both HIV-1 and HIV-2 cause AIDS, but HIV-1 is found world wide. HIV is one of the human T-cell lymphotropic retro viruses which infect and kills helper ($CD_4$) T lymphocytes, resulting in loss of cell mediated immunity and the host will develop opportunistic infections. While there is no permanent cure of AIDS without prevention or elimination of HIV infection, AIDS patients can prolong their life, if early diagnosed and treatment started.

### 3.2 Classification

#### I. Based on Mode of Action

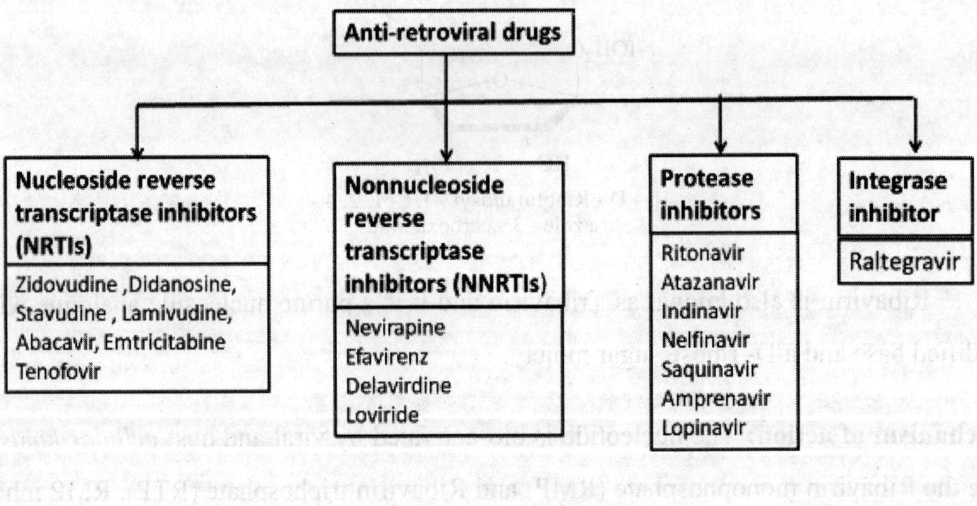

### Mechanism of Action

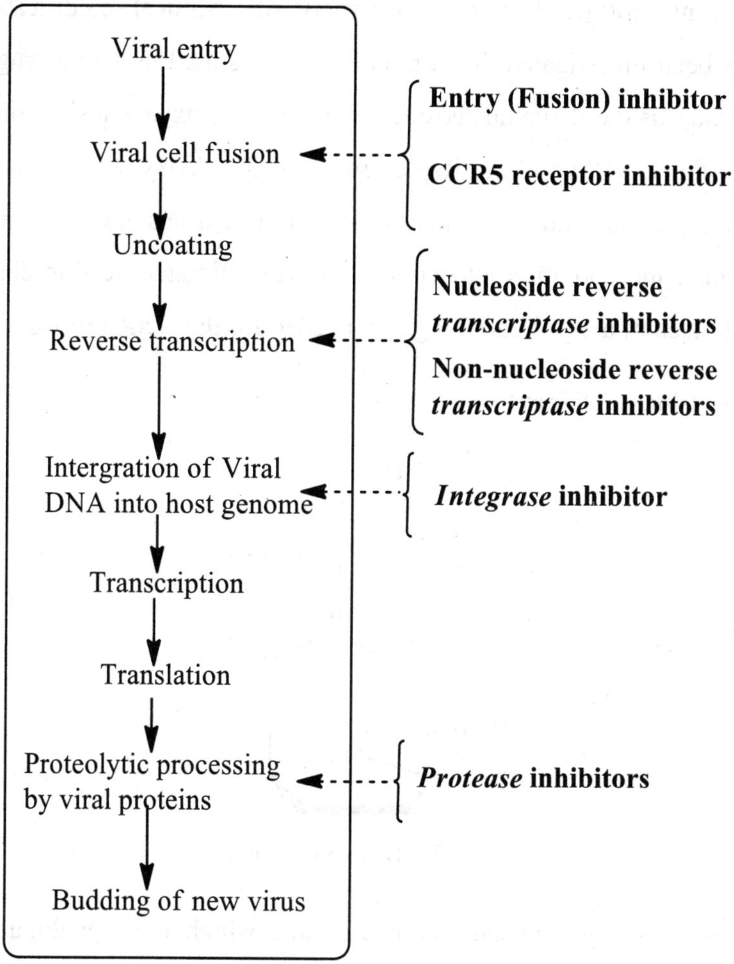


**Fig. 6.3 Mechanism of Action of Antiretroviral Drugs**

### 3.2.1 *Reverse Transcriptase* (RT) Inhibitors

*Reverse transcriptase* is RNA-dependent *DNA polymerase*. The drugs inhibiting RT interferes with replication of HIV and stops the synthesis of infective viral particle. They are further classified into nucleoside and non-nucleoside RT inhibitors.

At the early stage of HIV-1 is reverse transcription, whereby genomic RNA from the virus is converted into a cDNA-RNA complex, then into double stranded DNA ready for integration into the host chromosome. The enzyme that catalyzes this, set of reaction is *reverse transcriptase* (RT). To synthesis this complex RT, requires purine and pyrimidine nucleoside and nucleotide. Therefore, a variety of chemical modification of natural nucleoside has been investigated. Such modification resulted in active drugs. Removal of 3'- hydroxy group of the deoxynucleoside gave rise to deoxyadenosine; dideoxy cytidine and didehydro dideoxy thymidine. Replacement of 3'- deoxy with an azido group has given 3'- azido thymidine and 3'- azido uridine. All these drugs have similar mechanism of action in that their incorporation into viral DNA will ultimately lead to chain terminating blockage due to lack of a 3' – hydroxyl group needed for the DNA propagation.

**A. Didanosine (Dinosin, Dinex)**

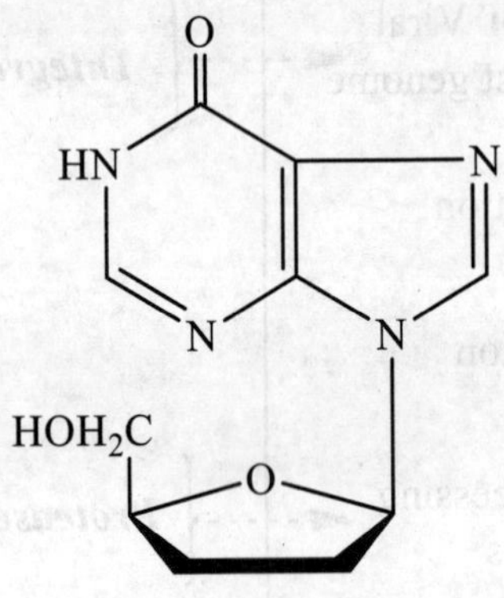

2', 3' - Dideoxyinosine

Didanosine is a purine dideoxy nucleoside, which is an analogue of Inosine. It differs from Inosine by having hydrogen atom in place of 2' and 3' hydroxy groups on the ribose ring.

**Mechanism of action:** It is a prodrug which is bio-activated to dideoxyadenosine triphosphate, which is a competitive inhibitor of *reverse transcriptase*. Due to the absence of 3'- hydroxyl group it causes chain termination. It inhibits HIV-RT and exerts a virustatic effect on the retroviruses.

**Use:** It is recommended for the treatment of patients with advanced HIV infections.

**B. Zidovudine (Zidine, Zilion)**

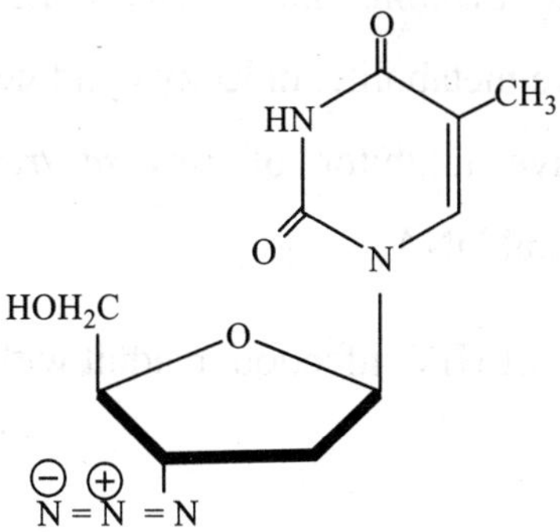

3' - Azido - 3' - deoxythymidine

It is an analogue of thymidine in which the azido group is substituted at the 3 - carbon atom of the dideoxyribose moiety.

**Mechanism of action:** It is phosphorylated by cellular *thymidine kinase. Thymidylate kinase* then converts monophosphate into di and triphosphate. Zidovudine triphosphate competitively inhibits *reverse transcriptase*. The 3'-azido group prevents the formation of 5', 3' - phosphodiester bond, which causes DNA chain termination.

**Use:** It is used for the treatment of AIDS and AIDS related complex. Because it crosses blood brain barrier, it has favourable effect on neurological symptoms of AIDS.

**C. Zalcitabine (Hivid)**

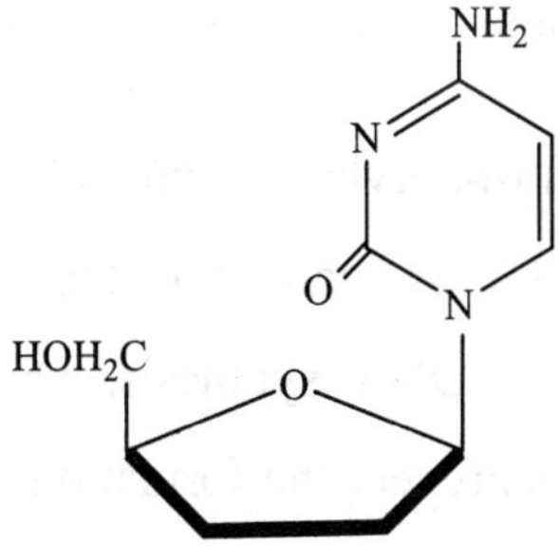

2', 3' - Dideoxycytidine

It is a synthetic pyrimidine nucleoside analogue. It differs from 2' - deoxycytidine in that the 3'- hydroxy group of 2' - deoxy ribose moiety is replaced with a hydrogen atom.

**Mechanism of action:** It enters human cells by carrier - facilitated diffusion and undergoes initial phosphorylation by *deoxy cytidine kinase*. The mono phosphorylated compound is further metabolized to the active metabolite, dideoxy cytidine - 5'- triphosphate by *cellular kinase* which is a competitive inhibitor of *reverse transcriptase*. This causes the termination of the elongating viral DNA.

**Use:** It is used for the treatment of HIV infection in adult with advanced disease, who is intolerant to Zidovudine.

**D. Lamivudine (Lamda, Lamivir)**

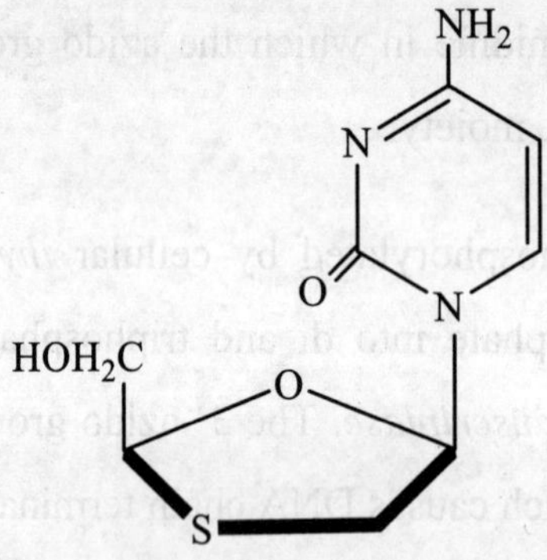


(-) - 1 - [(2R, 5S) - 2 - (hydroxy methyl) - 1, 3 - oxathiolan - 5 - yl] cytosine

Lamivudine is a synthetic nucleoside analogue that differs from 2', 3' - dideoxy cytidine (ddc) by the substitution of sulfur atom in place of methylene group at 3' position of the ribose ring. The (+) enantiomer is more active than (-) enantiomer.

**Mechanism of action:** It is phosphorylated, intracellular to its active 5'-triphosphate metabolite that competitively inhibits the activity of the *HIV reverse transcriptase* enzyme and act as a chain terminator of DNA synthesis. Due to the lack of 3'-OH group, incorporated nucleoside analogues prevent the formation of 5' to 3' phosphodiester linkage that is essential for DNA chain elongation.

**Use:** It is used for the treatment of HIV infection and chronic hepatitis.

### 3.2.2 Non-nucleoside *Reverse Transcriptase* Inhibitors (NNRTIs)

Non-nucleoside *reverse transcriptase* inhibitors (NNRTIs) are used with nucleoside drug to obtain synergistic activity. These drugs do not require bioactivation by *kinase* to yield phosphate esters. They are not incorporated into the growing DNA chain. Instead, they bind to an allosteric site that is distinct from the substrate-binding site of *reverse transcriptase*. The inhibitor can bind either free or substrate-bound enzyme, interfering with the action of both. Such binding inactivates the enzyme, so that it cannot form the enzyme-substrate complex at its normal rate.

**A. Delavirdine (Rescriptor)**

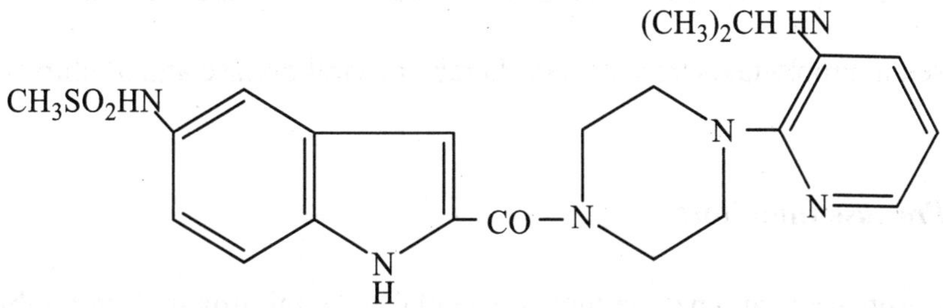


1- [3 - (Isopropyl amino) - 2 - pyridyl] - 4 - [(5 - methanesulfonamido indol - 2- yl) carbonyl] piperazine

Delaviridine, is a bis hetero aryl piperazine derivative and a potent non-nucleoside RT inhibitor specific for HIV-I.

**Mechanism of action:** It binds directly to viral reverse transcriptase (RT) and blocks the RNA-dependent and DNA-dependent *DNA polymerase* activities by disrupting the enzyme's catalytic site.

**Use:** It is used along with other anti-retroviral drugs for the treatment of human immunodeficiency virus infection.

**B. Loviride**

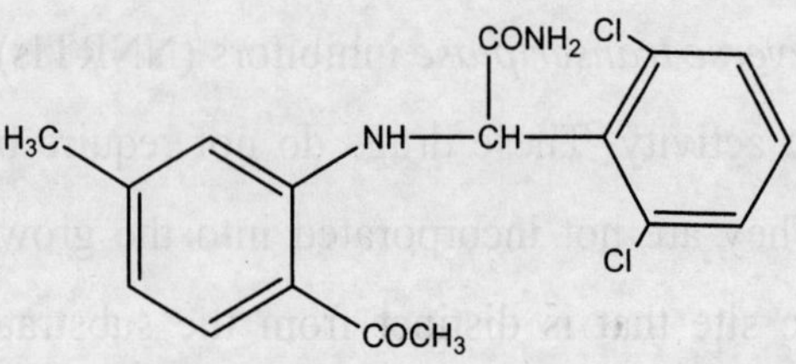


2 - (2 - Acetyl - 5 - methylanilino) - 2 - (2,6 - dichlorophenyl)acetamide

**Mechanism of action:** It acts by preventing viral replication by inhibiting viral *DNA polymerase* by binding to specific cell-surface receptors and inhibiting viral penetration or uncoating; inhibiting viral protein synthesis; or blocking late stages of virus assembly.

**Use:** It is used in prophylaxis treatment or therapy of viral disease and it inhibits HIV -1, HIV-2.

### 3.2.3 *HIV Protease* Inhibitors

*HIV protease* is an enzyme that is essential for viral growth. The inhibitors act on *HIV protease* and prevent post-translation processing and budding of immature viral particles from the infected cell.

**A. Saquinavir (Saquin)**

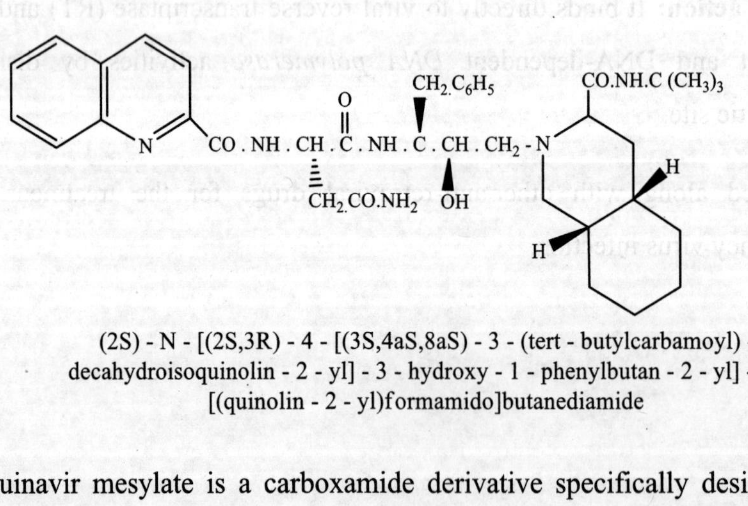


(2S) - N - [(2S,3R) - 4 - [(3S,4aS,8aS) - 3 - (tert - butylcarbamoyl) - decahydroisoquinolin - 2 - yl] - 3 - hydroxy - 1 - phenylbutan - 2 - yl] - 2 - [(quinolin - 2 - yl)formamido]butanediamide

Saquinavir mesylate is a carboxamide derivative specifically designed to inhibit *HIV protease.*

**Mechanism of action:** It is a protease inhibitor binds to the active site of the viral *protease* and prevents cleavage of viral polyproteins, preventing maturation of the virus. It inhibits both HIV-1 and HIV-2 *proteases.*

**Use:** It is used in the treatment of advanced HIV infection in selected patients.

**B. Indinavir (Indease, Indivan)**

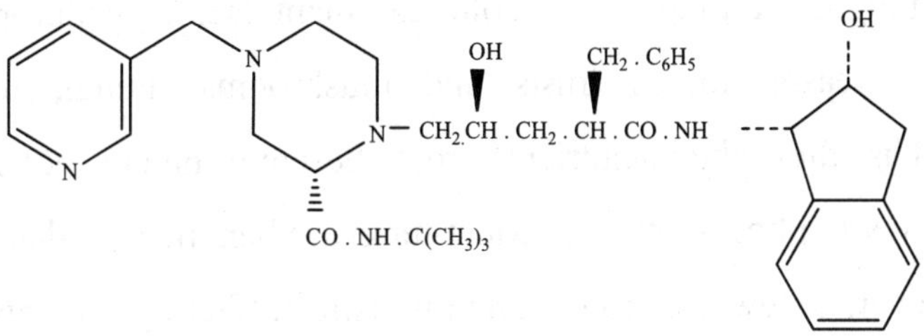

(2S) - 1 - [(2S,4R) - 4 - benzyl - 2 - hydroxy - 4 - {[(1S,2R) - 2 - hydroxy - 2,3 - dihydro - 1H - inden - 1 - yl]carbamoyl}butyl] - N - tert - butyl - 4 - (pyridin - 3 - ylmethyl)piperazine - 2 - carboxamide

Indinavir is a pentanoic acid amide derivative

**Mechanism of action:** It binds to the protease active site and inhibits the activity of the enzyme. This inhibition prevents cleavage of the viral polyproteins resulting in the formation of immature non-infectious viral particles.

**Use:** It is an antiretroviral drug for the treatment of HIV infection.

**C. Ritonavir (Ritomax, Norvir)**

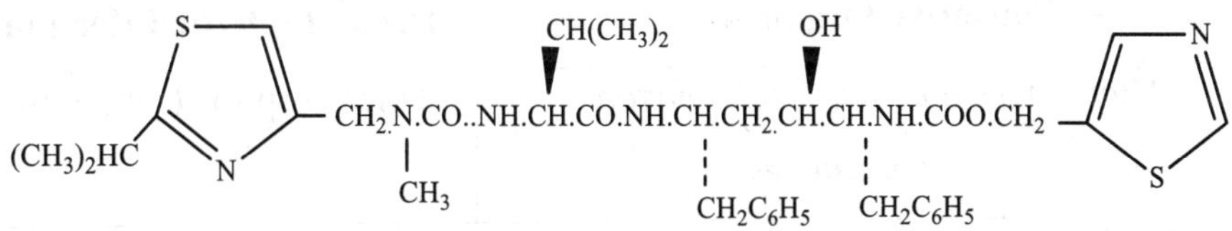

(1,3 - thiazol - 5 - yl)methyl - N - [(2S,3S,5S) - 3 - hydroxy - 5 - [(2S) - 3 - methyl - 2 - {[methyl({[2 - (propan - 2 - yl) - 1,3 - thiazol - 4 -yl]methyl})carbamoyl]amino}butanamido] - 1,6 - diphenylhexan - 2 - yl]carbamate

**Mechanism of action:** Same as Indinavir.

**Use:** It is used in combination with other antiretroviral drug for the treatment of HIV infection.

Chapter

# 7

# ANTIFUNGAL AGENTS

## 1. INTRODUCTION

Antifungal agents are drugs used to treat infections in various parts of the body that are caused by a fungus. A fungus is a colorless plant lacking chlorophyll. The fungal kingdom includes yeasts, molds, rusts and mushrooms. Fungi, like animals, are heterotrophic, that is, they obtain nutrients from the environment, not from endogenous sources (like plants with photosynthesis). Most fungi are beneficial and are involved in bio-degradation, however, a few can cause opportunistic (affecting patients only or chiefly when the immune system is depressed) infections, if they are introduced into the skin through wounds or into the lungs and nasal passages if inhaled. Fungi that cause disease in humans may be like yeast or hyphae (mould) and are called mycotic infections.

Fungal infections may be any one of the two types namely

**i) Superficial mycotic infections** are those occur on the surface or just below the skin or nail caused by dermatophytes in the Microsporum, Trichophyton or Epidermophyton genera. These dermatophytic infections are named for the site of infection rather than the causative organism.

**Table 7.1 Examples for Superficial Mycotic Infections and Causative Organism**

| Causative Organism | Dermatophytic Infections |
|---|---|
| *Microsporum canis, Trichophyton mentagrophytes* | Tinea corporis (ringworm) |
| *Trichophyton rubrum, Trichophyton mentagrophytes, Epidermophyton floccosum* | Tinea pedis (athlete's foot) |
| *Trichophyton rubrum, Trichophyton mentagrophytes, Epidermophyton floccosum* | Tinea cruris (jock itch) |
| *Microsporum canis, Trichophyton tonsurans* | Tinea capitis (scalp) |
| *Trichophyton rubrum, Trichophyton* | Tinea barbae (beard/hair) |

| | |
|---|---|
| *mentagrophytes* | |
| *Trichophyton rubrum, Trichophyton mentagrophytes, Epidermophyton floccosum* | Tinea unguium (nails) |

**ii) Systemic mycotic infections** are those occur inside the body, such as in lungs and other body organs. Many of the organisms that cause systemic fungal infections are confined to specific geographic locations due to favorable climates for their proliferation.

**Table 7.2 Examples for Systemic Mycotic Infections and Causative Organism**

| **Causative Organism** | **Systemic Infections** |
|---|---|
| *Coccidioides immitis* | Coccidioidomycosis |
| *Histoplasma capsulatum* | Histoplasmosis |
| *Paracoccidioides brasiliensis* | Brazilian blastomycosis |
| *Blastomyces dermatitidis* | Blastomycosis |

Fungi thrive in moist, dark places, including some parts of the body. Fungal infections are common, not only as primary disease but also secondary to therapy with oral antibiotics.

Individuals suffering from malignancy, diabetes mellitus, those on corticosteroids and immune compromised subjects are more prone to develop fungal infections. Organisms that cause opportunistic infections and their causative organism and target organs are given in Table 7.1

**Table 7.3 Fungal Infection and Causative Organism**

| **Causative Organism** | **Opportunistic Infections** | **Target organs** |
|---|---|---|
| *Candida albicans* | Candidiasis, Thrush, Vulvovaginitis | GI tract and vagina |
| *Cryptococcus neoformans* | Cryptococcal meningitis | Through inhalation, may cause mild lung infection. Mainly affects CNS |

| | | |
|---|---|---|
| *Aspergillus* sp | Aspergillosis | Lung, brain, sinuses and other organs |
| *Mucor* sp. | Mucormycosis | Sinuses, eyes, blood and brain |
| *Pneumocystis carinii* | Pneumocystis carinii pneumonia | Lungs (especially in HIV patients) |

## 1.1 Biochemical Targets for Antifungals

Antifungal chemotherapy depends on biochemical difference between fungi and mammals. The fungal cell wall is a unique organelle that fulfills the criteria for selective toxicity. At the cellular level, the greatest difference between fungal cells and mammalian cell is that fungal cell has cell walls but the mammalian cell does not. The fungal cell wall differs greatly from the bacterial cell wall and is not affected by antibacterial cell wall inhibitors.

a) **Fungal Cell Membrane**: Fungi and mammalian cells both contain a cell membrane that serves and play an important role in cell structure, division and metabolism. The mammalian cell contains cholesterol as sterol component, whereas fungi contain ergosterol which is important for proper functioning of many cell membrane enzymes and ion transport proteins. This difference in the sterol is the basis for most of the currently available antifungal drugs polyenes, azoles and allylamines. **Polyene antifungals** such as Amphotericin B act by binding to ergosterol in the fungal cell membrane. **Azole antifungals** inhibit the fungal enzyme *14α - demethylase*, thereby interrupting the synthesis of ergosterol. **Allylamines** act at an earlier step in the ergosterol synthesis pathway by inhibiting the enzyme *squalene epoxidase*.

b) **Fungal Cell Wall**: The fungal cell wall is a critical site for exchange and filtration of ions and proteins, as well as metabolism and catabolism of complex nutrients. Because mammalian cells lack a cell wall, it also represents an ideal and specific target for antifungal therapy. Structurally, the fungal cell wall is composed of a complex network of proteins and poly carbohydrates that varies in composition depending on the fungal species. Disruption of this protein/carbohydrate matrix results in a structurally defective cell wall, rendering the fungal cell sensitive to osmotic lysis. **Glucan synthesis inhibitors** block fungal cell wall synthesis by inhibiting the enzyme *1,3β - glucan synthase.* Inhibition of this enzyme results in depletion of glucan polymers in the fungal cell, resulting in an abnormally weak cell wall, unable to withstand osmotic stress.

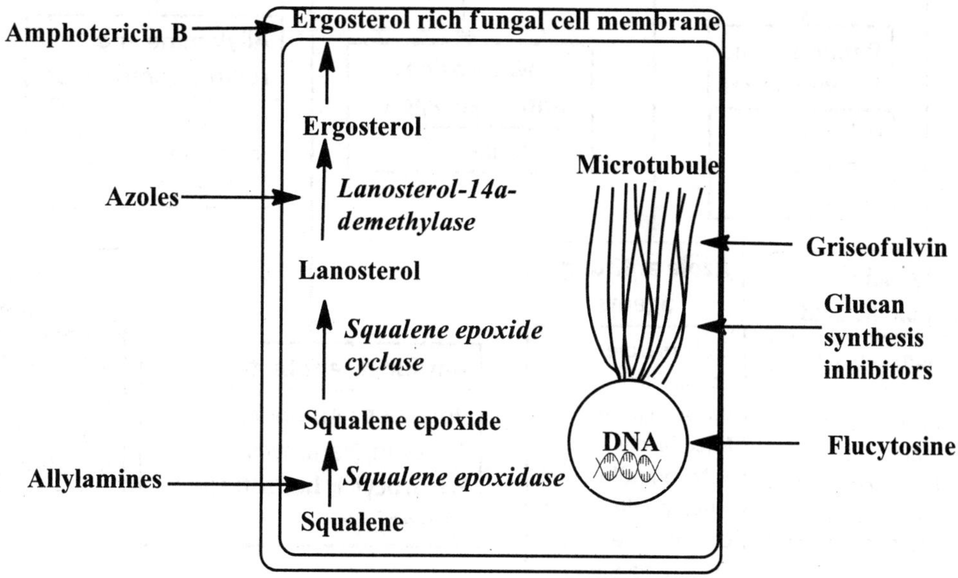


**Fig. 7.1 Mechanism of Antifungal Agents**

c) **Fungal Cell Division**: Nucleoside antifungal agents affect cell division by targeting the microtubule effect in forming the mitotic spindle or by inhibiting DNA transcription. Griseofulvin inhibits microtubule polymerization, thus inhibiting the formation of mitotic spindle. Flucytosine or 5-Fluorocytosine only one class of agents in clinical use targets DNA/RNA synthesis.

## 2. CLASSIFICATION

### I. Based on Chemical Structure

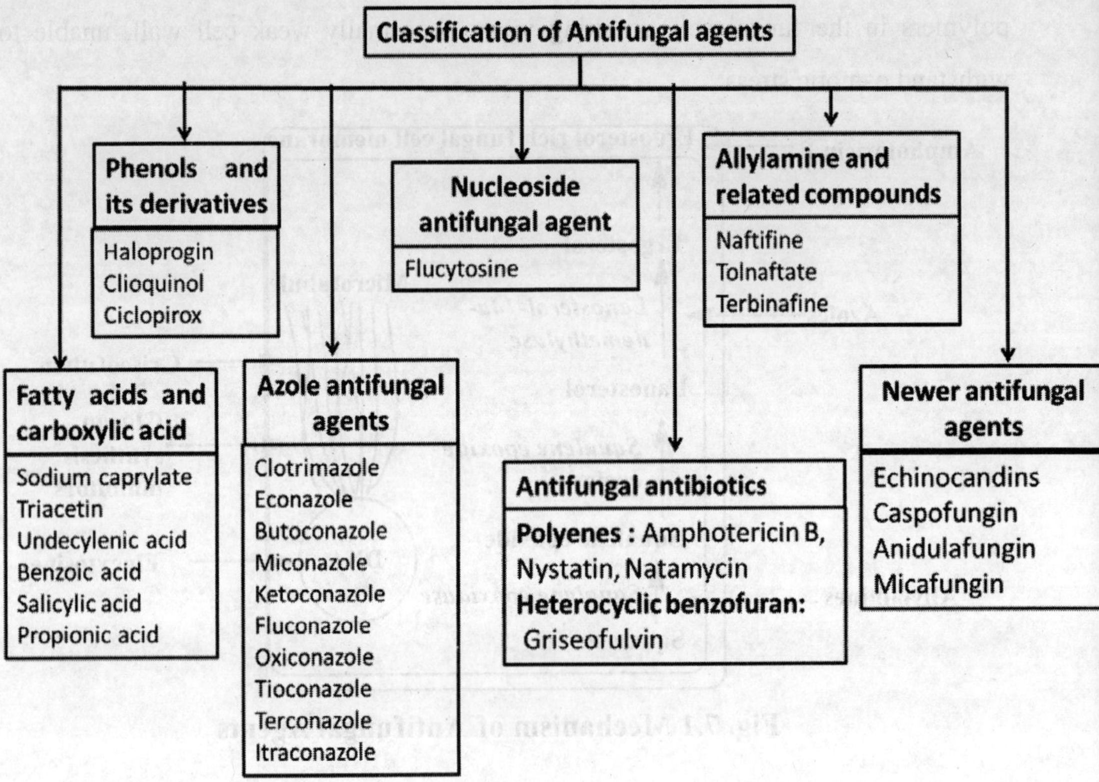


### II. Based on Mechanism of Action

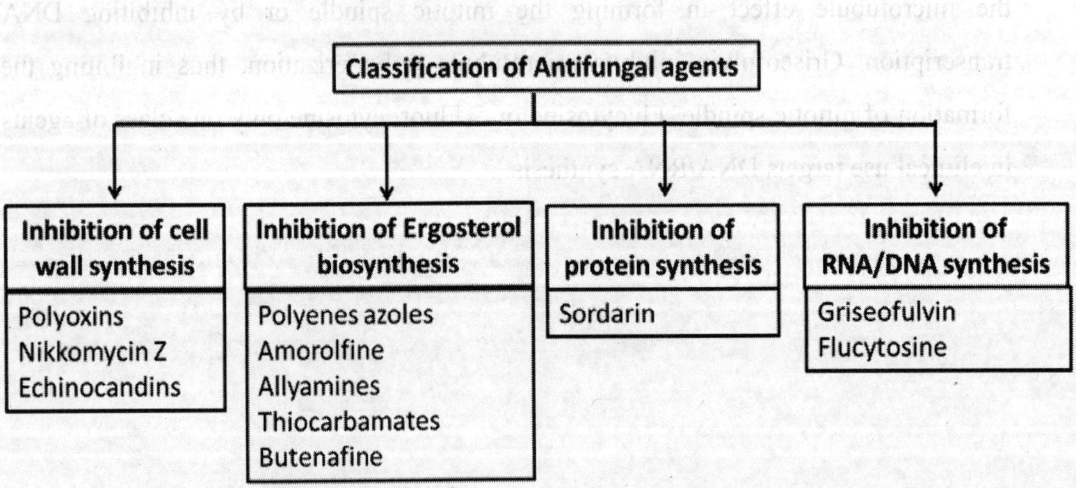

## 2.1 Antifungal Antibiotics

### 2.1.1 Polyenes

The polyene antifungals that are in current clinical use are Nystatin, Natamycin, and Amphotericin B. These complex antifungal antibiotics are isolated from soil bacteria of the genus *Streptomyces*. Polyenes are macrocyclic lactones with distinct hydrophilic and lipophilic region. The lipophilic region contains conjugated double bonds in macrocyclic lactone ring. Hence, they are called as polyene antibiotics. The hydrophilic region contains

(i) a hydroxy group on the acid derived portion of the ring.

(ii) a glycosidically linked deoxy amino hexose called mycosamine.

Polyenes are divided into two groups

(i) 26-membered ring polyene. eg. Natamycin.

(ii) 38-membered ring polyenes. eg. Amphotericin B, Nystatin.

### A. Amphotericin B (Amfotex, Mycol)

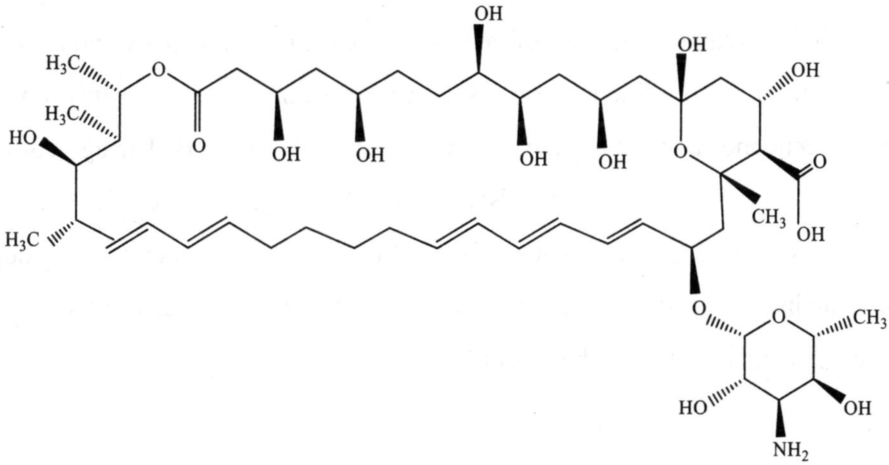


Amphotericin B is an antifungal agent obtained from *Streptomyces nodosus*, an actinomycetes found in the soil. It possess a broad spectrum of antifungal activity and is effective against several fungal organisms including Candida species, *Histoplasma capsulatum, Cryptococcus neoformans, Blastomyces dermatitidis* and *Coccidioides immitis*. It is a 38 membered polyene antibiotic, their structure contains a large lactone (macrolide) ring with numerous conjugated double bonds. The polar hydroxylated portion and the nonpolar hydrocarbon sequence lend an amphophilic character to the molecule. The polyenes are unstable in solution because of the unsaturated chromophore region, which is easily photo-oxidized.

**Mechanism of action:** It acts by binding to ergosterol in the fungal cell membrane. Binding result in depolarization of the membrane and formation of pores that increase permeability to proteins and monovalent and divalent cations, eventually leading to cell death

**Use:** It is the only polyene used in systemic infection. Topically it is used to treat mycoses caused by *Candida albicans*. The drug cannot cross the blood brain barrier and must be administered intrathecally for treatment of fungal infections of central nervous system.

**B. Nystatin (Mycostatin)**

Nystatin is a polyene antifungal drug that has broad-spectrum fungicidal and fungistatic activity against a number of yeasts and fungi, most notably Candida species. It is isolated from the strain of actinomycetes called *Streptomyces noursei*. It is a mixture of four different tetraenes namely Nystatin A, $A_2$, $A_3$ and polyfungin B. The aglycone portion of Nystatin called nystatinolide consists of a 38-membered macrolide lactone ring containing single tetracene and diene moieties separated by two methylene groups. The aglycone contains 8 hydroxyl groups, 1 carboxyl group and lactone ester functional group. This entire aglycone is linked to the glycone mycosamine.

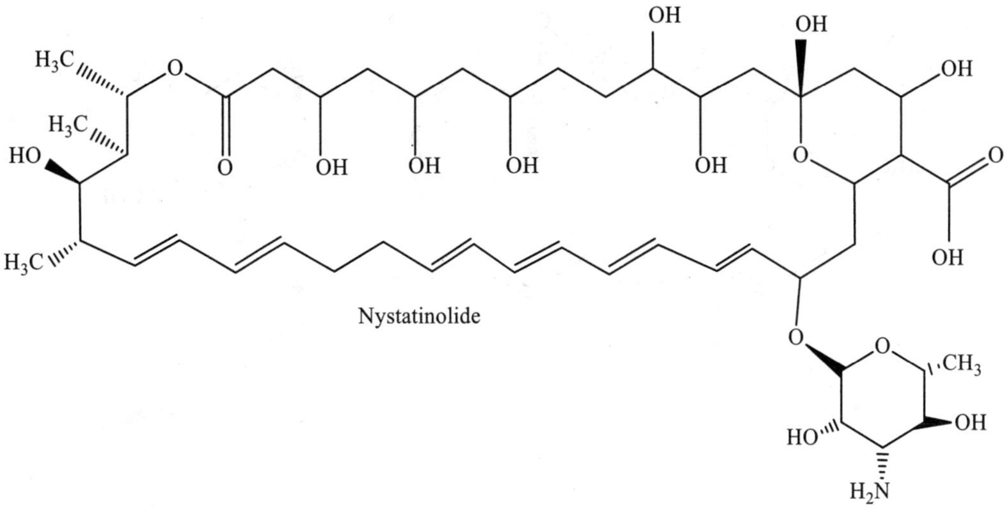


Nystatinolide

Mycosamine

**Mechanism of action:** It acts by binding to the fungal cell membrane. It binds to ergosterol in fungal cell membranes and causes a disturbance in the permeability of the cell membrane. Cells lose intracellular potassium and other cellular contents and eventually die.

**Use:** It is an effective topical antifungal agent. It is used for the treatment of local and gastro intestinal infection caused by *Candida albicans* and other *Candida* species. It is too toxic to be used systematically, but due to its poor absorption, used to treat mouth and GIT infections, fever, myalgia, hypotension and bronchospasm.

## C. Natamycin (Pimafusin)

Natamycin is also known as Pimaricin, is a polyene natural antibiotic obtained from the cultures of *Streptomyces natalensis*. The structure consists of 26-membered lactone ring containing a tetraene chromophore, a $\alpha$, $\beta$-unsaturated lactone carbonyl group, 3 hydroxyl groups, a carboxyl group, a *trans* epoxide and a glycosidically linked mycosamine.

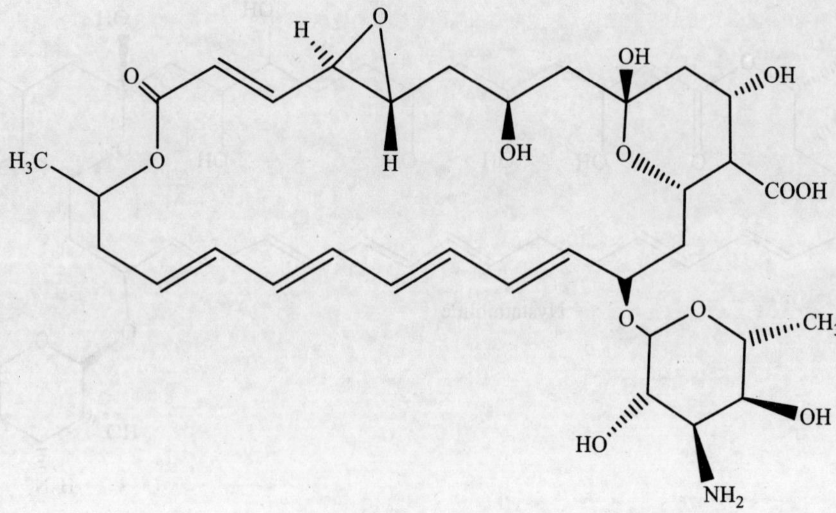

Mycosamine

**Mechanism of action:** It exerts its antifungal effects by binding to ergosterols in the fungal cell membrane thereby increasing membrane permeability. This leads to a leakage and loss of essential cellular constituents.

**Use:** It is active against yeast and fungi, including *Candida, Aspergillus, Cephalosporium, Penicillium* and *Fusarium spp*. It is used for fungal conjunctivitis, blepharitis and keratitis.

### 2.1.2 Heterocyclic Benzofuran

### A. Griseofulvin (Gris OD, Fluvin)

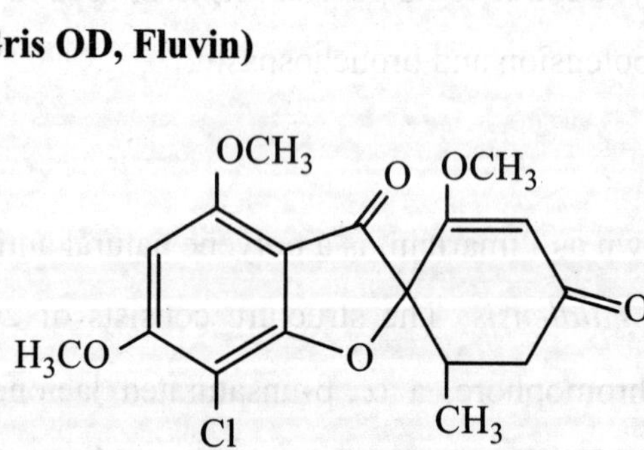

[7 - Chloro - 2', 4, 6 - trimethyoxy - 6'β - methylspiro - (benzofuran) - 2 - (3H) - 1' - [2- cyclohexen] - 3, 4' - dione

It is an example of spiro compound. It is isolated from the fungus *Penicillium griseofulvum.*

**Mechanism of action**: It inhibits fungal mitosis by disrupting the mitotic spindle through interaction with polymerized microtubules. By interfering with tubulin polymerization, Griseofulvin stops mitosis at metaphase. The destruction of cytoplasmic microtubules interferes with the transport of secretory material, which inhibits cell wall synthesis.

**Use:** It is used for the systemic infections caused by ringworm in body, hair and nail.

### 2.2 Allylamine and Related Compounds

#### A. Naftifine hydrochloride (Exoderil)

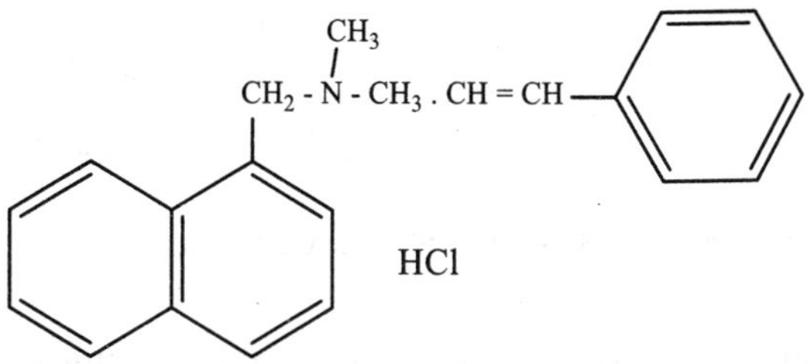


N - Methyl - N - (3 - phenyl - 2 - propenyl) - 1 - naphthalen methanamine hydrochloride

**Mechanism of action:** It interfere with sterol biosynthesis by inhibiting the enzyme *squalene 2,3-epoxidase* results in decreased amounts of ergosterol and a corresponding accumulation of squalene in the cells.

**Use:** It is a topical antifungal agent, effective against ring worm of skin, nail, beard, scalp and tinea versicolor.

#### B. Tolnaftate (Tinaderm-M, Tinactin)

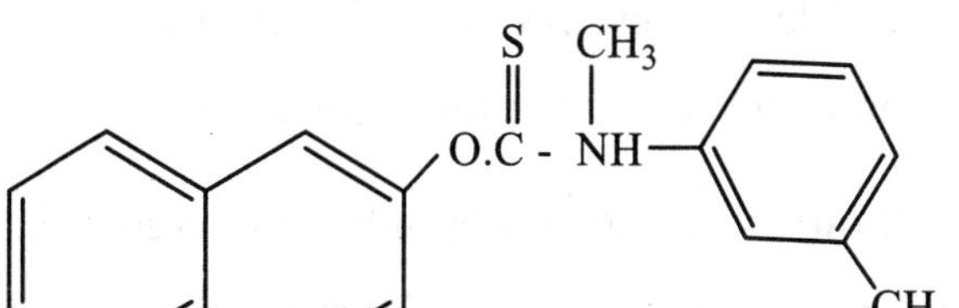


*N* - Methyl - N - (3 - methylphenyl) - 1 - naphthalen - 2 - yloxy methanethioamide

Synthesis

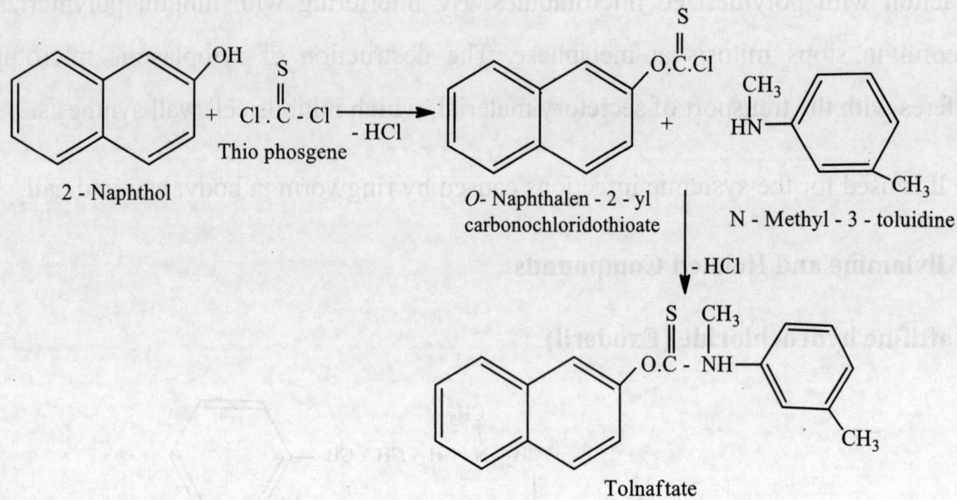


**Mechanism of action:** Same as Naftifine hydrochloride.

**Use:** It is a fungicidal, effective against dermatophytes, ring worm, jock itch and athlete's foot.

### 2.3 Azole Antifungal Agents

Azole antifungal agents are the largest class of antifungals available today with more than 20 drugs in the market. Azoles are five membered aromatic rings containing either two nitrogen (imidazole) or three nitrogen (triazole) with a side chain at N, containing at least one aromatic ring. The azoles with slow first pass metabolism like Ketoconazole, Fluconazole, Itraconazole and Posaconazole are used systematically. The other azoles (Clotrimazole, Oxiconazole, Terconazole, Econazole, Sulconazole and Ketoconazole) are available as creams and ointments for topical treatment of dermatophytic infection and intravaginal use for vaginal yeast infections.

**2.3.1 Mechanism of Action:** All azoles act by inhibiting ergosterol biosynthesis through the inhibition of *14α-demethylase*. Inhibition of this enzyme, results in accumulation of sterol bearing 14α-methyl group. This results in permeability changes and leaky membrane-imbedded protein, together causes fungal cell death.

### 2.3.2 Classification

**Classification of Azole antifungal agents**

**Imidazole derivatives**
- Clotrimazole
- Oxiconazole
- Lanoconazole
- Ketoconazole
- Miconazole
- Sulconazole
- Isoconazole
- Tioconazole
- Econazole
- Butoconazole

**Triazole derivatives**
- Fluconazole
- Voriconazole
- Terconazole
- Itraconazole
- Posaconazole

#### 2.3.2.1 Imidazole Derivatives

**A. Clotrimazole (Canesten)**

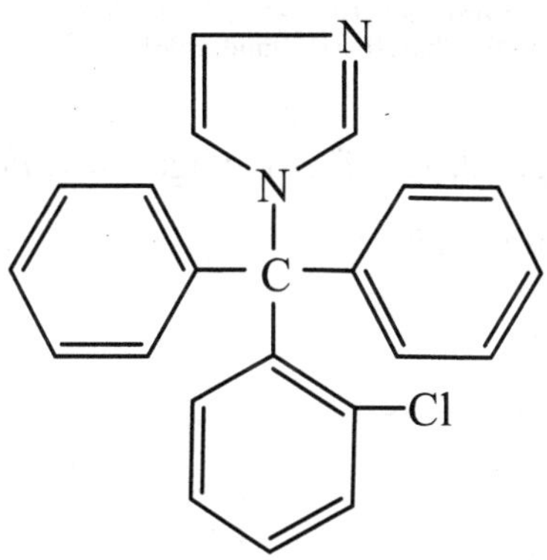


1 - (2 - Chloro - α, α - diphenyl benzyl) imidazole

**Use:** It is effective against *Tinea pedis, Tinea cruris, Tinea capitis, Tinea versicolor, Cutaneous candidiasis* and *Vulvovaginal candidiasis.*

**B. Econazole (Ecoza, Spectazole)**

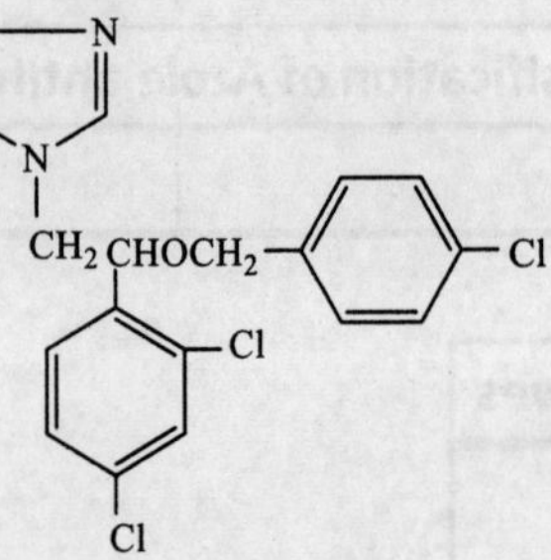

1 - [2 - [(4 - Chloro phenyl) methoxy] - 2 - (2, 4 - dichloro phenyl)ethyl] - 1H - imidazole

**Use:** It is used for the topical Tinea infection and C*utaneous candidiasis*.

**C. Butoconazole (Femstat)**

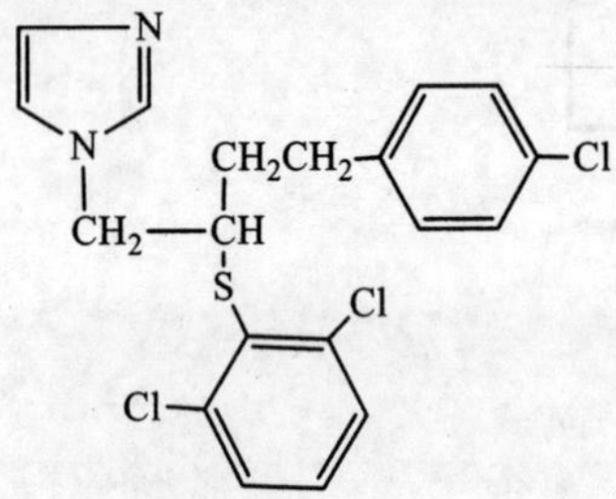

1 - [4 - (4 - Chloro phenyl) - 2 - [(2, 6 - dichloro phenyl)thio]butyl] -1H - imidazole

**Use:** It is a broad-spectrum antifungal drug, effective against *Candida albicans.* It is also used for the treatment of *Vaginal candidiasis*.

**D. Oxiconazole (Oxistat)**

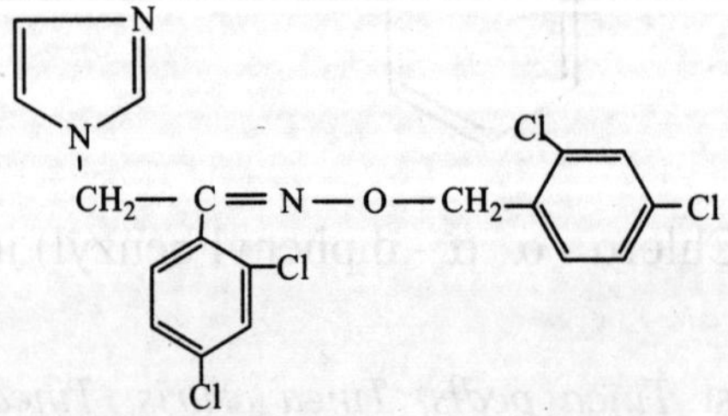

(Z) - 1 - (2, 4 - Dichloro phenyl) - 2 - (1H - imidazol - 1 - yl) ethanone - o - [(2, 4 - dichloro phenyl) methyl] oxime

**Use:** It is used for the treatment of *Tinea pedis, Tinea corporis* and *Tinea capitis.*

## E. Tioconazole (Vagistat)

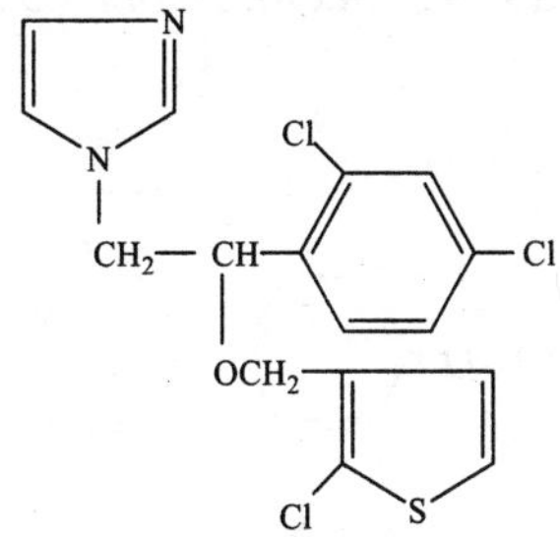

1 - [2 - [(2 - Chloro - 3 - thienyl) methoxy] - 2 - (2, 4 - dichloro phenyl) ethyl] - 1H - Imidazole

**Use:** It is effective against *Vulvovaginal candidiasis.*

## F. Miconazole (Oravig, Monistat)

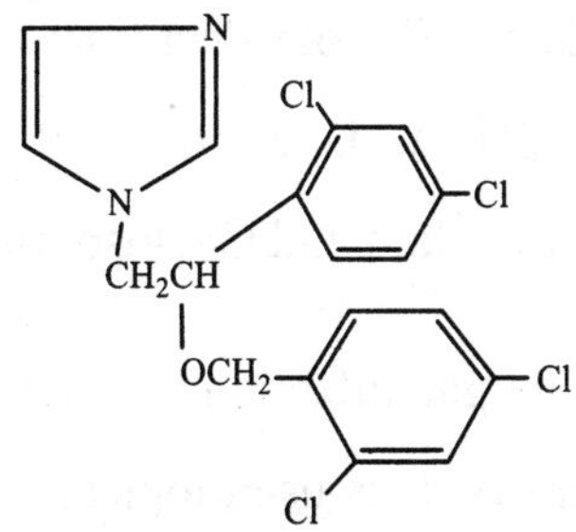

1- [2 - (2, 4 - Dichloro phenyl) - 2 - [2, 4 - dichloro phenyl] methoxy] ethyl] - 1H - imidazole

Synthesis

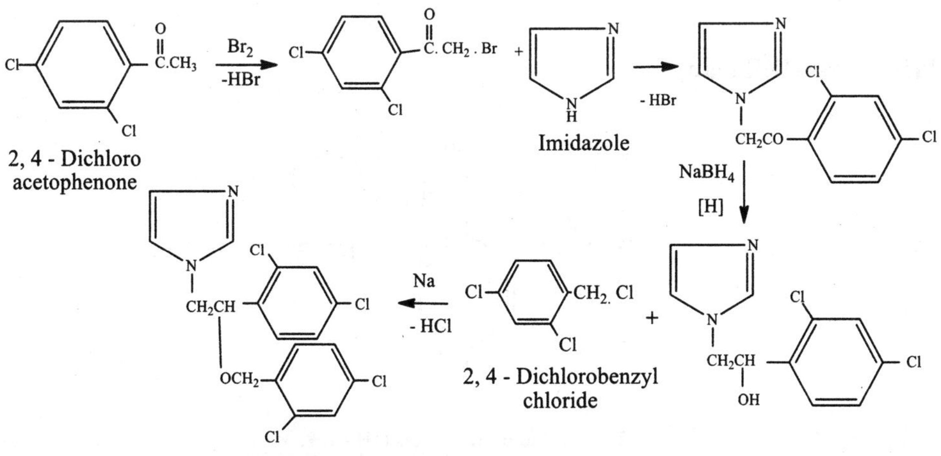

**Use:** It is used in systemic fungal infections such as C*andidiasis, Coccidioidomycosis, Cryptococcosis, Petriellidiosis* and *Paracoccidioidomycosis.*

## G. Ketoconazole (Nizoral)

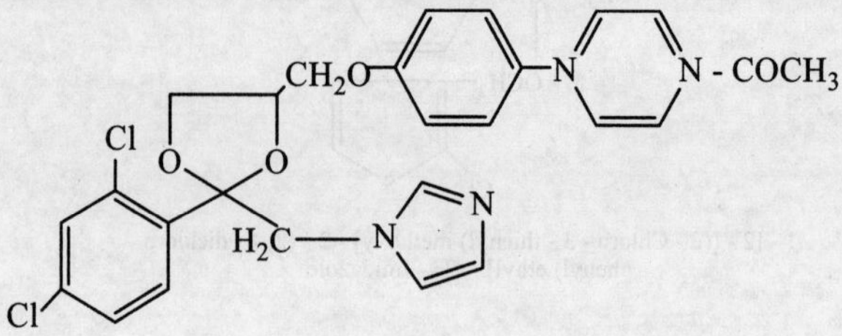


cis - 1- Acetyl - 4 - [4 - [[2 - (2, 4 - dichloro phenyl) - 2 - (1H - imidazole - 1- ylmethyl) - 1, 3 - dioxolan - 4 - yl] methoxy] phenyl] piperazine

It is a broad-spectrum imidazole antifungal agent used for systemic fungal infection. Bioavailability of Ketoconazole decreases when administered with antacid or drugs which raises stomach pH. It is a powerful inhibitor of CYP3A4 and causes interaction with other drugs (Triazolam and Cyclosporine)

**Use:** It is used for systemic fungal infections namely C*andidiasis, Coccidioidomycosis, Blastomycosis* and H*istoplasmosis*. It is used topically in the form of cream and shampoo for the management of *Cutaneous candidiasis* and T*inea* infection. It has little effect on *Aspergillus or Cryptococcus*.

## 2.3.2.2 Triazole Derivatives

## A. Fluconazole (Diflucan)

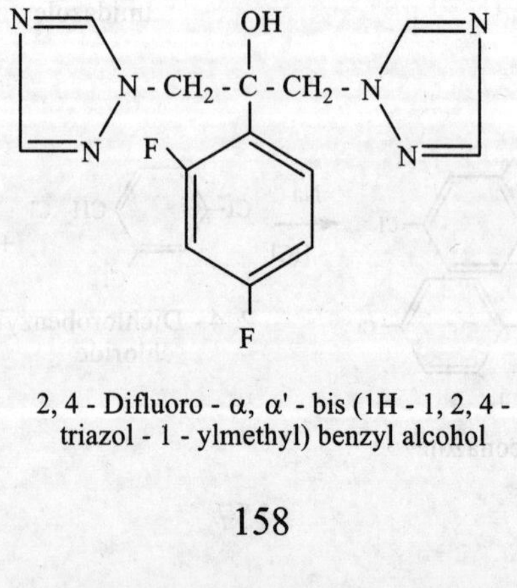


2, 4 - Difluoro - α, α' - bis (1H - 1, 2, 4 - triazol - 1 - ylmethyl) benzyl alcohol

It has two advantages over other antifungal agents: (a) It can cross the blood brain barrier and (b) It has efficacy against *Cryptococcus neoformans.*

**Use:** It is used to control oesophageal and *Oropharyngeal candidiasis.*

**B. Terconazole (Terazol)**

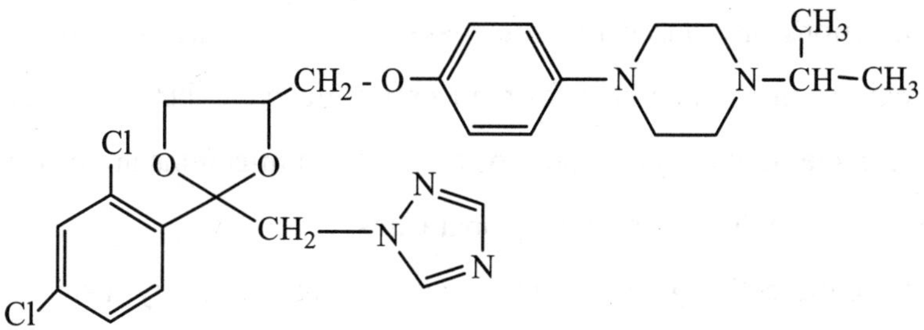

*cis* - 1 - [4 - [[2 - (2, 4 - Dichloro phenyl) - 2 - (1H - 1, 2, 4 - triazol - 1 - ylmethyl)-1, 3 - dioxolan - 4 - yl) methoxy] phenyl] - 4 - (1 - methyl ethyl) piperazine

**Use:** It is used for the control of *Vulvovaginal moniliasis* caused by *Candida albicans.*

**C. Itraconazole (Sporanox)**

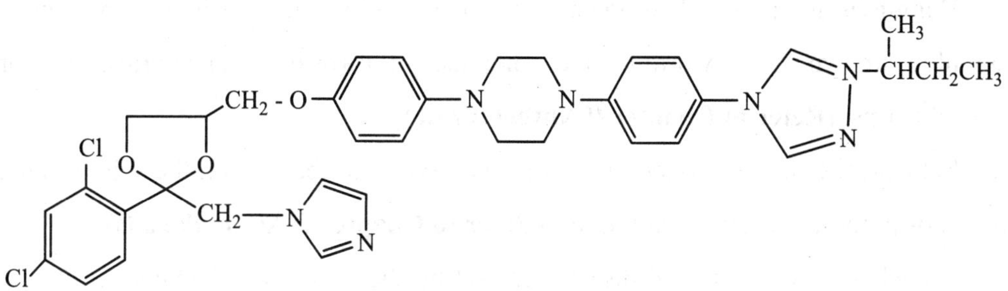

4 - {4 - [4 - [4 - [[2 - (2, 4 -Dichloro phenyl) - 2 - 1H - 1, 2, 4 - triazol - 1- ylmethyl) - 1, 3 - dioxolan - 4 - yl] methoxy] phenyl] - 1- piperazinyl]phenyl} - 2, 4 - dihydro - 2 - (1 - methyl propyl) - 3H -1, 2, 4 - triazol - 3 - one

**Use:** It is an orally active, broad spectrum antifungal agent used to treat a number of fungal infections that includes aspergillosis, blastomycosis, coccidioidomycosis, histoplasmosis, and paracoccidioidomycosis.

Chapter

8

# ANTIPROTOZAL AGENTS

## 1. INTRODUCTION

Protozoal infections are caused by protozoans, a type of parasitic infection. These organisms may remain in the human host for their entire life cycle, but many carryout part of their reproductive cycle in insects or other hosts. Parasitic infections are caused by three types of organisms: protozoa, helminths and ectoparasites.

Protozoa are single-cell organisms, which can live and multiply inside of humans. Some infections caused by protozoa include amoebiasis, giardiasis, leishmaniasis, trypanosomiasis etc., They are able to multiply in humans, which contributes to their survival and also permits serious infections to develop from just a single organism. Transmission of protozoa that live in a human's intestine to another human typically occurs through a fecal-oral route (eg. contaminated food or water or person-to-person contact).

Helminths are multi-celled organisms, which can live alone or in humans. These are commonly known as worms and include flatworms, tapeworms, ringworms, and roundworms. **(Refer to Chapter-9 Anthelmintic)**

Ectoparasites are multi-cell organisms that live in or feed off on the skin of humans, such as mosquitoes, fleas, ticks and mites. **(Refer to Chapter-3 Antimalarials)**

Amoebiasis is a protozoal disease, caused by the protozoan *Entamoeba histolytica*. Amoebic infections generally remain confined to the intestine, where they may give rise to dysentery, but in an appreciable fraction of cases the amoebae may locate elsewhere, especially in the liver. The chemotherapy of amoebiasis thus must provide drugs to treat both the intestinal and extra-intestinal forms of the disease.

## 2. CLASSIFICATION

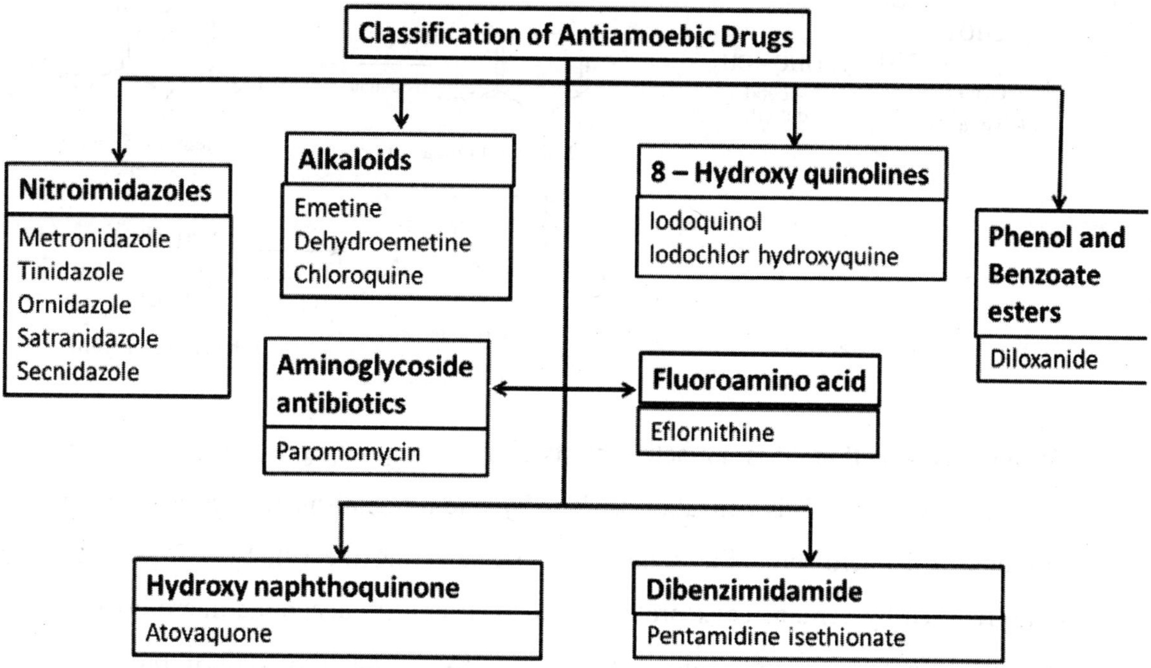


### 2.1 Nitroimidazoles

### A. Metronidazole (Flagyl, Metrogyl)

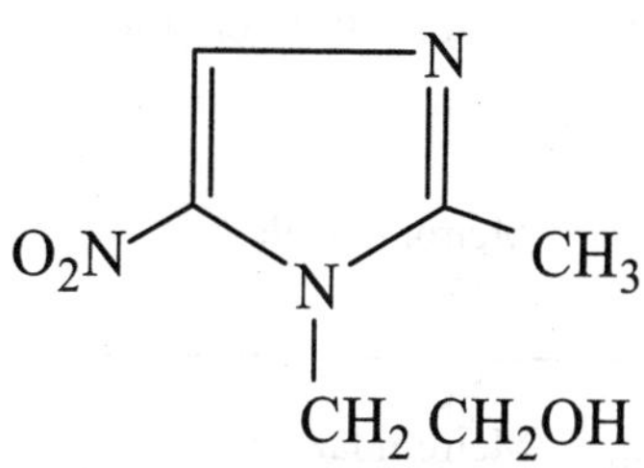


2 - Methyl - 5 - nitroimidazole - 1- ethanol

Synthesis

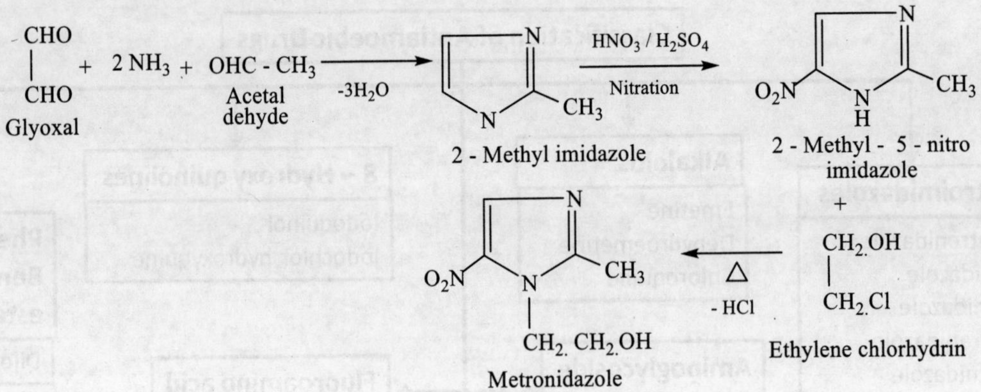


**Mechanism of action:** It is not active by itself; its nitro group gets activated to convert it into the active form. This activation is done by micro-organism. It is selectively toxic to anaerobic and micro-aerophilic pathogens. After entering the cell by diffusion its nitro group reduced by certain redox proteins functional only in anaerobic micro-organisms to extremely reactive nitrogen radical that is cytotoxic. The nitro radical present in the Metronidazole acts as an electron sink, which competes with the biological electron acceptors of the anaerobic organism for the electrons produced by the *pyruvate-ferredoxin oxidoreductase* (PFOR) enzyme pathway of pyruvate oxidation. The energy metabolism of anaerobes is, thus disturbed and replication, transcription and repair process of DNA is hindered leading to cell death.

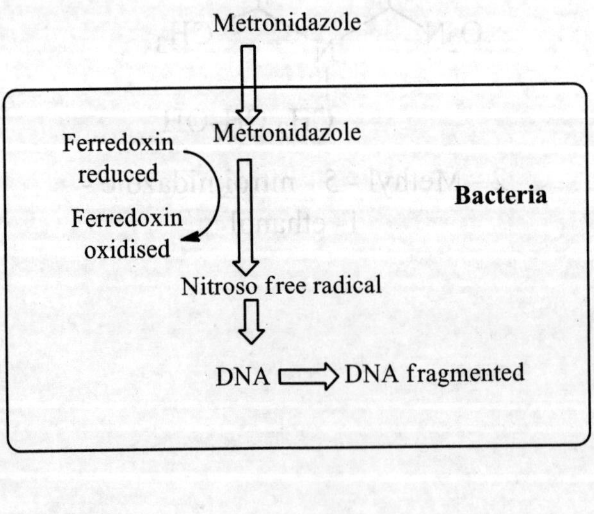

**Use:** It is an antibacterial and antiprotozoal agent used against protozoa such as *Trichomonas vaginalis*, amoebiasis and giardiasis. It is effective against anaerobic bacterial infections and is also used to treat Crohn's disease and antibiotic-associated diarrhoea.

**B. Ornidazole (Dazolic, Ornida)**

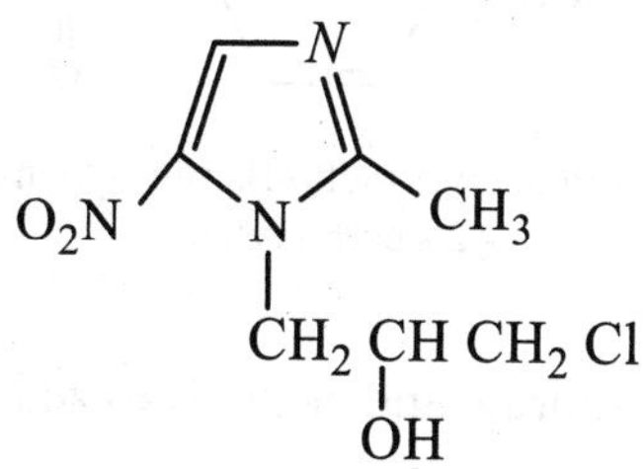


1 - (3 - Chloro - 2 - hydroxypropyl) - 2 - methyl - 5 - nitroimidazole

**Mechanism of action:** Same as Metronidazole.

**Use:** It is used in the treatment of amoebiasis, giardiasis, trichomoniasis, Crohn's disease and anaerobic infections.

**C. Tinidazole (Fasigyn)**

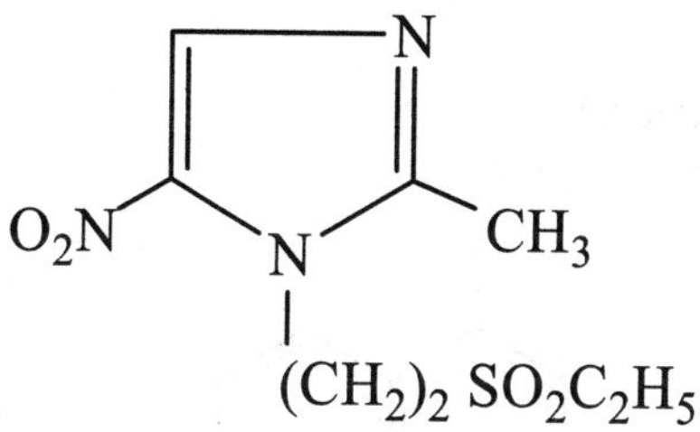


1- [2 - (Ethyl sulfonyl) ethyl] - 2 - methyl - 5 - nitro - 1H - imidazole

**Mechanism of action:** It damages DNA's helical structure and breaks its strands, which inhibits bacterial nucleic acid synthesis and causes cell death.

**Use:** It is used in the treatment of intestinal and hepatic amoebiasis.

## 2.2 Phenol and Benzoate esters

### A. Diloxanide (Amicline)

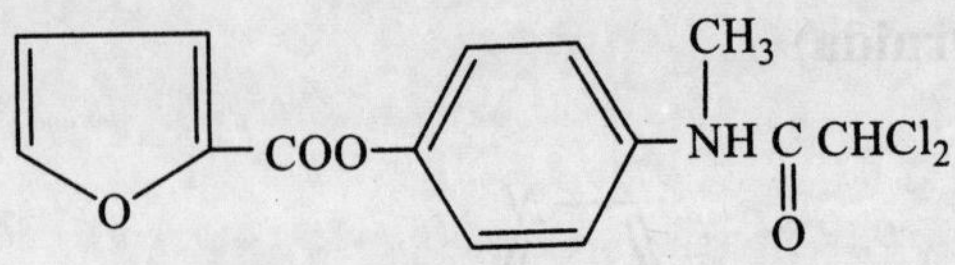

4 - [(Dichloroacetyl)(methyl)amino]phenyl furan - 2 - carboxylate

Diloxanide furoate is a prodrug and is hydrolyzed in the gastrointestinal tract to produce diloxanide the active drug. It destroys the trophozoites of *Entamoeba histolytica* that eventually form cysts. The cysts are then excreted by person infected with asymptomatic amoebiasis.

**Mechanism of action:** It acts by inhibiting protein synthesis.

**Use:** It is used in the treatment of extra-intestinal amoebiasis. It is used along with Metronidazole in the treatment of invasive or extra-intestinal amoebiasis.

## 2.3 8-Hydroxy quinolines

### A. Iodoquinol (Diquinol, Yodoxin)

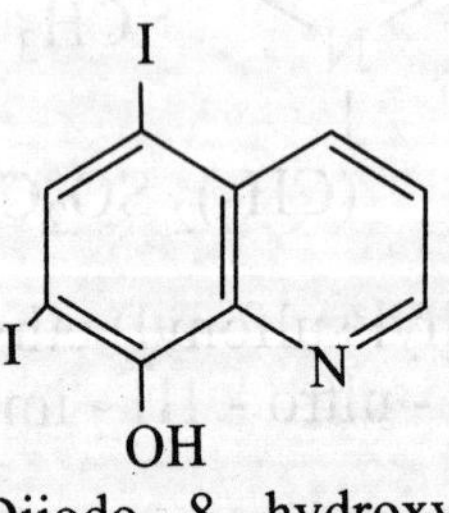

5, 7 - Diiodo - 8 - hydroxy quinoline

**Mechanism of action:** It acts by chelation of ferrous ions essential for metabolism.

**Use:** It is the used in the treatment of symptomatic infections caused by *Entamoeba histolytica*. In symptomatic intestinal disease, it is combined with Metronidazole to treat mild to moderate infections. It is not effective in the treatment of extra-intestinal amoebiasis such as hepatic abscess.

## 2.4 Dibenzimidamide

### A. Pentamidine isethionate (Nebupent)

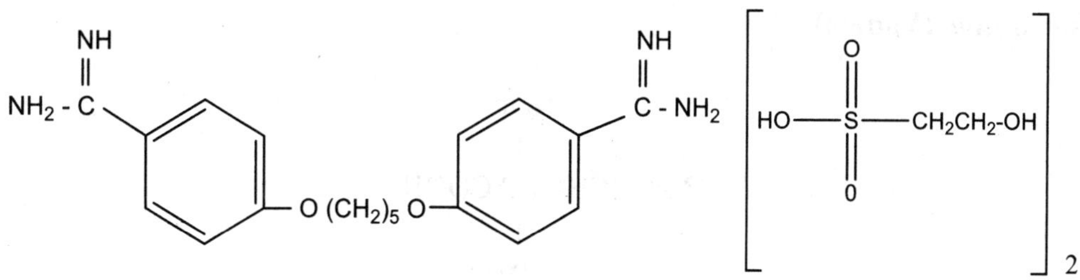

4,4 '- (Pentane - 1, 5 - diylbis (oxy)) dibenzimidamide bis (2 - hydroxy ethanesulfonate)

**Mechanism of action:** It acts by interfering with nuclear metabolism producing inhibition of the synthesis of DNA, RNA, phospholipids and proteins.

**Use:** It is used as antiprotozoal (*Trypanosoma, Leishmania*) and anti-pneumocystis.

## 2.5 Hydroxy naphthoquinone

### A. Atovaquone (Mepron)

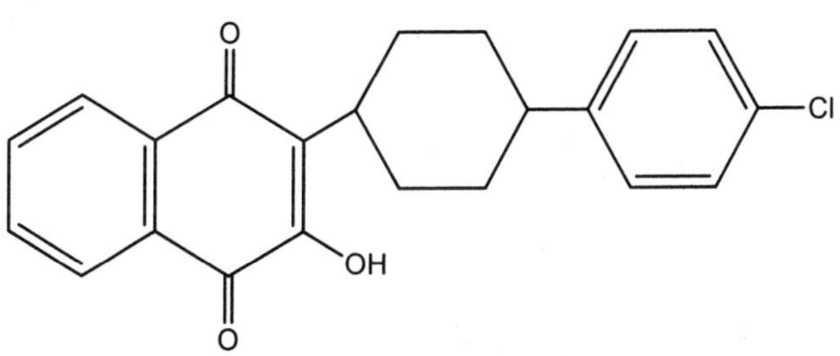

2 - (4 - (p - Chlorophenyl) cyclohexyl) - 3 - hydroxy -1, 4 - naphthoquinone

It is recommended, alternative to Trimethoprim-Sulfamethoxazole for the treatment and prophylaxis of *Pneumocystis carinii* patient intolerance to this combination.

**Mechanism of action:** It selectively inhibits the malarial Cytochrome bc1 complex in the parasitic electron transport chain, collapsing the mitochondrial membrane potential.

**Use:** It is used to treat pneumonia caused by a fungal infection called *Pneumocystis carinii.*

### 2.6 Fluoro amino acid

#### A. Eflornithine (Vaniga)

$$\begin{array}{c} HCF_2 \\ | \\ NH_{2.}\ (CH_2)_3\ C\ COOH \\ | \\ NH_2 \end{array}$$

2 - (Difluromethyl) - DL - ornithine

**Mechanism of action:** It inhibits the enzyme *ornithine decarboxylase* which is needed for protozoal cell division and differentiation.

**Use:** It is used for the treatment of West African sleeping sickness caused by *Trypanosoma brucei gambiense.*

# ANTHELMINTIC

Chapter 9

## 1. INTRODUCTION

The term anthelmintic is restricted to drugs acting locally to expel parasites from the GIT. There are several types of worms which penetrate other tissues; drugs which act on these parasitic infections are known as anthelmintic.

The worm parasites of man belong to two phyla: Nemathelminthes (round-worms) and Platyhelminthes (flatworms). The roundworms include hookworm, roundworm, whipworm, pinworm, *Strongyloides stercoralis*, *Trichinella spiralis* and *Wuchereria bancrofti.* Anthelmintics are defined as drugs used to combat any type of helminthiasis.

## 2. CLASSIFICATION

### I. Based on Chemical Structure

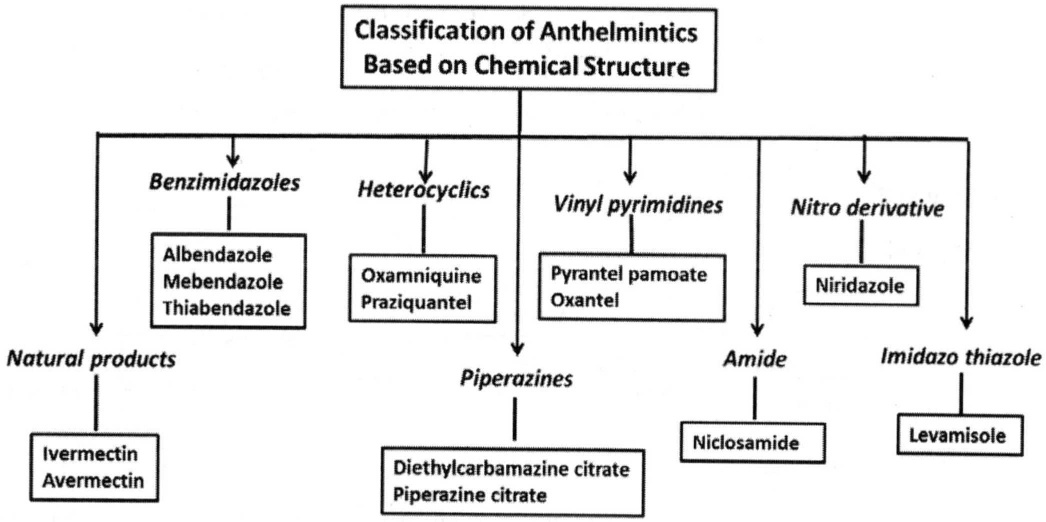

## II. Based on Therapeutic use

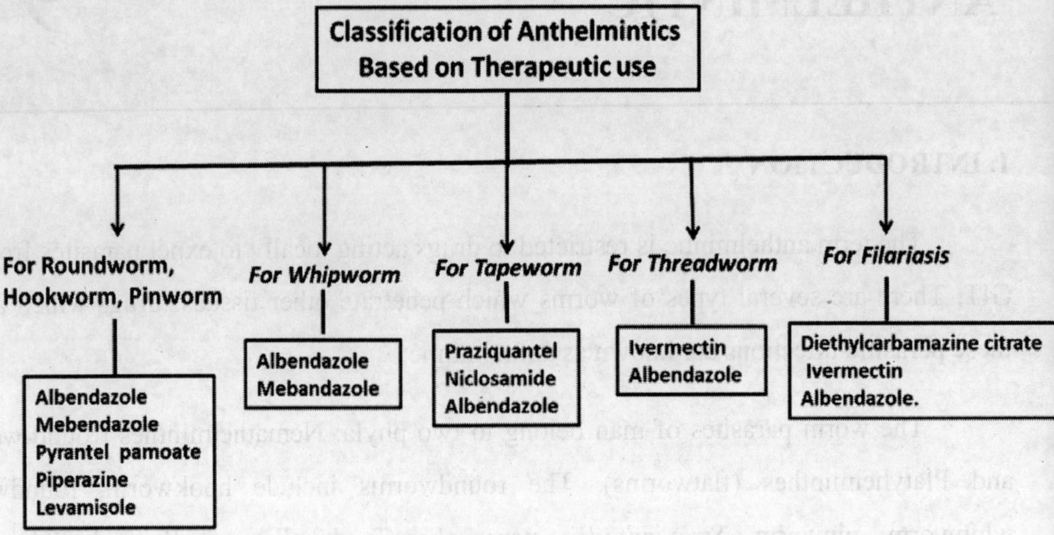


## 2.1 Piperazine Derivatives

### A. Diethylcarbamazine citrate (Hetrazan)

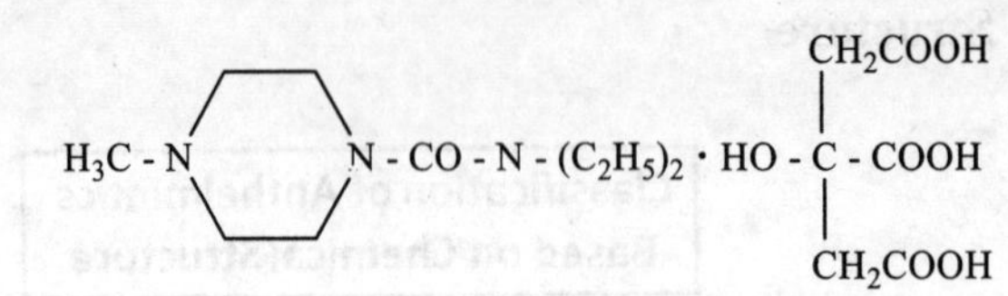


N, N' - Diethyl - 4 - methyl -1- Piperazine carboxamide citrate

Synthesis

Method - I

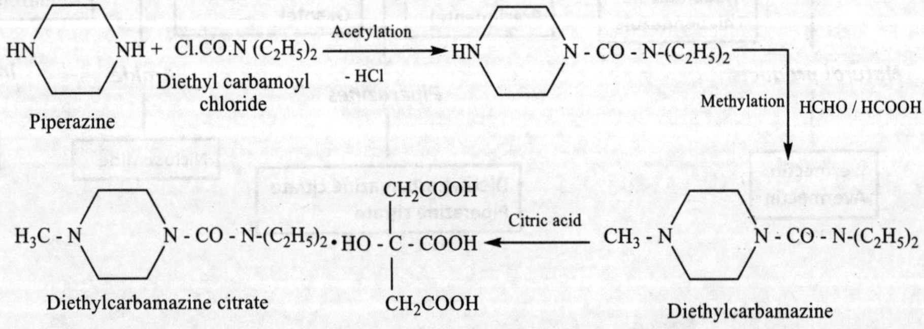

Method - II

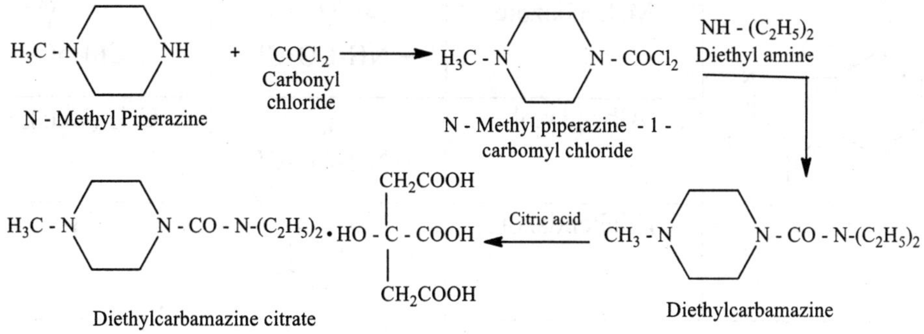


Method - III

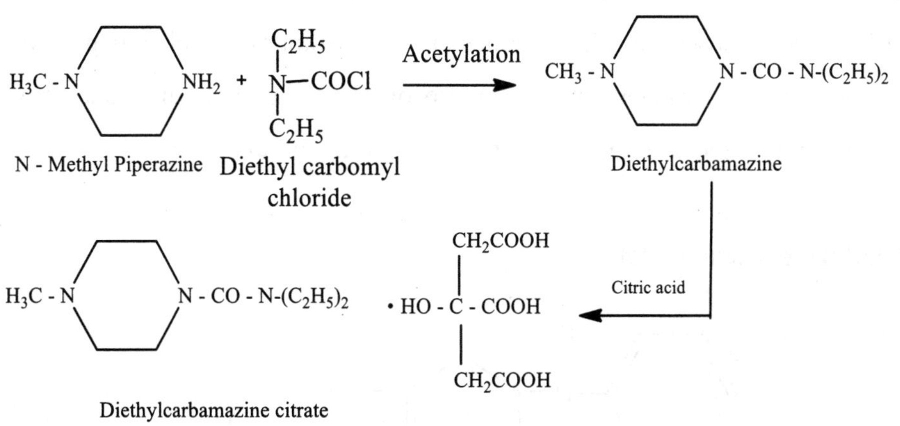


**Mechanism of action:** It has a highly selective effect on microfilariae, act by inhibiting the arachidonic acid metabolism of filarial microfilaria. This makes the microfilaria more susceptible to immune attack.

**Use:** It is the drug of choice for filariasis (*Wuchereria bancrofti, Brugia malayi* and *Acanthocheilonema perstans*).

### 2.2 Benzimidazoles

Thiabendazole was the first highly effective broad spectrum anthelmintic belongs to benzimidazole derivative produced.

| Structure | Name | R | R1 |
|---|---|---|---|
| 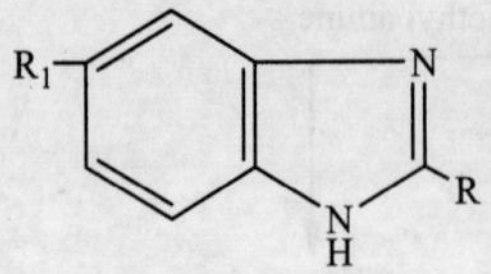 | Mebendazole | $-NH-CO-CH_3$ | $C_6H_5C(O)-$ |
| | Albendazole | $-NH-CO-CH_3$ | $CH_3(CH_2)_2S-$ |
| | Thiabendazole | 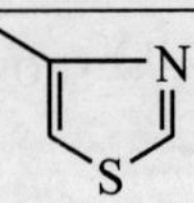 | H- |

All benzimidazole have similar mode of action and differ only in its bioavailability. The benzimidazole drugs bind selectively to β-tubulin of nematodes, cestodes and fluke and inhibit microtubule formation. Microtubules are intracellular organelles that serve a variety of functions including movement of chromosomes during cell division, providing the structural skeleton to the cell, movement of intracellular and exocytosis.

### A. Mebendazole (Mendazole)

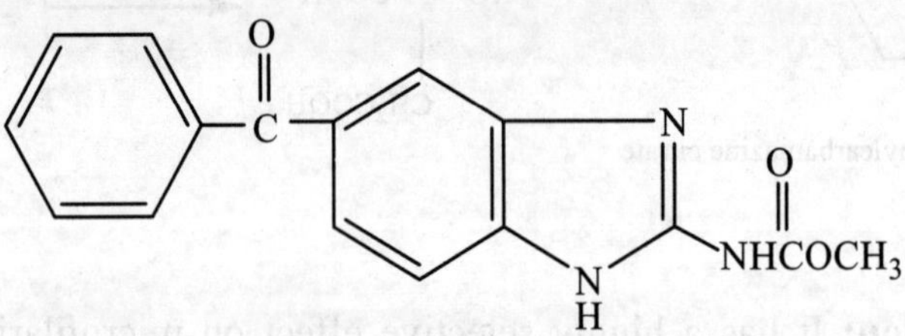

Methyl - 5 - benzoyl -2 - benzimidazole carbamate

Synthesis

Step - I: Synthesis of Methyl - S - methyl thiourea carboxylate (MMTC)

$$H_2N-C(=NH)-S.CH_3 + ClCOOCH_3 \xrightarrow[-HCl]{NaOH / pH8} H_2N.C(=N.COOCH_3)-S.CH_3$$

S - Methyl isothio urea + Methyl chloro formate → Methyl - S - methyl thiourea carboxylate (MMTC)

Step - II: Synthesis of 3, 4 - Diamino benzophenone

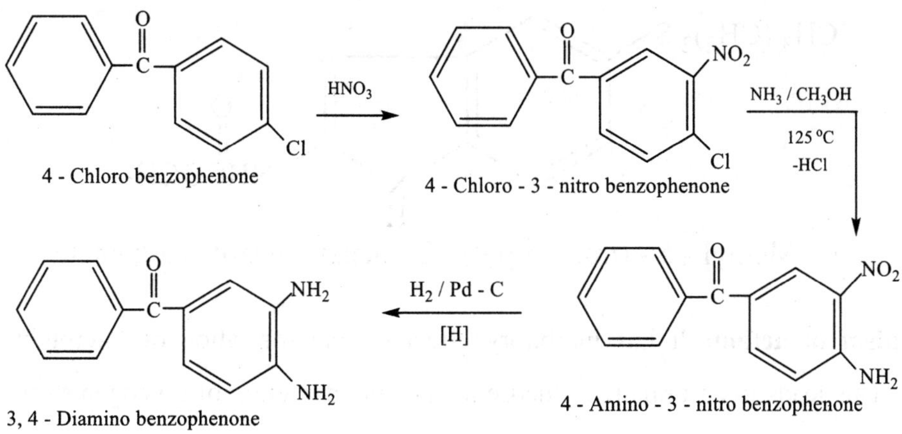


Step - III: Condensations of Step I and Step II Products

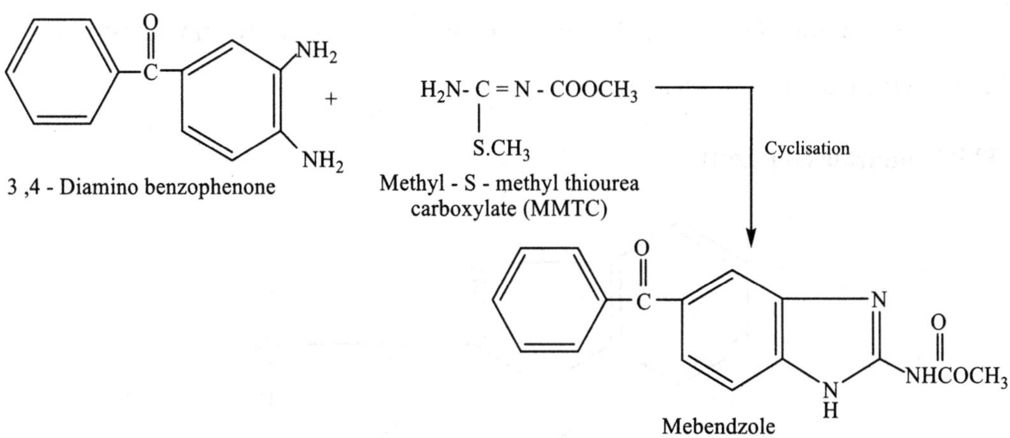


**Mechanism of action:** It selectively inhibits the synthesis of microtubules via binding to colchicine binding site of β-tubulin, thereby blocking polymerization of tubulin dimers in intestinal cells of parasites.

**Use:** It is used in the treatment of hookworm, pinworm, round worm and whipworm infestation.

**B. Albendazole (Albucid)**

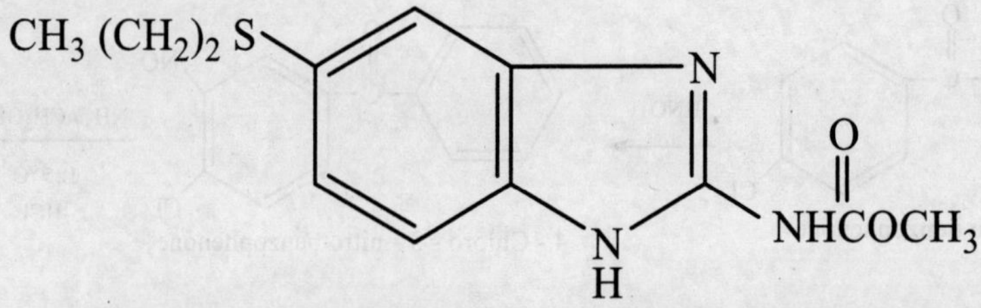


Methyl - 5 - (thio propyl) - 2 - benzimidazole carbamate

**Mechanism of action:** It has inhibitory effect on the formation of microtubules from tubulin. This leads to an impaired glucose uptake and depletion of glycogen stores leads to worm's death.

**Use:** It is useful in the treatment of intestinal nematode infection and echinococcosis. It is effective against roundworm, hookworm, whipworm and threadworm infestations. It is effective in the treatment of ascariasis.

**C. Thiabendazole (Bovizol)**

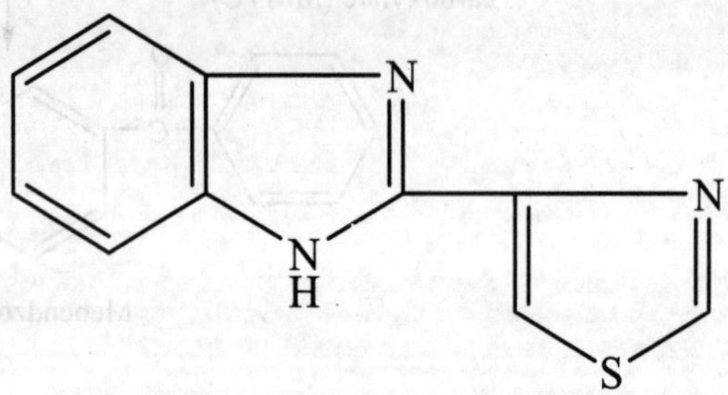


2 - (4 - Thiazolyl) - benzimidazole

**Mechanism of action:** It inhibits the helminth-specific enzyme *fumarate reductase*.

**Use:** It is a broad spectrum anthelmintic. It is effective against threadworm, roundworm, hookworm and whipworm infestation.

## 2.3 Heterocyclics

### A. Oxamniquine

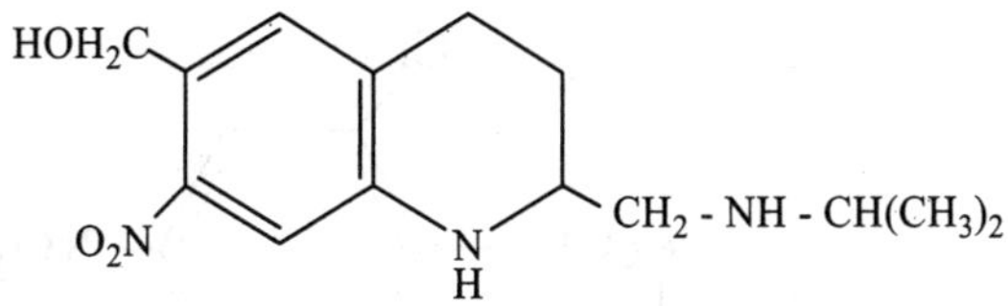


1, 2, 3, 4 - Tetrahydro - 2 - [(isopropyl amino) methyl] - 7 - nitro - 6 - quinoline methanol

**Mechanism of action:** It acts by binding with DNA, which results in contraction and paralysis of the worms and eventual detachment from terminal venules in the mesentery and death.

**Use:** It is a drug of choice for infection caused by *Schistosoma mansoni*. (Antischistosomal agent)

### B. Praziquantel (Cysticide)

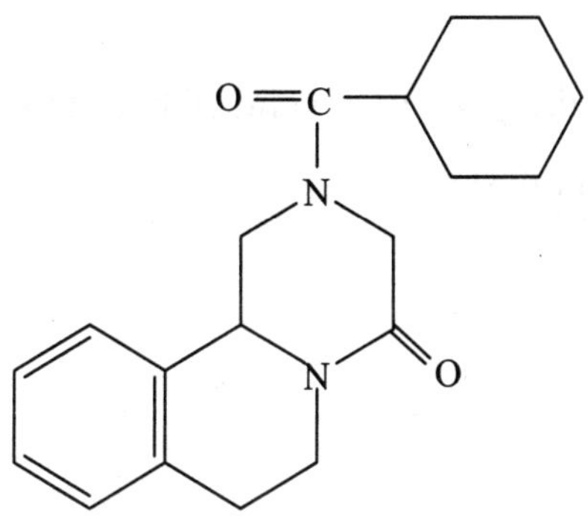


2 - (Cyclohexyl carbonyl) -1, 2, 3, 6, 7, 11b - hexahydro - 4H - pyrazino - [2, 1-a] - isoquinolin - 4 - one

**Mechanism of action:** It increases $Ca^{2+}$ permeability of parasite muscle and/or tegumental membranes. This causes severe spasms and paralysis of the worms. The worms are then either completely destroyed in the intestine or passed in the stool.

**Use:** It is considered as drug of choice for the treatment of *Schistosoma japonicum*, (blood fluke) fasciolopsiasis (intestinal flukes) clonorchiasis (Chinese liver fluke) and opisthorchiasis (liver fluke).

### 2.4 Amide

#### A. Niclosamide (Niclosan)

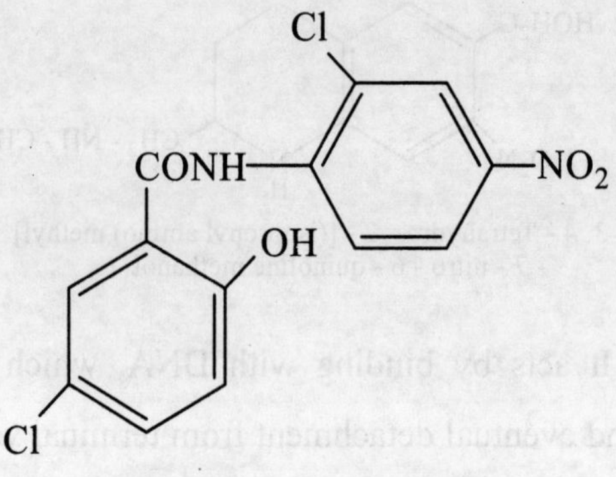

N - (2 - Chloro - 4 - nitrophenyl) - 5 - chloro - 2 - hydroxy benzamide

**Mechanism of action:** It has three major mechanism of action affecting tapeworm: inhibition of glucose uptake, inhibition of energy production by anaerobic metabolism and inhibition of inorganic phosphate incorporation into ATP.

**Use:** It is the first choice of drug for treatment of beef tapeworm, fish tapeworm, pork tapeworm and dwarf tapeworm infestations.

### 2.5 Natural Products

#### A. Ivermectin (Imectin)

Ivermectin is usually extracted from the soil of actinomycete *Streptomyces avermitilis*, the natural Ivermectin is 16-membered macrocyclic lactones, with broad anti-nematicidal activity. It is a mixture of 22, 23 - dihydro derivative of Avermectins $B_1A$ and $B_1B$.

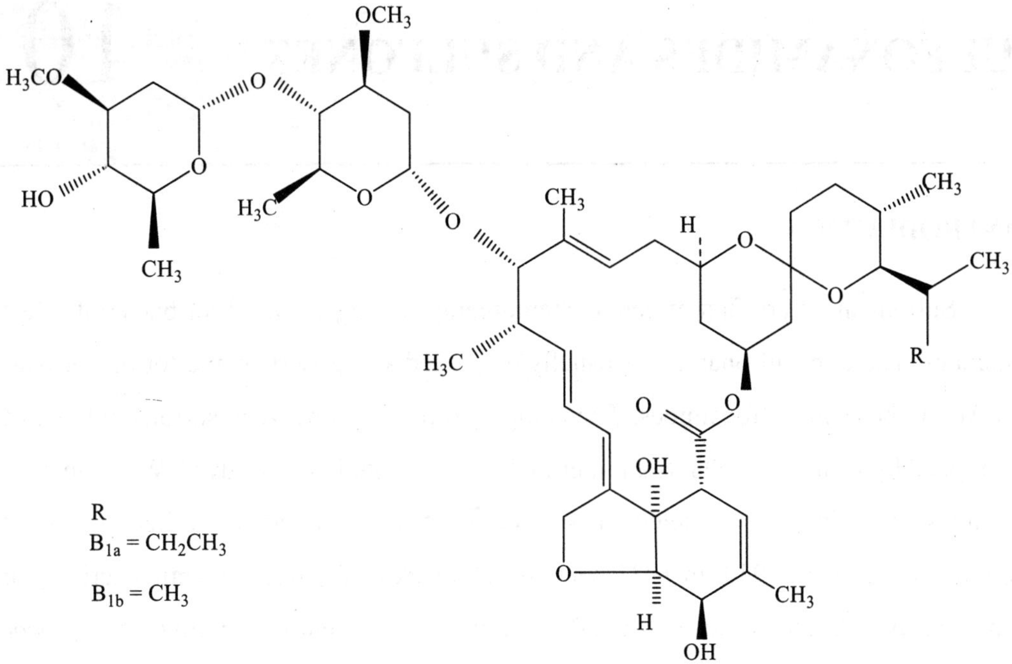


R
$B_{1a} = CH_2CH_3$
$B_{1b} = CH_3$

**Mechanism of action:** It causes an influx of Cl- ions through the cell membrane of invertebrates by activation of specific Ivermectin-sensitive ion channels. The resultant hyperpolarization results in paralysis and death of the parasite either directly or by causing the worms to starve.

**Use:** It is widely used in veterinary practice for the control of endoparasites and exoparasites in domestic animals. It is also used to treat onchocerciasis (river blindness) in humans caused by the round worm *Onchocerca volvulus,* head lice and scabies.

Chapter 10

# SULFONAMIDES AND SULFONES

## 1. INTRODUCTION

Sulfonamides are first effective chemotherapeutic agents used for bacterial infection in humans. The term sulfonamide is usually employed as a generic name for the derivatives of p-Amino benzene sulfonamides. The compound p-Amino benzene sulfonamide was first synthesized by Gelmo in 1908 as an intermediate in the study of azo dyes. Work on azo dye containing a sulfonamide nucleus has been started by research workers of the I.G. Farbenindustrie about 1930. In 1932, Gerhard Domagk recognized the antibacterial activity of the azo dye, Prontosil red. It was effective in the treatment of hemolytic S*treptococcal* infection. Prontosil is totally inactive *in vitro* but possesses excellent activity *in vivo*. In 1935, Trofouel at Pasteur Institute discovered that Prontosil breaks down in the tissues into p-Amino benzene sulfonamide and suggested that antibacterial characteristic of the drug reside in this part of the molecule.

This discovery leads to the synthesis of at least 5500 Sulfonamides, but only few are in clinical practice. The rapid development of widespread resistance to the Sulfonamides and an increasing use of the broad-spectrum Penicillin's in the treatment of infectious disease diminished the usefulness of Sulfonamides. The development of combination of Trimethoprim and Sulfonamide in the treatment and prophylaxis on certain opportunistic microbial infection, reawaked interest in Sulfonamides.

Sulfonamides inhibit Gram-positive and Gram-negative bacteria, *Nocardia,* C*hlamydia trachomatis* and some *Protozoa*. Some enteric bacteria such as *E. coli,* Klebsiella, *Salmonella, Shigella* and *Enterobacter* are inhibited. Sulfonamides are used in the treatment of tonsillitis, septicemia, meningococcal meningitis, bacillary dysentery and number of infections of urinary tract.

## 1.1 Nomenclature of Sulfonamides

Sulfonamides are considered as derivatives of p-Amino benzene sulfonamide. The nitrogen atom of - $SO_2NH_2$ is numbered as 1 and that of the - $NH_2$ group as 4.

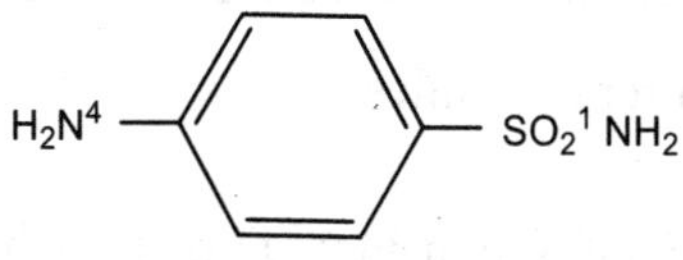

Sulphanilamide

## 1.2. General Properties

Sulfonamides are white crystalline powder, sparingly soluble in water. The sulfonamide group - $SO_2NH_2$ loses a proton and form salts, which is more soluble than the free sulfonamides. The negative charge on nitrogen after the loss of proton gain stability by resonance.

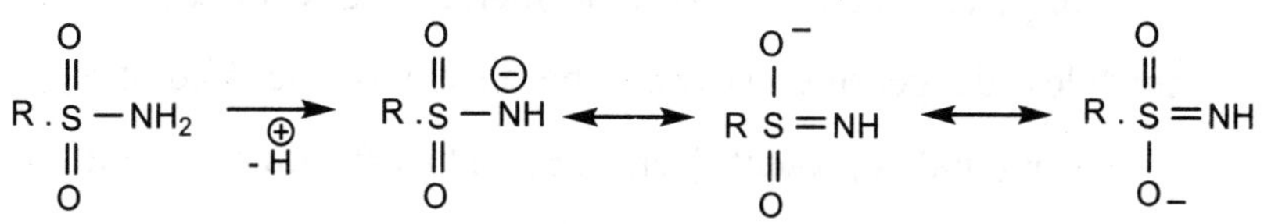

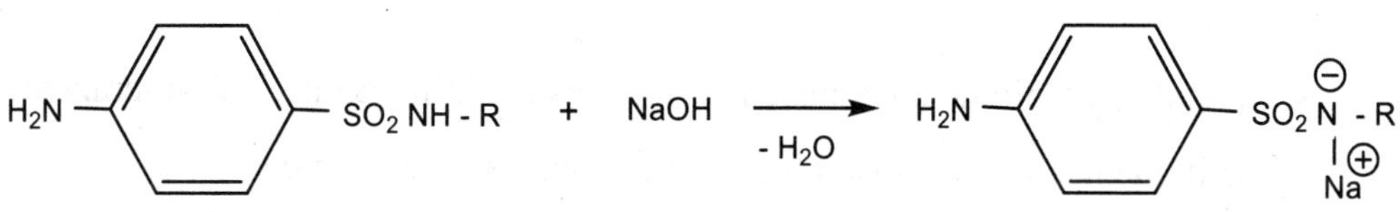

## 1.3 Crystalluria and pKa

The sulfonamides and their metabolites are excreted almost in the urine. The sulfonamides are not water soluble; they crystallize in the kidney and cause crystalluria. The pKa of sulfonamide group of sulfanilamide is 10.4, that the pH at which 50% of the drug is ionized. Because the urine pH is 6, essentially, all the sulfonamides are unionized and occur as insoluble form in the kidney. The sulfonamide coming out of solution in urine and kidney causes crystalluria.

Various approaches to adjust the solubility of sulfonamide in urine were done. They are:

i) Greatly increasing the urine flow by taking plenty of fluids, so that glomerular filtration rate could be increased there would be less opportunity to form crystals in renal tubules.

ii) Increasing the pH of the urine: This is achieved by giving oral sodium bicarbonate before to sulfonamide dose, so that the urine pH will be closure to 10.4.

iii) Mixed sulfonamides: Mixing different sulfonamide to achieve an appropriate total dose. When several sulfonamides are administered together, the antibacterial activity is the summation of the total sulfonamide concentration present, but the solubility is independent of each other. Thus, by giving a mixture of sulfonamide the same therapeutic level can be maintained with much less danger of crystalluria, because only one-third of the amount of any one compound is present. Hence, mixed sulfonamides are in current practice now. For example,

- Trisulfapyrimidine contains equal weights of Sulfadiazine, Sulfamerazine and Sulfamethazine. It is available as oral suspension and tablets.

- Sulfadoxine and Pyrimethamine: This combination is used for the treatment of *Plasmodium falciparum* malaria.

(iv) A newer sulfonamide has been synthesized whose pKa is closer to pH of urine. This is brought about, by introducing an electron with drawing, hetero cyclic ring at $N^1$ position which donates a proton and lowers the pKa value.

### 1.4 Mechanism of Action

Sulfonamides are bacteriostatic in nature. The sulfonamide sensitive micro-organisms require p-Amino benzoic acid (PABA) for the synthesis of folic acid which is essential for the synthesis of DNA and RNA. Various folate derivatives like folinic acid, $N^5$, $N^{10}$ - Methylene tetrahydro folic acid and $N^{10}$ - formyl tetrahydro folic acid acts as co-enzymes in transport of one carbon unit in several biochemical reactions in humans and micro organisms. The one carbon transfer reaction is necessary for the synthesis of purines, thymidine and some amino acids. One of the products of these folate dependent biochemical reactions is deoxy thymidine mono phosphate, which is an important precursor to DNA. Sulfonamides block the biosynthesis of this folate coenzyme resulting into the arrest of bacterial growth and cell division. The sulfonamides are structural analogues to PABA that competitively inhibit the action of *dihydropteroate synthase,* preventing the addition of PABA to pteridine diphosphate and blocking the net biosynthesis of folate coenzymes.

Folate coenzymes are biosynthesized from dietary folic acid in human and other cells. Bacterial and protozoa must biosynthesis it *de novo* from PABA and pteridine diphosphate. Microbes cannot take up the folic acid from the growth medium or from the host (bacterial cell wall may be impermeable to folic acid). Hence sulfonamides does not affect mammalian cell.

The conversion of dihydrofolic acid to tetrahydrofolic acid is catalyzed by the enzyme *dihydrofolate reductase*. Trimethoprim is a selective competitive inhibitor of microbial *dihydrofolate reductase*. So, when combined with sulfa drug, it appears to be most active agent (Fig. 10.1) that exerts a synergistic antibacterial activity. Trimethoprim does not have high affinity for malarial protozoan's *folate reductase*. In antimalarial therapy, Pyrimethamine and sulfa combination yields synergistic effect.

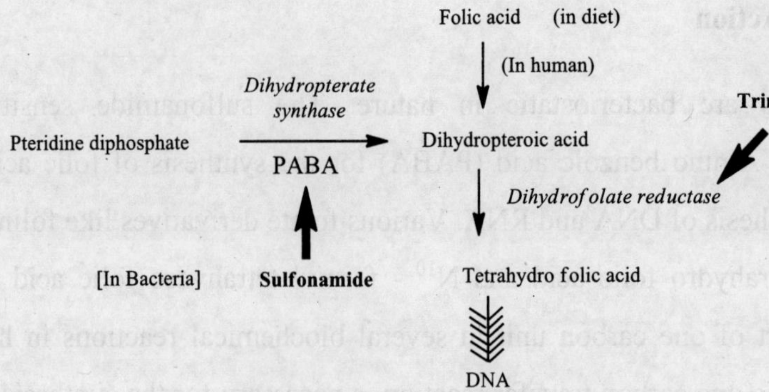


**Fig. 10.1 Mechanism of Action of Sulfonamide**

## 1.5 Structure Activity Relationship

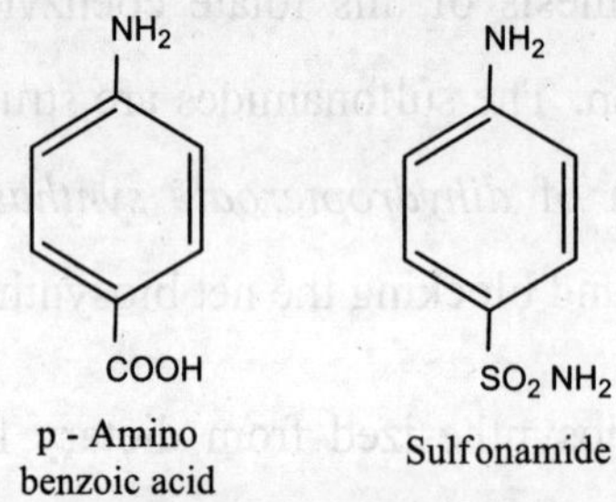


- The sulfanilamide skeleton is the minimal structural requirement for antibacterial activity.
- The free amino group (- $NH_2$) is essential for activity. However, it can be replaced by groups which can be reconverted it back to free amino group eg. succinyl amido, acetamido and phthalyl amido group.
- Sulfur should be directly linked to the benzene ring.
- The amino and sulfonyl radical should be 1, 4 position; 1, 2 and 1, 3 isomers are therapeutically less active.
- Any substitution on aromatic ring or replacement of benzene ring by other ring decreases or abolishes the activity.

- Substitution of hetero cyclic aromatic nucleus in N[1] position yields highly potent compound
- N[1] disubstitution in general, leads to inactive compound because one hydrogen is essential for ionization.
- Maximum antibacterial activity is exhibited by sulfonamides having pKa value between 6.6 to 7.4.
- The lipid solubility influences the pharmacokinetic and antibacterial activity. In general as the lipid solubility increases, the half life and antibacterial activity *(in vitro)* also increases.

## 1.6 Therapeutic Uses

Sulfonamides may be used systemically, topically or orally for local effects depending upon its solubility. Some uses of sulfonamides are:

- Pneumocystis carinii pneumonia: eg. Trimethoprim and Sulfamethoxazole
- Cerebral toxoplasmosis: eg. Pyrimethamine and Sulfadiazine
- Urinary tract infection: eg. Sulfamethizole
- Nocardiosis: eg. Sulfadiazine, Sulfisoxazole
- Respiratory tract infection: eg. Sulfalene
- Dermatitis herpetiformis: eg. Sulfapyridine
- Menincoccal infection: eg. Sulfadiazine
- Burn therapy: eg. Silver sulfadiazine
- Conjunctivitis and superficial ocular infections: eg. Sulfacetamide
- Traveler's diarrhea (or) GIT infection: eg. Sulfaguanidine

- Chloroquine resistant malaria: eg. Sulfadoxine with Pyrimethamine
- Treatment of leprosy: eg. Dapsone

## 1.7 General Method of Synthesis

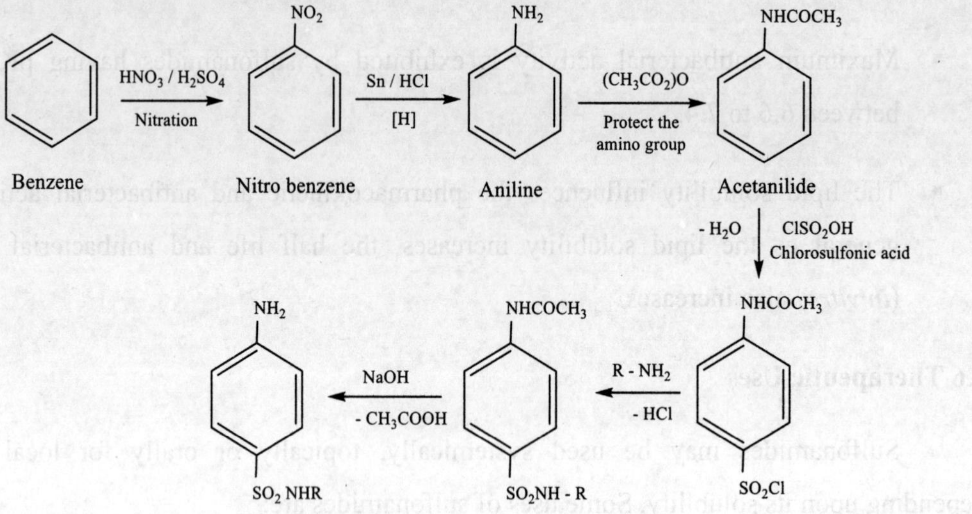


### Table 10.1 Antibacterial Sulfonamides

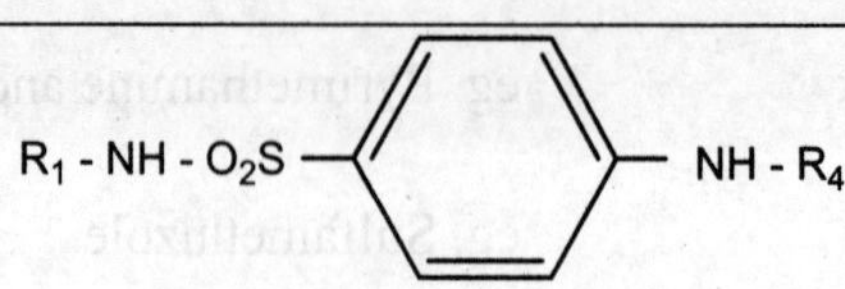


N' - Subsituted sulfonamides

| S. No | Generic Name | $R_1$ | $R_4$ | Therapeutic uses |
|---|---|---|---|---|
| 1. | Sulfacetamide | $-COCH_3$ | - H | Ophthalmologic use |
| 2. | Sulfapyridine | 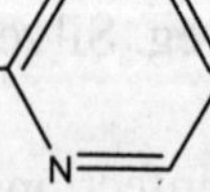 | - H | Dermatitis herpetiformis |

| | | | | |
|---|---|---|---|---|
| 3. | Sulfamethazine | 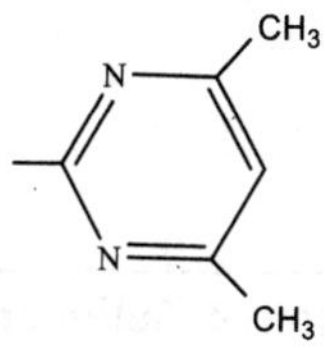 | - H | Used in meningitis |
| 4. | Sulfadiazine | 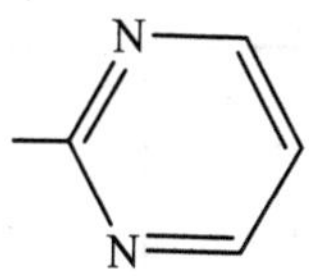 | - H | Used in meningitis and nocardiosis |
| 5. | Sulfamethizole | 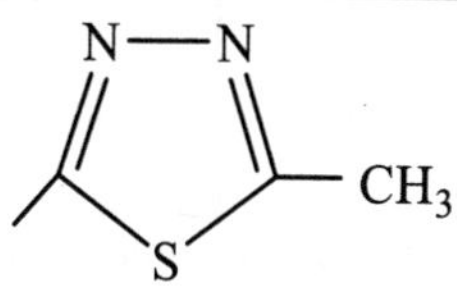 | - H | UTI infection |
| 6. | Sulfamethoxazole | 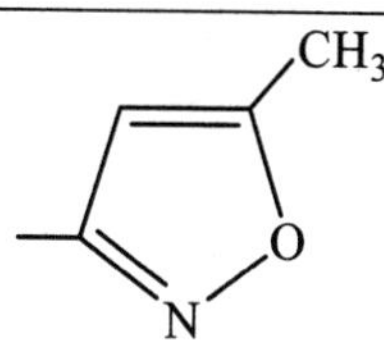 | - H | UTI infection |
| 7. | Sulfisoxazole (Sulfafurazole) | 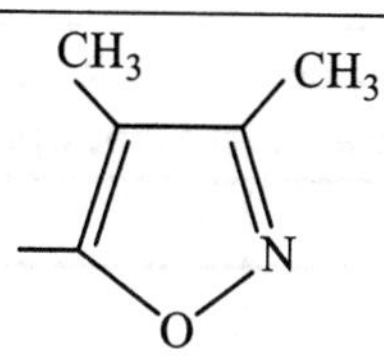 | - H | Rheumatic fever, UTI infection |
| 8. | Sulfathiazole | 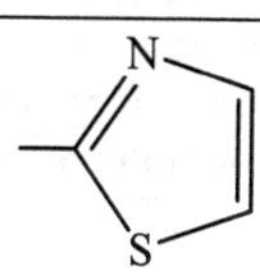 | - H | Systemic sulfonamides |

## 2. CLASSIFICATION

### I. Based on Site of Action

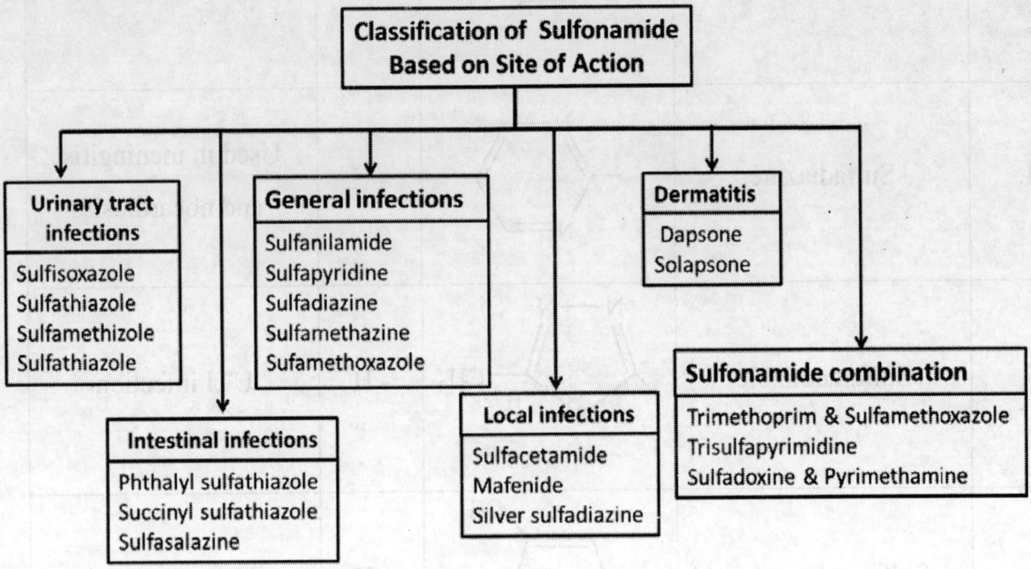


### II. Based on Pharmacokinetic Properties

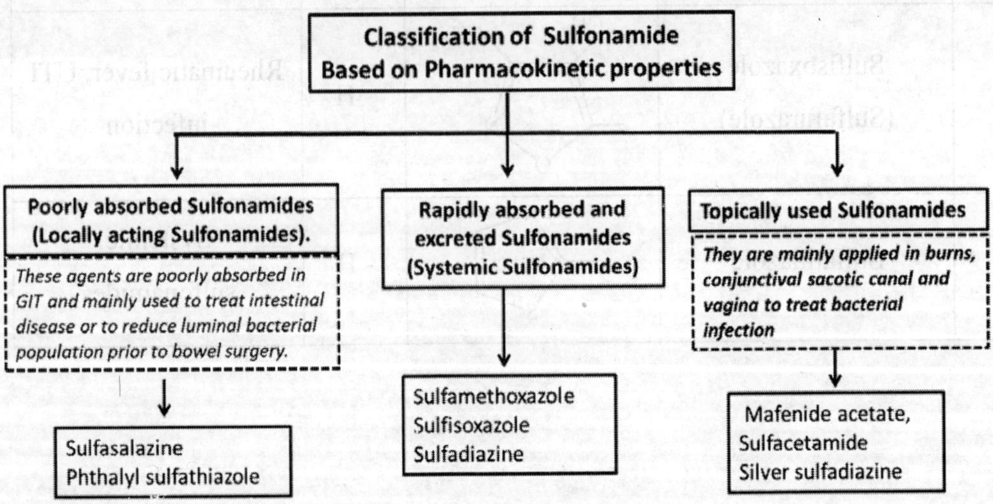

## III. Based on Chemical Structure

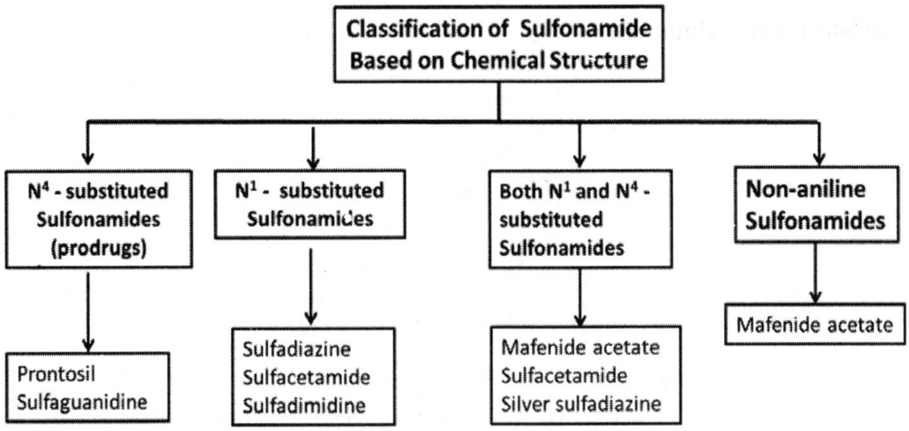


## IV. Based on Pharmacological Activity

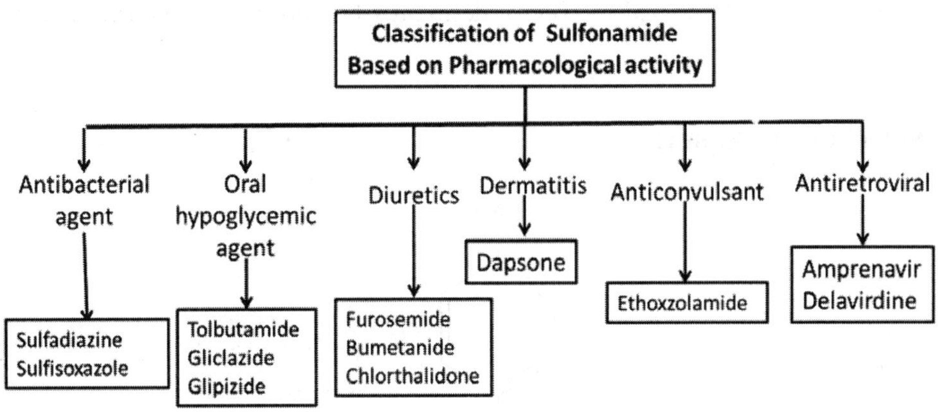


## V. Based on Duration of Action

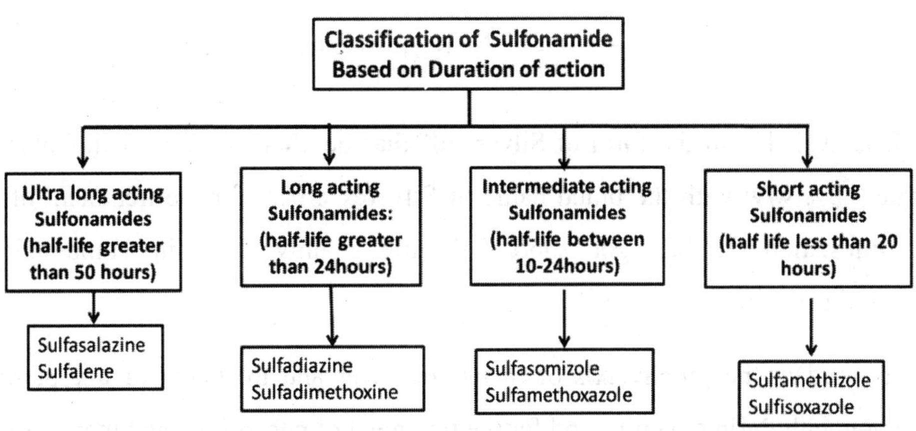

## 2.1 Sulfonamides for General Infections

### A. Sulfapyridine (Dagenan)

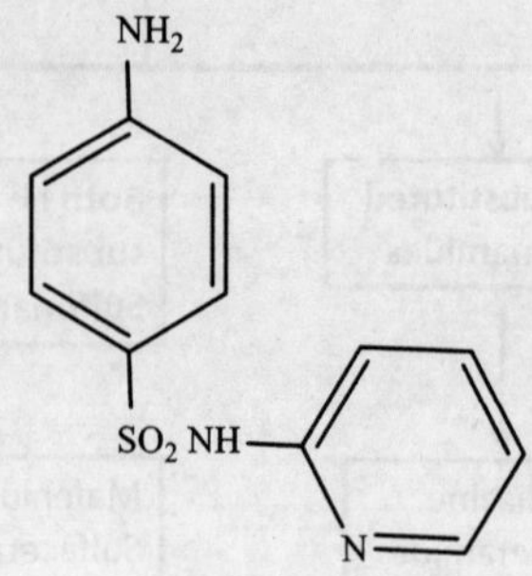

4 - Amino - N - 2 - pyridinyl benzene sulfonamide

**Use:** It was the first drug to have a curative effect on pneumonia, because of high toxicity it is not in use now. It is used to control dermatitis herpetiformis (Duhring's disease), a skin problem.

### B. Sulfadiazine (Duplex)

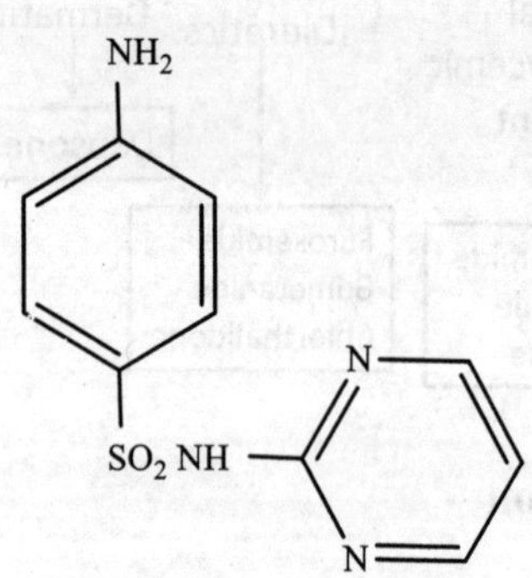

4 - Amino - N - [2 - pyrimidinyl] benzene sulfonamide

It is available in the form of Silver sulfadiazine 1%w/w along with Chlorhexidine gluconate 0.2% w/w with the brand name of Silverex cream for the treatment of burning wound infestation. It has got short half life mainly used in combination with Pyrimethamine.

**Use:** It is used in the prophylaxis of rheumatic fever and treatment of toxoplasmosis in combination with Pyrimethamine and for the treatment of nocardiosis and meningitis.

**C. Sulfamethoxazole (Gantanol)**

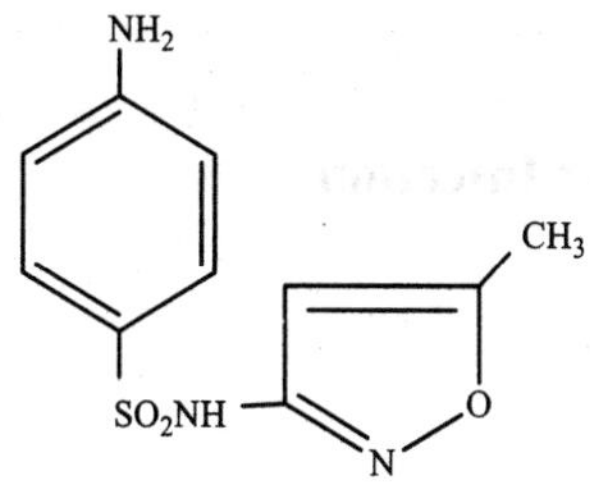


4 - Amino - N - (5 - methyl - 3 - isoxazol - yl) benzene sulfonamide

Synthesis

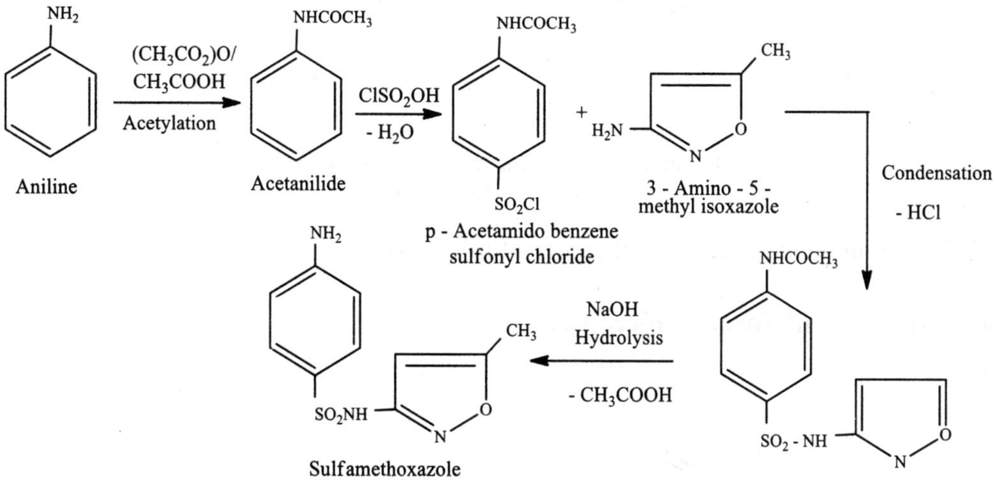


**Use:** It is used in the treatment of meningitis, toxoplasmosis, trachoma, lower urinary tract infection caused by *Escherichia coli* and *Proteus mirabilis.*

**D. Sulfamethazine/ Sulfadimidine (Bovibol)**

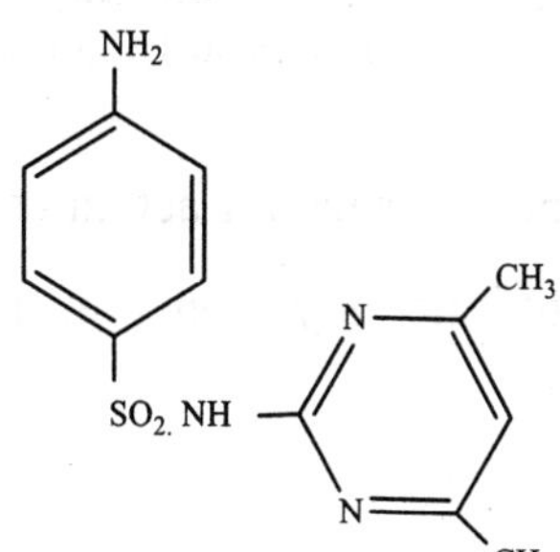


4 - Amino - N - (4, 6 - dimethyl - 2 - pyrimidinyl) benzene sulfonamide

**Use:** It is less effective in meningeal infection, because of its poor penetration into cerebrospinal fluid.

## 2.2 Sulfonamides for Urinary Tract Infection

### A. Sulfamethizole (Sulfuno)

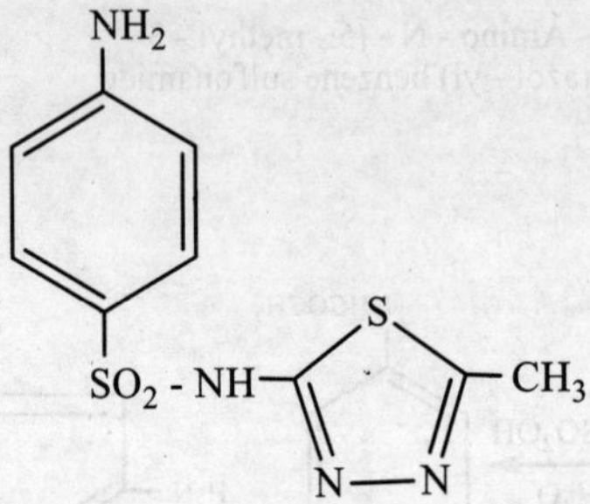


4 - Amino - N - (5 - methyl - 1, 3, 4 - thiazol - 2 - yl) benzene sulfonamide

**Use:** It is used in the treatment of urinary tract infection.

### B. Sulfisoxazole/Sulfafurazole (Gantrisin)

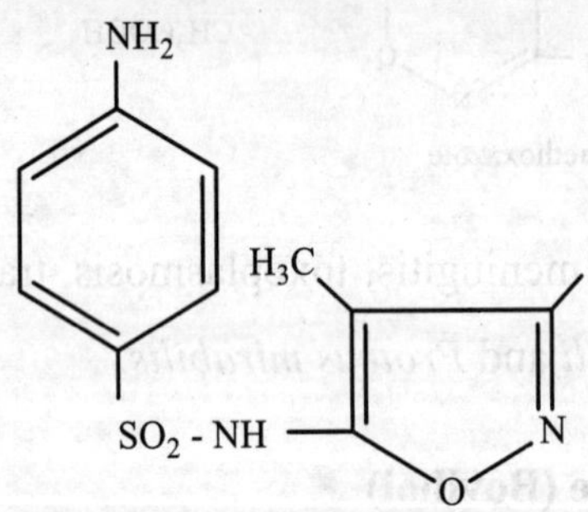


4 - Amino - N - (3, 4 - dimethyl - 5 - isoxazoly) benzene sulfonamide

**Use:** It is effective in the treatment of urinary tract infection caused by Gram-negative bacteria. In combination with antibiotic Erythromycin it is used to treat middle ear infections in children.

## 2.3 Sulfonamides for Intestinal Infections

### A. Sulfasalazine (Salazar)

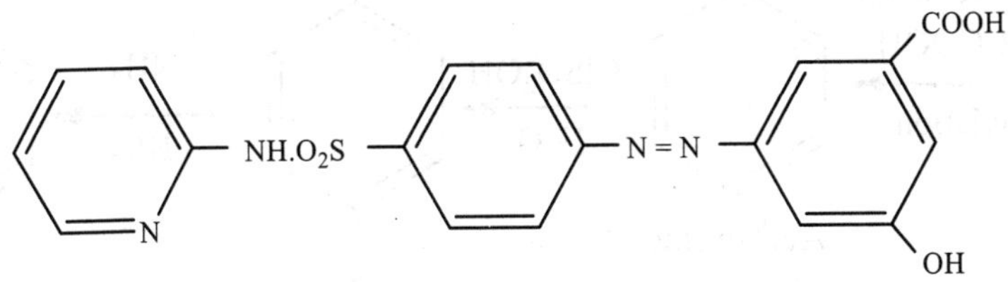

2 - Hydro - 5{[4 - (2 - pyridinyl amino) sulfonyl] phenyl} azo benzoic acid

Sulfasalazine is a prodrug, which cleaved at $N^4$ position in large intestine to m-Amino salicylic acid and Sulfapyridine by *azo reductase*. Sulfapyridine acts as antibacterial and amino salicylic acid has anti-inflammatory effect on the colon. The advantage of this prodrug is the release of amino salicylic acid, which prevents the absorption of the agent (prevents the systemic absorption) so that duration of action increases (concentrates the drug in active site) mainly used in intestinal infections.

**Use:** It is used in the treatment of inflammatory bowel disease, including ulcerative colitis and Crohn's disease. It is also used in rheumatoid arthritis and in other types of inflammatory arthritis like psoriatic arthritis and reactive arthritis.

## 2.4 Sulfonamides for Local Infections

### A. Sulfacetamide (Albucid)

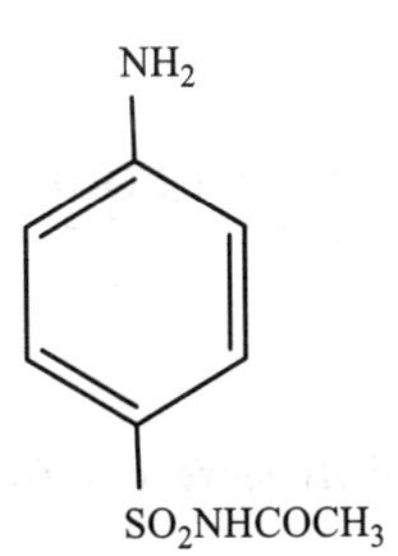

N - sulphanilyl acetamide

It is available in the form of sodium salt in various dosage forms like tablet, capsule, syrup, cream, gel, ointment, liquid and injection.

Synthesis

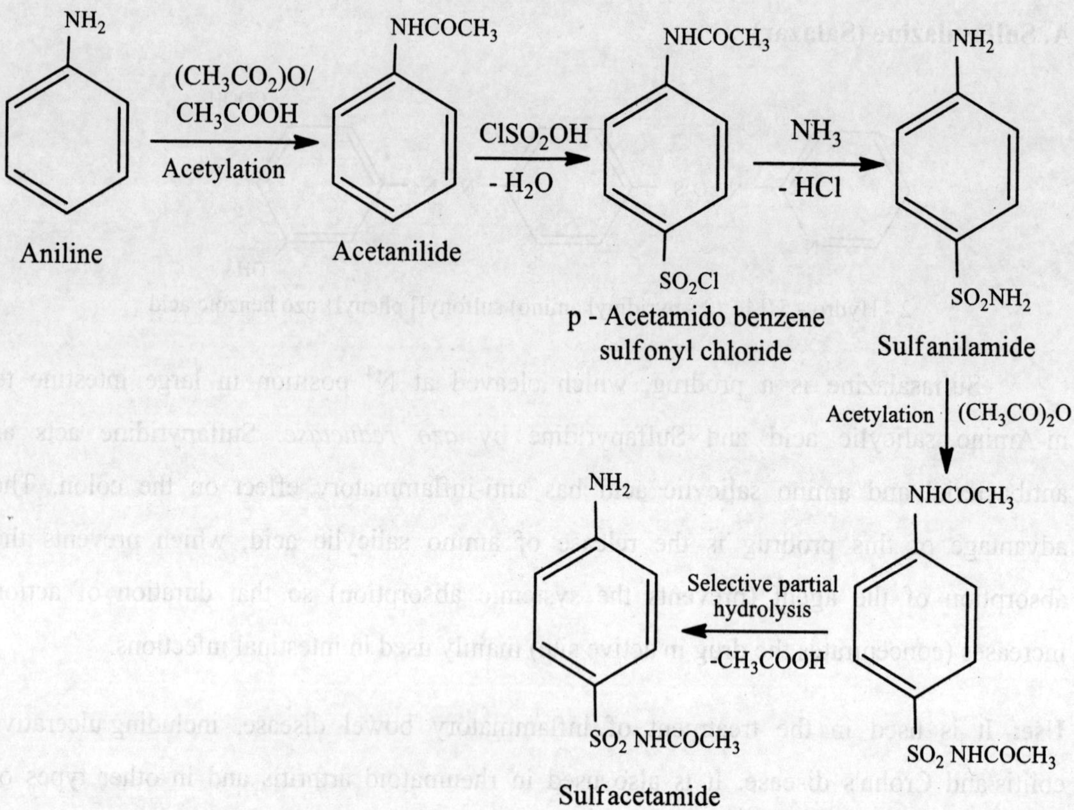


**Use:** It is used to treat infection or injuries of eye.

**B. Mafenide acetate (Sulfamylon)**

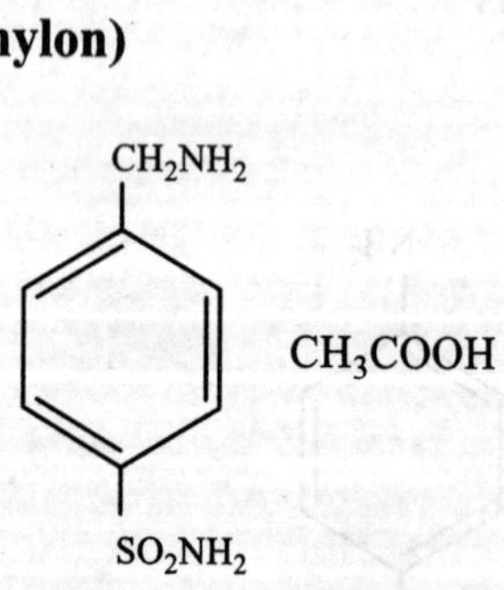


4 - (Aminomethyl) benzene sulfonamide acetate

It is not a true sulfonamide type compound, as it does not inhibit PABA.

**Mechanism of action:** It acts by reducing the bacterial population present in the burn tissue and promotes healing of deep burns.

**Use:** It is used in the treatment and cure of gas gangrene. It is useful for the treatment of infections caused by P*seudomonas aeruginosa* in second- and third-degree burns. It is also effective against C*lostridium welchii* in topical application.

## 2.5 Sulfonamide for Dermatitis

### A. Dapsone (Acnesone)

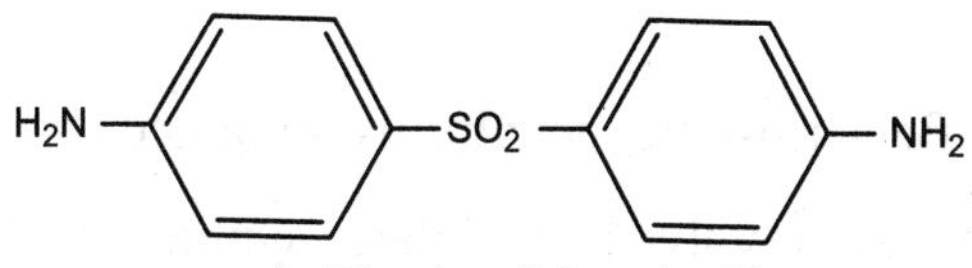


p, p' - Diamino diphenyl sulfone

Synthesis

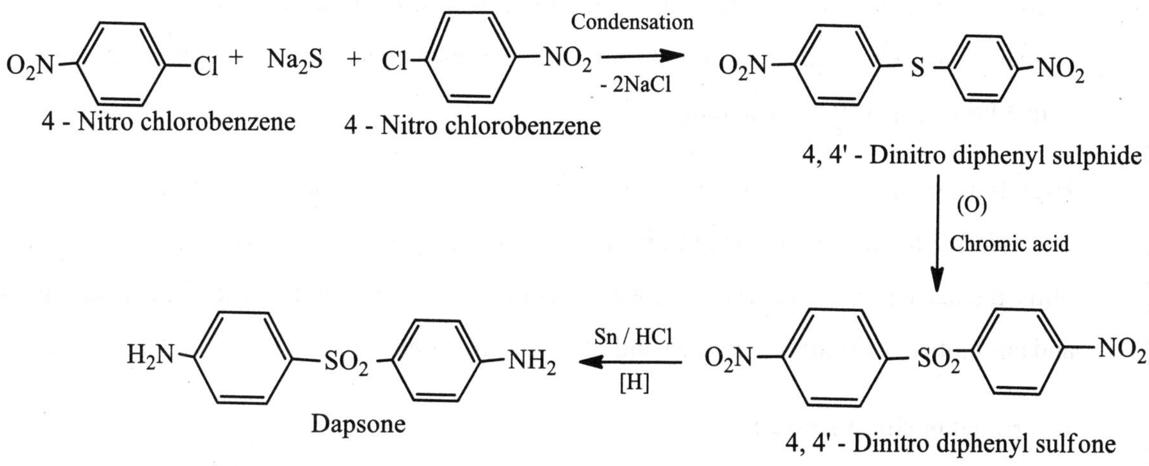


**Mechanism of action:** It acts against bacteria and protozoa in the same way as sulfonamides, by inhibiting the synthesis of dihydrofolic acid through competition with p-Aminobenzoate for the active site of *dihydropteroate synthase*.

**Use:** It is used in combination with Rifampicin and Clofazimine for the treatment of leprosy and in combination with Pyrimethamine for the prevention of malaria.

## 2.6 Sulfonamide Combinations

### A. Cotrimoxazole (Septran, Bactrim)

Cotrimoxazole is a combination of Trimethoprim and Sulfamethoxazole which is very widely used in antibacterial therapy. It consists of one part of Trimethoprim and five parts of Sulfamethoxazole. The synergy between Trimethoprim and Sulfamethoxazole was first described in the late 1960s.

**Mechanism of action:** Bacteriostatic activity is obtained by two prominent steps in bacterial enzymatic pathway involved in folate synthesis. Sulfamethoxazole inhibits utilization of PABA in the formation of dihydrofolate, while Trimethoprim is a selective inhibitor of the enzyme that catalyses the conversion of dihydrofolate to tetrahydrofolate. Sulfamethoxazole was selected from the systemic Sulfonamide on the basis that it has similar pharmacokinetic features to that of Trimethoprim. It is co-administered with Trimethoprim in a fixed dose ratio of 5:1.

**Use:** It is used in the treatment of urinary tract infection, cholera, methicillin resistant *Staphylococcus aureus,* intestinal and lower respiratory tract. It is also effective in acute otitis media, chronic bacterial prostates, meningococcal infection, gonorrhea, nocardiosis and antibiotics resistant *Salmonella* and *Shigella* infections.

### B. Trimethoprim (Primsol)

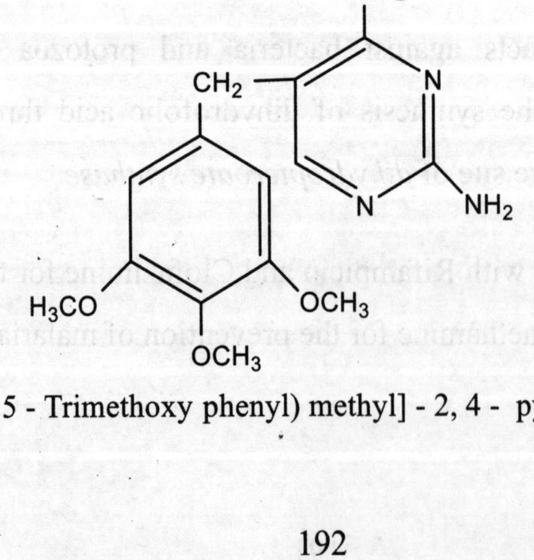


5 - [(3, 4, 5 - Trimethoxy phenyl) methyl] - 2, 4 - pyrimidine diamine

Synthesis

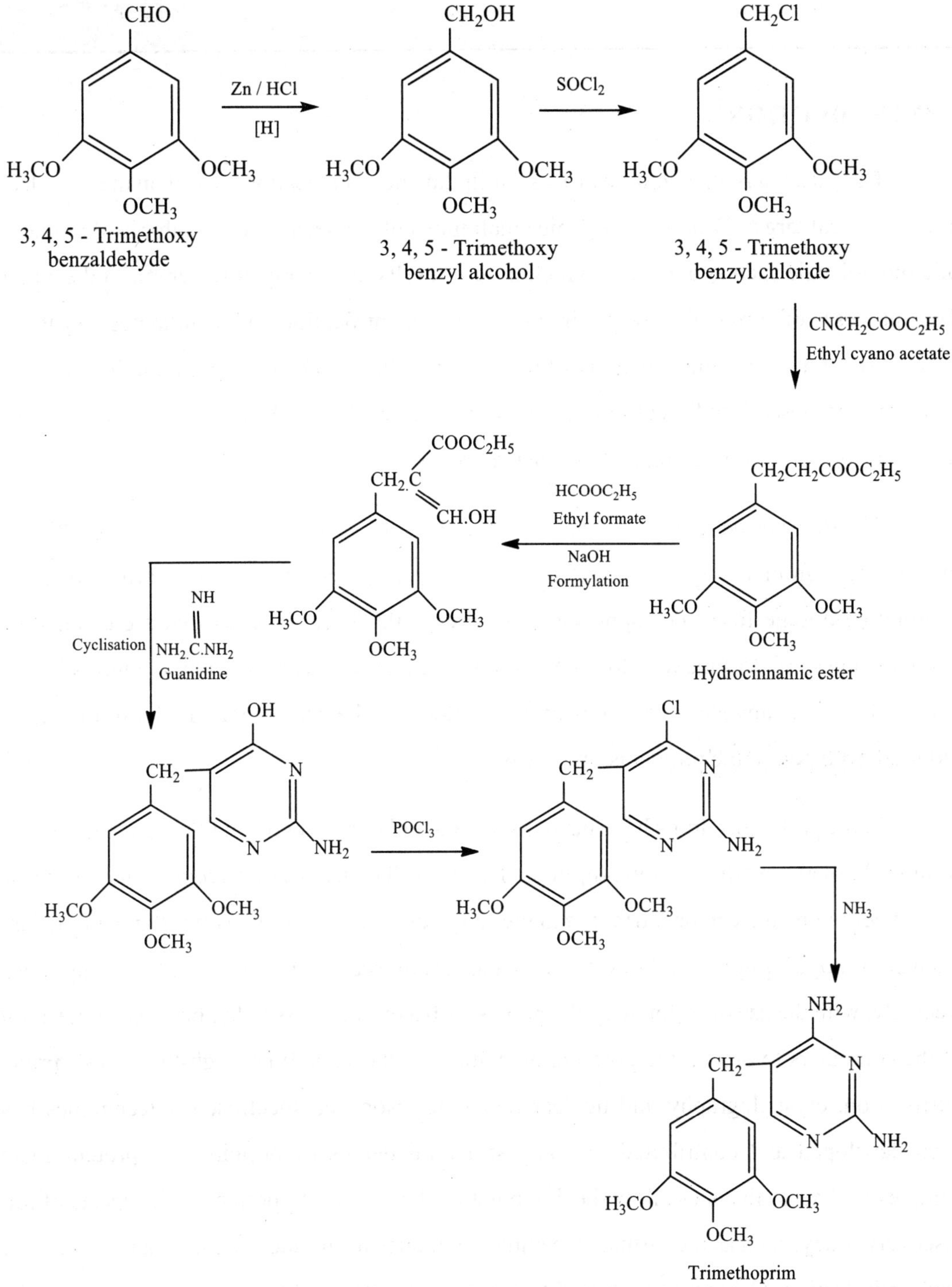
CHO
H3CO
OCH3
OCH3
3, 4, 5 - Trimethoxy benzaldehyde
Zn / HCl
[H]
CH2OH
3, 4, 5 - Trimethoxy benzyl alcohol
SOCl2
CH2Cl
3, 4, 5 - Trimethoxy benzyl chloride
CNCH2COOC2H5
Ethyl cyano acetate
CH2CH2COOC2H5
Hydrocinnamic ester
HCOOC2H5
Ethyl formate
NaOH
Formylation
COOC2H5
CH2.C
CH.OH
Cyclisation
NH
NH2.C.NH2
Guanidine
OH
CH2
N
NH2
POCl3
Cl
NH3
NH2
Trimethoprim

**Mechanism of action:** It binds to *dihydrofolate reductase* and inhibits the reduction of dihydrofolic acid (DHF) to tetrahydrofolic acid (THF). THF is an essential precursor in the thymidine synthesis pathway and interference with this pathway and inhibits bacterial DNA synthesis.

**Use:** It is effective against Chloroquine and Pyrimethamine resistant strains of *Plasmodium falciparum*.

Chapter

# DRUG DESIGN

11

## 1. INTRODUCTION

Drug design is an inventive process of finding new medications based on the knowledge of a biological target. Drug is an organic small molecule that activates or inhibits the function of a biomolecule such as a protein, which in turn results in a therapeutic benefit to the patient. The process of drug discovery involves the identification of candidates, synthesis, characterization, screening and assay of therapeutic efficacy. Once a compound has shown its value in these tests, it will begin the process of drug development prior to clinical trial. Drug discovery is a time consuming and expensive process.

The time period to bring a drug to market is 12-15 years at an average cost of $800-900 million right from the synthesis to its clinical development and finally formulating it to appropriate dosage form. For approximately every 10,000 compounds that are evaluated in animal studies, 10 will make it to human clinical trials in order to get one compound on the market. Failure at any stage would mean a huge loss for the company and a lot of planning is required even before the project is underway.

In the past, most drugs have been discovered either by identifying the active ingredients from traditional remedies or serendipitous discovery. The leaves of *Ocimum sanctum* for the cure of common cold can be attributed to the religious believers of the Hindus and antimalarial plant *Dichroa febrifuga*, also known in china as C*hang shan* were discovered serendipitously. Recently, with the use of technology the process is becoming a less risky, because of the ability of the computers to predict the possible outcomes. At the same time, high-throughput protein purification, crystallography and nuclear magnetic resonance spectroscopy techniques have been developed and contributed to many structural details of proteins and protein–ligand complexes. These advances allow the computational strategies to permeate all aspects of drug discovery today, such as the virtual screening techniques for hit identification and methods for lead optimization. Compared with traditional experimental, virtual screening techniques is a more direct and rational drug discovery approach and has the advantage of low cost and

effective screening. Virtual screening of databases is gaining increasing importance in drug discovery because it is a reliable and a low-cost method for identifying lead molecules. In the pharmaceutical industry, which is under ever increasing pressure to increase its success rate to bring drugs to the market. The advances in computational techniques make a significant impact on the drug discovery process.

## 1.1 Various Approaches of Drug Design

Virtual screening techniques can be classified into two major types

- Ligand-based drug design
- Structure-based drug design

### (a) Ligand-based Drug Design

It is otherwise known as indirect drug design. Many of the naturally occurring molecules are found to be very potent and also the endogenous chemicals give a lot of information for drug designing. The use of such ligands to generate and design newer ligands is called ligand-based drug design. In other words, biologically active target model is designed based on the information of binding molecules. When a set of active ligand molecule is known and little or no structural information is available for targets, the ligand-based methods, such as pharmacophore modelling and quantitative structure activity relationship (QSAR) methods can be employed.

### (b) Structure-based Drug Design

Structure-based drug design (or direct drug design) relies on knowledge of the three-dimensional structure of the biological target obtained through methods such as x-ray crystallography or NMR spectroscopy. As to structure-based drug design, molecular docking is the most common method which has been widely used ever since early 1980s. Computational docking (also called *in silico* molecular docking or just docking) is a computational science aiming at predicting the optimal binding orientation and conformation of interacting molecules in space and to estimate the stability of their complex.

# 2. MOLECULAR DOCKING

## 2.1 Introduction

Docking is an automated computer algorithm that determines how a compound will bind in the active site of a protein. Molecular docking classifies biomolecules into three categories: small molecules (also called "ligands"), proteins and nucleic acids. The most important types of docking systems are: protein-ligand, protein-protein and nucleic acid-protein. The interactions between a small molecule and a protein are by far much better understood than those between a protein and a nucleic acid. In a simple definition, docking is a molecular modelling technique that is used to predict how a protein (enzyme) interacts with small molecules (ligands).

The ability of a protein (enzyme) to interact with small molecules to form a supramolecular complex plays a major role in the dynamics of the protein, which may enhance or inhibit its biological function. The behaviour of small molecules in the binding pockets of target proteins can be described by molecular docking.

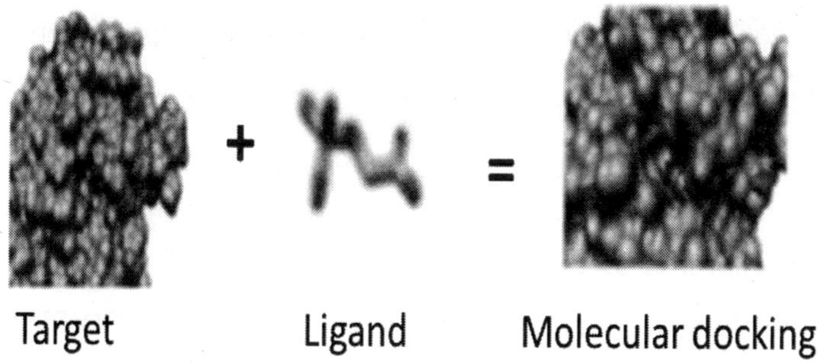


Although each docking program operates slightly differently, they share common features that involve ligand and receptor, sampling and scoring. It comprises two major tasks for which separate algorithms are used.

- The sampling algorithm predicts many confirmations, referred as poses, which the ligand can assume within the binding or active pocket. A "pose" is a term widely adopted for describing the geometry of a particular complex (also called "binding mode"). It refers to a precise configuration which is characterized not only by the relative orientation of the docked molecules but also their respective conformations.
- A scoring function then predicts the binding energies between the ligand and receptor for each predicted pose. The generated binding poses are then ranked based on their binding energies, where the top-ranked pose should correspond to the correct confirmation of the ligand.

The small molecule, known as ligand usually fits within protein's cavity which is predicted by the search algorithm. These protein cavities become active when they come in contact with any external compounds and are thus called as active sites. The method aims to identify correct poses of ligands in the binding pocket of a protein and to predict the affinity between the ligand and the protein. The results are analysed by a statistical scoring function which converts interacting energy into numerical values called as the docking score and the interacting energy is calculated. The 3D pose of the bound ligand can be visualized using different visualizing tools like Pymol, Rasmol etc which could help in inference of the best fit of ligand. Predicting the mode of protein-ligand interaction can assume the active site of the protein molecule and further help in protein annotation.

Practical application of molecular docking requires data bank for the search of target with proper PDB format and a methodology to prepare ligand as a PDB file. To do this, there are various software's available from where the ligand can be made in PDB format. These tools provide the organization to ligands based upon their ability to interact with given target proteins/DNA. Molecular docking of small molecules to a target includes a pre-defined sampling of possible conformation of ligand in the particular groove of target in order to establish the optimized conformation of the complex. This can be made possible using scoring function of software.

## 2.2 Docking Software Description

There are many algorithms available to assess and rationalize ligand-protein or protein-protein interactions and their number is constantly increasing. Speed and accuracy are key features for obtaining successful results in docking approaches. Several algorithms share common methodologies with novel extensions focused on obtaining a fast method with accuracy as high as possible. The most common docking programs include Auto Dock, DOCK, FlexX, GOLD, ICM, Glide, ADAM, DARWIN, DIVALI, FTDOCK, QXP, FLOG FRED Slide, Surflex, Swiss Dock and Dock Vision.

## 2.3 Molecular Docking Approaches

Two types of approaches are used in molecular docking

- Simulation approach and
- Shape complementarity approach

### 2.3.1Simulation Approach

In this approach, the protein and the ligand are separated by some physical distance and then ligand is allowed to bind into groove of target after "definite times of moves" in its conformational space The moves involve variations to the structure of ligand either internally (torsional angle rotations) or externally (rotations and translations). The ligand in every move in the conformational limit releases energy, as "Total Energy". This approach is more advantageous in the sense that it is more compatible to accept ligand flexibility. Additionally, it is more real to assess the molecular recognition between ligand and target. However, this approach takes longer duration to estimate optimal docked conformer due to the large energy dissipating for each conformation. Recently, fast optimization method and grid-based tools have significantly overcome these drawbacks to make simulation approach more user friendly.

### 2.3.2 Shape Complementarity Approach

This approach employs ligand and target as surface structural feature that provides their molecular interaction. These features may include molecular surface/ complementary surface descriptors. In this case, the receptors molecular surface is described in terms of its solvent-accessible surface area and the ligands molecular surface is described in terms of its matching surface description. The complementary between the two surfaces amounts to the shape matching description that may help in finding the complementary pose of docking the target and the ligand molecules.

Another approach is to describe the hydrophobic features of the protein using turns in the main-chain atoms and a Fourier shape descriptor technique. The shape complementarity approach is rather quick and involves the rapid scanning of numerous thousands of ligands in a few seconds to find out the possible binding properties of ligand on target molecular surface. They are also much more amenable to pharmacophore-based approaches, since they use geometric descriptions of the ligands to find optimal binding.

## 2.4 Types of Docking

The protein-ligand docking procedure can be typically divided into three parts:

**2.4.1 Rigid body docking**: It ignores the flexibility of the molecules and treats them like rigid objects. When the ligand and receptor are both treated as rigid bodies, the search space is very limited, considering only three translational and three rotational degrees of freedom. The early versions of DOCK, FLOG and some protein-protein docking programs, such as FTDOCK, adopted such a method

**2.4.2 Rigid receptor-flexible ligand docking**: In which only the ligand is treated as flexible, receptor is rigid. The rigid-body docking approaches are often not sufficient to predict the structure of a protein complex from the separate unbound structures. The incorporation of molecular flexibility into docking algorithms requires to add conformational degrees of freedom to translations and rotations. It is of vital importance to consider the flexibilities of both the ligand and receptor since both the ligand and receptor change their conformations to form a minimum energy perfect-fit complex. Incorporating protein flexibility into molecular docking software involving a huge number of degrees of freedom that represent the receptor flexibility and optimization is difficult. However, the cost is very high when the receptor is also flexible. Thus, the common approach, is treating the ligand as flexible while the receptor is kept rigid during docking. Almost all the docking programs have adopted this methodology, such as Auto Dock. Many methods have been developed for incorporating flexible small molecules into docking software; they include: Ligand-ensemble docking method, Fragmentation method and Stochastic conformational search method.

**2.4.3 Flexible receptor-flexible ligand docking**: In which both protein and ligand are treated as flexible. Incorporating the receptor flexibility is significant challenge in the field of docking. Various methods are currently available to implement the receptor flexibility. The simplest one is so-called "soft-docking", decreases the van der Waals repulsion energy term in the scoring function to allow for a degree of atom-atom overlap between the receptor and ligand. Side-chain flexibility is another way to provide receptor flexibility. Side chains are critical for the binding of the ligand to proteins. The most efficient method for considering the full flexibility of the protein is the "Multiple Protein Structure" (MPS) approach (also called "multiple receptor structure" or "ensemble approach" or "multiple copy approach"). The MPS approach is based on the use of multiple structures of the target protein as obtained either from experimental (X-ray, NMR) determinations or generated by theoretical simulations (molecular dynamics).

## 2.5 Theories of Docking

Docking protocols can be categorised based on the following criteria:

- Molecular representation - a way to represent structures and properties

- Searching algorithm prediction of the ligand conformation as well as its position and orientation within these sites (usually referred to as pose)
- Scoring method - a method to assess the binding affinity.

### 2.5.1 Molecular Representation

The protein structure and a database of ligands serves as an inputs to a docking program. There are three representations commonly used in docking programs:

- the atomic representation
- the surface representation
- the grid representation

The most common is atomic representation, each atom is characterized by its co-ordinates and atom-type.

### 2.5.2 Search Algorithms

The search algorithm positions molecules in various locations, orientations and conformation within the active site. Some of the earliest docking programs positioned a molecule in the active site, holding it rigid with respect to conformational changes, but all modern docking algorithms include ligand conformational changes. The choice of search algorithm determines how thoroughly the program checks possible molecule positions and how long it takes to run. They can also calculate the energy of the resulting complex and of each individual interaction. With six degrees of translational and rotational freedom as well as the conformational degrees of freedom of both the ligand and protein, there are a huge number of possible binding modes between two molecules. Unfortunately, it would be too expensive to computationally generate all the possible conformations. Some common searching algorithms include molecular dynamics, Monte Carlo methods, genetic algorithms, fragment-based, point complementary and distance geometry methods, Tabu and systematic searches.

Molecular dynamics is widely used as a powerful simulation method in many fields of molecular modelling. Molecular dynamics process is based on the simulation of molecular motion by solving Newton's equations of motion for each atom and incrementing the position and velocity of each atom by use of a small-time increment. Molecular dynamics simulation represents the flexibility of both the ligand and protein more effectively than other algorithms. However, the disadvantage of Molecular dynamics simulations is that they progress in very small steps and thus have difficulties in stepping over high energy conformational barriers, which may lead to inadequate sampling.

The Monte Carlo simulation is based on statistical mechanics and generates sufficient different configurations of a system by computer simulation to allow the desired structural, statistical and thermodynamic properties to be calculated as a weighted average of these properties over these configurations. Monte Carlo methods generate poses of the ligand through bond rotation, rigid-body translation or rotation. The conformation obtained by this transformation is tested with an energy- based selection criterion. If it passes the criterion, it will be saved and further modified to generate next conformation, until the predefined quantity of conformations is collected. The main advantage of Monte Carlo method is that the change can be quite large, allowing the ligand to cross the energy barriers on the potential energy surface, a point that not easily achieved by molecular dynamics-based simulation methods.

### 2.5.3 Scoring Function

A scoring function then predicts the binding energies between the ligand and receptor for each predicted pose. The generated binding poses are then ranked based on their binding energies, where the top-ranked pose should correspond to the correct confirmation of the ligand. Scoring functions are, therefore, also capable of filtering through and ranking, large databases of compounds in virtual screening, where the highest-ranked binding energies should correspond to a potential lead.

Mathematical methods used to predict the strength of the non-covalent interaction called as binding affinity, between two molecules after they have been docked. Scoring functions have also been developed to predict the strength of other types of intermolecular interactions, for example between two proteins or between protein and DNA or protein and drug. The binding process that leads to the formation of a complex between a ligand and its receptor is controlled by several factors including:

(i) **Interaction energies between the two molecules** such as electrostatic interactions, hydrogen bond interactions, van der Waals interactions and hydrophobic forces

(ii) **Desolvation and solvation energies associated with the interacting molecules**: The binding of a ligand to a protein is a complex process influenced by desolvation and solvation phenomena, where the interacting entities become partially desolvated. This thermodynamically driven chain of events leads to the formation of favourable interactions between the ligand and the protein where hydrophobic contacts are the driving forces: hydrophobic moieties associate together to reduce the interactions with the surrounding water. Another important energy term is electrostatic interaction between charged atoms and water molecules.

(iii) **Entropic factors that occur upon binding**: The flexibility of the molecules and the consequences in terms of entropy can have a significant impact on the binding energy of a ligand

## 2.6 Calculation of Binding Energy

The binding energy $\Delta G_{binding}$ is the energy required to separate a complex into two parts (protein and ligand). It is defined as the difference between the energy of the associated (bound) form (E complex) and that of the separated (unbound) molecules ($E_{protein}$ and $E_{ligand}$). A complex has a lower potential energy than its constituent parts and this keeps them together.

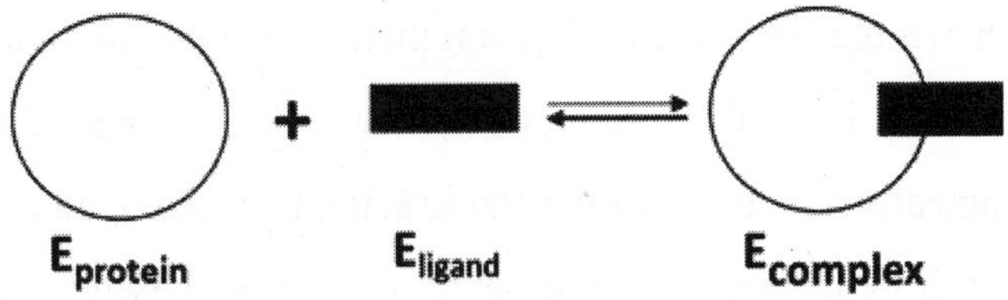


$$\Delta G_{binding} = E_{complex} - E_{protein} - E_{ligand}$$

Scoring functions can be divided into force-field-based, empirical, knowledge-based scoring functions and consensus scoring. Force field scoring functions predict binding free energy of a protein-ligand complex by adding up individual contributions from different types of interactions (electrostatics and van der Waals) between all atoms of the two molecules in the complex using a force field. The total energy of a system is described as the sum of the independent terms of the force field. The energies obtained by force field methods can be used directly to approximate free energies of binding.

Binding Energy $\Delta G$ bind = $\Delta$Gvdw + $\Delta$Ghbond + $\Delta$Gelect + $\Delta$Gconform + $\Delta$Gtor + $\Delta$Gsol

Software programs, such as DOCK, GOLD and Auto Dock uses such functions.

## 2.7 The Docking Process

The setup for a ligand docking approach requires components a target protein structure, the molecules of interest or a database containing existing or virtual compounds for the docking process and a computational framework that allows the implementation of the desired docking and scoring procedures.

**(i) Protein preparation**: The Protein Data Bank (PDB), National Centre for Biotechnology Information (NCBI), Research Collaboratory for Structural Bioinformatics (RCSB) and the Biological Magnetic Resonance Bank (BMRB) are some database. The database contains structures of biomolecules produced by X-ray crystallography, NMR, electron microscopy of a hybrid approach which can be downloaded. After selecting the model, it must be prepared by removing the water molecules from the cavity, stabilizing charges, filling the missing residues, and generating the side chains, all according to the available parameters. The receptor should be at this point biologically active and in the stable state. Homology modelling is a technique which builds a 3D structure from a protein sequence of interest, based on the 3D structure of a similar protein. In the absence of an available crystal structure for a protein of interest, a homology model can provide an alternative for subsequent receptor-ligand analyses such as molecular docking or dynamics as long as a three-dimensional structure exists for a similar protein.

**(ii) Ligand Preparation**: The type of ligands chosen for docking will depend on the goal. It can be obtained from various databases, e.g. ZINC or/and PubChem, or it can be sketched (using suitable software like ACD ChemSketch or MarvinSketch). Often it is necessary to apply filters to reduce the number of molecules to be docked. Examples include the net charge, molecular weight, polar surface area, solubility, commercial availability, similarity thresholds, pharmacophores, synthetic accessibility and absorption, distribution, metabolism, excretion, and toxicology properties.

**(iii) Building the Ligand**: Docking programs offer several options for creating ligands and placing them in the active site. At the most automated end of the spectrum, some docking programs can take a database of ligands, place each one in the active site and do the docking run. This completely automated approach allows thousands of compounds to be analysed without manual intervention from the user. These poses can then be automatically read in and a docking score computed without any automated movement of the ligand. Storing all of the poses can take up significant disk space, because of this, most docking programs take a single pose as an input, generate many thousands of poses, but only store the best ones as the final results.

**(iv) Setting the Bounding Box:** The entire protein is read into the computer in order to obtain a correct geometry for the structure. However, docking calculations can take a significant amount of time and anything that speeds them up without loss of accuracy is utilized. Protein residues far from the active site do not generally have any measurable effect on the scoring results. In order to speed the calculation, a cut off distance is set and no interactions are computed for residues beyond that distance from the ligand. For ease of coding, this cut off is usually a rectangular box, called a bounding box. In the case of grid potentials, the grid is only computed for points within the cut off distance. Many dockings packages default to setting the bounding box far enough out from the ligand or active site that there is no need to alter it.

**(v) Docking Options:** When setting up the inputs to a docking calculation, there will be an option for flexible active sites, scoring method, search method, solvation, handling encapsulated active sites, etc. Some packages may have an option to do a fast-initial check and then continue only if the first check criterion is satisfied. Nearly always, the docking results will be more accurate with the calculation running more slowly, if an optimization is performed for each pose.

**(vi) Running the Docking Calculation:** Once the inputs have been set, the docking calculation can be run. Most docking programs allow individual docking runs to be started from the graphical interface. A few docking programs can run many docking calculations in a batch mode. These calculations are sometimes run on the same computer where the graphical interface is used and sometimes can be sent off to a different server.

**(vii) Analysis of Results:** The most important result from a docking calculation is the binding energy of the ligand to the active site. The scoring function generates a score depending on the best selected ligand. This is the value that is compared between different compounds to determine which will be the best inhibitor. The pose of the ligand in the active site associated with a few of the best binding energy is examined visually to ensure that it looks reasonable. Validating a docking program for the specific target and class of ligands being designed is often the most important criterion for selecting a docking program. It is commonly accepted that there is no "first-in-class" algorithm or molecular docking software for the prediction of correct ligand-binding pose or relative free energy of binding.

Molecular docking algorithms are often calibrated on a training set of experimental ligand-protein complexes and accuracy of these docking program is often highly dependent on the training set used. This highlights the importance of confirming that the docking software used for virtual screening is capable of replicating the binding mode of known, experimental inhibitors for the class of receptor studied. To improve ligand enrichment in a virtual screening setting, the docking algorithm selected must be properly validated for the class of receptor under investigation. Actually, in a virtual screen, where hundreds of thousands to millions of compounds are potentially being screened, validating for each class of potential inhibitor would be impossible. The success of docking algorithms in predicting a ligand binding pose is normally measured in terms of the root-mean-square deviation (RMSD) between the experimentally-observed heavy-atom positions of the ligands and the one(s) predicted by the algorithm. A good performance is usually considered when the RMSD is less than 2Å.

## 2.8 Applications of Docking

Docking is most commonly used in the field of drug design and applied to:

- **Hit identification**-docking combined with a scoring function can be used to quickly screen large databases of potential drugs *in silico* to identify molecules that are likely to bind to protein target of interest.
- **Lead optimization**-docking can be used to predict the relative orientation of a ligand that binds to a protein (also referred as the binding mode or pose). This information may in turn be used to design more potent and selective analogues.
- **Bioremediation**-protein ligand docking can also be used to predict pollutants that can be degraded by enzymes

# 3. QUANTITATIVE STRUCTURE ACTIVITY RELATIONSHIP

## 3.1 Introduction

Quantitative structure-activity relationship (QSAR) studies are very important in *in silico* methods in rational drug design. Drug discovery and development is a process aims to design safe and effective medications to improve life's quality and to reduce suffering to minimum. However, the process is very complex, time consuming and resource intensive, requiring multi-disciplinary expertise and innovative approaches. Rational drug design methods minimize the time and cost needed in drug designing process in comparison to traditional drug discovery methods.

QSAR analysis is a ligand-based drug design method developed more than 50 years ago by Hansch and Fujita (1964). Since then and until now, QSAR remains an efficient method for building mathematical models, which attempts to find a statistically significant correlation between the chemical structure and continuous (pIC50, pEC50, Ki, etc.,) or categorical/binary (active, inactive, toxic, non-toxic, etc.,) biological/toxicological property. In 1968 Crum-Brown and Fraser published an equation which is considered to the first general formulation of QSARs.

QSAR attempts to correlate structural, chemical, statistical and physical properties with biological activity by various approaches. It is a mathematical relationship between a biological activity of a molecular system and its geometric and chemical characteristics. QSAR's general mathematical form is represented by the following equation.

$$\text{Biological Activity} = f\,(\text{Physicochemical Property})$$

In which, activity is expressed as log ($^1/c$) c is the minimum concentration required to cause a defined biological response.

QSARs mean computerized statistical method which helps to explain the observed variance in the structure changes caused by the substitution. In this concept it is assumed that the biological activity exhibited by a series of congeneric compound is a function of various physio-chemical analysis is performed it shows that certain physio-chemical properties are favourable to the concern activity, the latter can be optimized by choosing such substituent's which would enhance such physiochemical properties. A major goal of QSAR study is to find a mathematical relationship to find consistent relationship between the activity under investigation and one or more descriptors related to the structure of the molecule, so that these "rules" can be used to evaluate the activity of new compounds.

**3.2 QSAR Development Process**

**(i) Selection of Data set and Extraction of Structural/Empirical Descriptors**: The first major step in a QSAR study is the entry of the molecular structures and generation of the 3-D models. The 3-D molecular models are needed for geometric descriptor calculations. There are a lot of software available for QSAR development and they are either commercial or free. These include specialized software for drawing chemical structures, interconverting chemical file formats, generating 3D structures, calculating chemical descriptors, developing QSAR models, and general-purpose software that have all the necessary components for QSAR development. For Structure Drawing or File Conversion the most common programs are ChemDraw, ACD/ChemSketch and Open Babel software. Soft wares for 3D Structure Generation are CORINA, Concord, Frog, smi23d. Descriptor calculation can be made by using Dragon, Molconn-Z, PaDEL-Descriptor software.

**(ii) Variable Selection:** The second major step is the generation and selection of the most important descriptors.

**(iii) Model Construction**: The next step is the generation of the QSAR models using the descriptor sets.

**(iv) Validation Evaluation**: The last step is to validate the model by predicting the activity of compounds in the external prediction set. The results obtained by the predictions should be compared to those achieved for the training set and cross validation set to easily understand model's fitness level.

### 3.3 Descriptors (or) Parameters

The QSAR approach uses parameters which have been assigned to the various chemical groups that can be used to modify the structure of the drug. The parameter is a measure of the potential contribution of its group to a particular property of the parent drug. Molecular descriptors are final products of mathematical procedures transforming chemical information encoded within a molecular structure to a numerical representative. Dimensionality of molecular descriptors can identify QSAR model type as described below:

(a) 0D QSAR- These are descriptors derived from molecular formula eg. molecular weight, number and type of atoms etc.,

(b) 1D QSAR: A substructure list representation of a molecule can be considered as a one-dimensional (1D) molecular representation and consists of a list of molecular fragments (eg. functional groups, rings, bonds, substituents etc.,).

(c) 2D QSAR: A molecular graph contains topological or two dimensional (2D) information. It describes how the atoms are bonded in a molecule, both the type of bonding and the interaction of particular atoms (eg. total path count, molecular connectivity indices etc.,).

(d) 3D QSAR: These are calculated starting from a geometrical or 3D representation of a molecule. These descriptors include molecular surface, molecular volume and other geometrical properties. There are different types of 3D descriptors. eg. electronic, steric, shape etc.,

(e) 4D QSAR: Four dimensional information is described in this type of models and the fourth dimension is an ensemble of conformation of each ligand.

The various parameters used in QSAR studies are

i) Lipophilic parameters: Partition coefficient, Chromatographic parameters and $\pi$–Substitution constant.

ii) Polarizability parameters: Molar refractivity, Molar volume, Parachor.

iii) Electronic parameters: Hammett constant, Field and resonance parameters, Parameters derived from spectroscopic data, Charge-transfer constant, Dipole moment, Quantum-chemical parameters.

iv) Steric parameters: Taft's steric constant, van der Waals radii.

v) Miscellaneous parameters: Molecular weight, Geometric parameters, Conformational entropies, Connectivity indices, other topological parameters.

### 3.3.1 Partition Coefficient

A drug has to pass through a number of biological membranes in order to reach its site of action. Consequently, organic / aqueous system partition coefficient is the obvious parameters used to measure the movement of drug through these membranes. Partition coefficient is generally given as,

$$P = \frac{[C]_{org.}}{[C]_{aqu.}}$$

It is a ratio of concentration of substance in organic and aqueous phase of a two compartment system under equilibrium conditions. For easily ionisable drug, correlation must be made as follows

$$P = \frac{[C]_{org}}{[C]_{aqu}(1-\alpha)} \qquad \alpha = \text{degree of ionization}$$

The accuracy of the correlation of drug activity with partition coefficient will depend on the solvent system used as a model for the membrane. Both pure water and buffered solution are used for the aqueous medium. The n-octanol/water system is frequently chosen, because it appears to be a good mimic of lipid polarity; however more accurate results may be obtained if the organic phase is matched to the area of biological activity being studied. For example, n-octanol usually gives more consistent result for drugs absorbed in GI tract while less polar solvents such as olive oil give more consistent correlation for drugs crossing the blood-brain barrier. More polar solvents such as chloroform give more consistent value for buccal absorption. n-octanol/ water system has more advantages over other systems:

- It is a suitable model of the lipid constituents of biological membrane due to its long alkyl chain and the polar hydroxyl group.
- n-octanol has a low vapor pressure, allowing reproducible measurements
- n-octanol is UV transparent over a large range, making the quantitative determination of a compound is relatively easy.

The nature of the relationship between P and drug activity depends on the range of P values obtained in the compounds used. If this range is small the result may be expressed as a straight line equation having the general form:

$\log {}^{1}/_{c} = K_1 \log P + K_2$ Where $K_1$ and $K_2$ are constants.

This equation indicates a linear relationship between the activity of the drug and its partition coefficient. Over large ranges of P values the graph of $\log {}^{1}/_{c}$ against log P often has a parabolic form with a maximum value ($\log P^{o}$). The existence of this maximum value implies that there is an optimum balance between aqueous and lipid solubility for maximum biological activity. Below $P^0$ the drug will be reluctant to enter the membrane while above $P^0$ the drugs will the reluctant to leave the membrane. This means that analogues with partition coefficient near this optimum value are likely to be most active and worth further investigation. The parabolic relationship could be represented by equation of the form:

$$\log ({}^{1}/_{c}) = -K_1 (\log P)^2 + K_2 \log P + K_3$$

Where

$K_1$, $K_2$ and $K_3$ are constants that are normally determined by regression analysis.

Experimental determination of Partition Coefficient

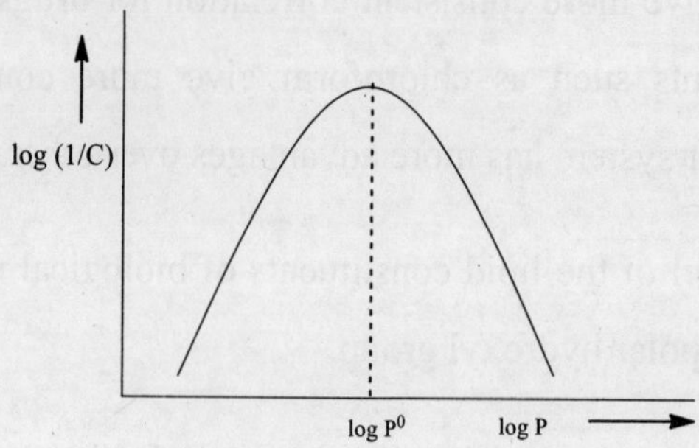


**Fig. 11.1 A Parabolic Plot for log (1/C) against log P**

The log P is measured by the following method

(i) Shake Flask Method

Weighed amount of the substance is shaken in a flask containing a measured amount of buffer pH - 7.4 or water and n-octanol. The amount of chemical in one or both the phase is determined by appropriate analytical technique and the partition coefficient is calculated. The method is tedious, time consuming, messy and smelly but is the only method that can be used in case of very low log P value.

(ii) Chromatographic Method

Compounds with known log P values are injected into a $C_{18}$ reverse phase high performance liquid chromatography (RPHPLC) column to create a calibration curve. Unknown compound are then injected to predict log P. The chromatographic method suffers the disadvantage that the retention time is linearly related to partition coefficient ie. for doubling of log P, there is a tenfold increase in the retention. This often requires different length column to be used, short one for high log P and long ones for low values.

### 3.3.2 The Hammett Constant (σ)

The distribution of electron in a drug molecule has a considerable influence on the distribution and activity of the drug. In general, non-polar and polar drug in their unionized forms are more readily transported through membranes than polar drugs and drugs in their ionized form. If the drug reaches the target site, the distributed electron will control the type of bond that it forms with the target site, which in turn affects its biological activity. The first attempt to quantify the electronic effect of groups on the physicochemical properties of compound was made by Hammett.. The distribution of electrons within a molecule depends on the nature of the electron withdrawing and donating group found in the structure. Hammett used this concept to calculate what now known as Hammett constant ($\sigma$) for a variety of mono-substituted benzoic acids. He used these constants to calculate the equilibrium and rate constants for chemical reactions.

However, they are now used as electronic parameters in QSAR relationships. Hammett constant are defined as:

$$\sigma_x = \log \frac{K_{Bx}}{K_B}$$

ie. $\sigma_x = \log K_{Bx} - \log K_B$

and so as $pKa = -\log Ka$

$$\boxed{\sigma_x = pK_B - pK_{Bx}}$$

Where $K_B$ and $K_{BX}$ are the equilibrium constants for benzoic acid and mono substituted benzoic acids respectively.

Hammett substitution constant ($\sigma$) is a measure of the electron withdrawing or electron donating ability of a substituent and has been determined by comparing the dissociation of series of substituted acid with that of parent or unsubstituted acid. A negative value of $\sigma_x$ indicates that the substituent is acting as an electron donor and the positive value indicates that it is acting as electron withdrawing group.

Hammett constant takes into account both resonance and inductive effect. Therefore the values of $\sigma$ for a particular substituent will depend on whether the substituent is *meta* or *para*. The *meta* and *para* σ value are commonly used and indicated by a subscript m or p after the symbol σ ortho σ are often unreliable due to steric hindrance and other effects such as intra molecular hydrogen bonding. Hammett constant suffer from the disadvantage that they only apply to substituents directly attached to benzene ring. Most QSAR studies start off by considering σ and if there is more than one substituent, the values are summarized (Σσ). Hammett substitution has been unsuccessful to relate biological activity since electron distribution is not the only factor involved.

### 3.3.3 Taft's Substituent Constant

Taft's substituent constant (σ *) are a measure of the polar effects of substituent in aliphatic compound when the group in question dces not form part of a conjugated system. They are based on the hydrolysis of ester and calculated from the following equation.

$$\sigma^* = \frac{1}{2.48}\left[\log\left(k/_{K_O}\right)_B - \log\left(k/_{K_O}\right)_A\right]$$

Where, k represents the rate constants for the hydrolysis of the substituted compound &

$K_0$ those of methyl derivative.

The bracketed term with subscript B represent basic hydrolysis and A as acid hydrolysis respectively. The factor 2.48 brings the constant on to the same scale as the Hammett constant. Only the basic term is influenced by polar effect, so that by subtracting the acid term from the basic term only the polar effect remain. In Taft's substituent constant only methyl group is the standard for which the constant is zero. However, that can be compared with other constant by writing the methyl group in the form $CH_2 - H$ and identifying it as the group for H. Taft's and inductive substituent constants are related as:

$$\sigma^* = 2.51\,\sigma_i$$

## 3.4 2D QSAR MODELS

1. Free energy models: Hansch analysis
2. Mathematical models
   i) Free Wilson analysis
   ii) Fujita-Ban modification
3. Other statistical methods
   i)) Discriminant Analysis (DA)
   ii)) Principle Component Analysis (PCA)
   iii) Cluster Analysis (CA)
   iv) Combine Multivariate Analysis (CMA)
   v) Factor Analysis (FA)
4. Quantum mechanical methods

### 3.4.1 Hansch Analysis (The Extra thermodynamic approach)

This is the most popular approach to QSAR introduced by Corwin Hansch. It is based on the fact that the drug action could be divided into two stages.

i) Transport of drug to its site of action. It is related to partition coefficient log P (lipophilic).

ii) Binding of drug to the target site which in turn depends on, a) Bulk of substituent groups (steric) b) Electron density on attachment group (electronic)

Each of these stages dependent on the chemical and physical properties of the drug and its target site. All the parameters used in Hansch analysis are linear free energy related (ie.

derived from equilibrium constant) so it is known as "linear free energy approach" or "extra thermodynamic approach".

The most commonly used physio-chemical parameters for Hansch analysis are log p, π, σ and steric parameters as practically. He suggested linear and non-linear dependence of biological activity on different parameters. If the hydrophobicity values are limited to a small range then the equation will be linear as follows:

$$\log (^1/c) = k_1 \log p + k_2\sigma + K_3E_3 + K_4 \quad \text{linear}$$

where, $K_1$, $K_2$ and $K_3$ are constant obtained by least square procedure,

c is the molar concentration that produce certain biological action.

The molecules which are too hydrophilic or too lipophilic will not be able to cross the lipophilic or hydrophilic barriers respectively. Therefore, the p value is spread over a large range, then the equation will be parabolic and given as,

$$\log (1/c) = -K (\log p)^2 + K_2 \log p + K_3\sigma + K_4\varepsilon_s + K_5 \quad \text{non-linear}$$

The constant $K_1$ - $K_5$ are obtained by least square method. Not all the parameters are necessarily significant in a QSAR model for biological activity. To derive an extra thermodynamic equation following rules are formulated by Hansch:

i) Selection of independent variables. A wide range of different parameters like log p, π, σ, MR, steric parameters etc., should be tried. The parameters selected for the `best equation' should be essentially independent ie. the inter correlation coefficient should not be larger than 0.6 - 0.7.

ii) All the reasonable parameters must be validated by appropriate statistical procedure ie. either by stepwise regression analysis or cross-validation. The "best equation" is normally one with lower standard deviation and higher F value.

iii) If all the equations are equal then one should accept the simplest one.

iv) Number of terms or variable should be at least 5 or 6 data point per variable to avoid chance correlations.

v) It is important to have a model which is consistent with known physical- organic and bio-medical chemistry of the process under consideration.

### 3.4.1.1 Applications of Hansch Analysis

Hansch equation may be used to predict the activity of an as yet unsynthesized analogue. This enables the medicinal chemist to make a synthesis of analogue which is worthy. However these predictions should only be regarded as valid, if they are made within the range of parameter values used to establish the Hansch equation. Hansch analysis may also be used to give an indication of the importance of the influence of parameters on the mechanism by which a drug acts.

Example:

The adrenergic blocking activity of series of analogue of β-Halo aryl amine was observed. It was found that only π and σ values only related to the activity and not the steric factor, from the following Hansch equation.

$$\log {}^{1}/c = 1.78\,\pi - 0.12\sigma + 1.674.$$

The smaller the value of coefficient of σ relative to that of π in the above equation shows that electronic effect do not play an important role in the action of drug.

The accuracy of Hansch equation depends on:

i) The number of analogues (n) used. The greater the number, the higher the probability of obtaining an accurate Hansch equation.
ii) The accuracy of biological data used in the derivation of the equation.
iii) The choice of parameters

### 3.5 QSAR Model Validation

Validation methods are needed to establish the predictiveness of a model. There are two types of validation methods: Internal and external validation.

Internal methods depend on training datasets like $Q^2$ (squared correlation coefficient), $R^2$ (coefficient of determination or the coefficient of multiple determination for multiple regression), chi-squared ($X^2$) and root-mean squared error (RMSE). The major disadvantage of this approach is the lack of predictability of the model, when it is applied to a new data set. However, external methods depend on the testing set and it is considered as best validation method. It was reported that, in general, there is no relationship between internal and external predictivity.

### 3.6 Advances in QSAR

Classical QSAR studies include ligands with their binding sites, inhibition constants, rate constants and other biological points, in addition molecular properties such as lipophilicity, polarizability, electronic and steric properties. These types of descriptors often fail to take into account the three-dimensional nature of chemical structures which obviously play a part in ligand-receptor binding and hence activity.

It is logical to model these potential interactions to find the location in space around the molecule that are both acceptable and forbidden. The preceding QSAR methods usually do not take into account the 3D structure of the molecules or their targets such as enzymes and receptors. So, efforts have been made to explore structure-activity studies of ligands that take into account the known X-ray structures of proteins and enzymes, as well as the interaction of drugs with models of their receptors. 3D-QSAR has emerged as a natural extension to the classical Hansch and Free–Wilson approaches, which exploit the three-dimensional properties of the ligands to predict their biological activities using statistical correlation methods. 3D-QSAR uses probe-based sampling within a molecular lattice to determine three-dimensional properties of molecules and can then correlate these 3D descriptors with biological activity.

After the introduction of 3D-QSAR different advanced tools like COMFA, COMSA, WHIM etc., extensively assist to study multiple 3D descriptors of a chemical compounds establishing correlation between structure and biological activity. More advanced QSAR approaches like 4D, 5D and 6D-QSAR have been evolved to overcome the limitations of 3D-QSAR. The recent advancement in QSAR developed two approaches, namely receptor independent (RI-QSAR) and receptor dependent (RD-QSAR) might serve as an important tool in drug discovery.

## 4. PHARMACOPHORE MODELLING

### 4.1 Introduction

A pharmacophore is defined as a descriptor of molecular features that are necessary for molecular recognition of a ligand by a biological molecule. A pharmacophore model can be used prior to a docking study to reduce the size of a ligand library or it can be used to filter hits following a virtual screen. The concept of pharmacophore was first introduced in 1909 by Ehrlich, who defined the pharmacophore as 'a molecular framework that carries (phoros) the essential features responsible for a drug's (pharmacon) biological activity'. After a century's development, the basic pharmacophore concept still remains unchanged, but its intentional meaning and application range have been expanded considerably.

According IUPAC, pharmacophore is defined as '**an ensemble of steric and electronic features that is necessary to ensure the optimal supramolecular interactions with a specific biological target and to trigger (or block) its biological response**'. Often the long definition is simplified to "A pharmacophore is the pattern of features of a molecule that is responsible for a biological effect," which captures the essential concept that a pharmacophore is built from features rather than defined chemical groups. A pharmacophore-based search of 3D databases can be carried out even in the absence of information on the receptor structure. In many cases, the receptor structure is difficult to obtain, because the receptor is embedded in the transmembrane that poses an obstacle for crystallization, for example, the G-protein coupled receptors (GPCRs). A ligand or a set of ligands that bind to a particular receptor can be utilized efficiently to search a database for molecules with similar properties.

According to definition, the interaction patterns of bioactive molecules with their targets are represented via a three-dimensional (3D) arrangement of abstract features that define interaction types rather than specific functional groups. Every type of atom or group in a molecule that exhibits certain properties related to molecular recognition can be reduced to a pharmacophore feature.

## 4.2 Pharmacophoric Features

Hydrophobic moieties, hydrogen bond donors and acceptors, aromatic rings, cations, and anions or any possible combinations are pharmacophore features. These molecular patterns can be labelled. For example the pharmacophore features of dopamine D1receptor agonists are basic amine nitrogen (:N), a hydroxyl group (OH) and an aromatic ring (Ar) with the distances between N – O (6.8 – 8.3 Å), Ar – O (2.7 – 2.9 Å) and Ar – N (4.2 – 4.8 Å). This model led to the discovery highly selective for the D1 receptor

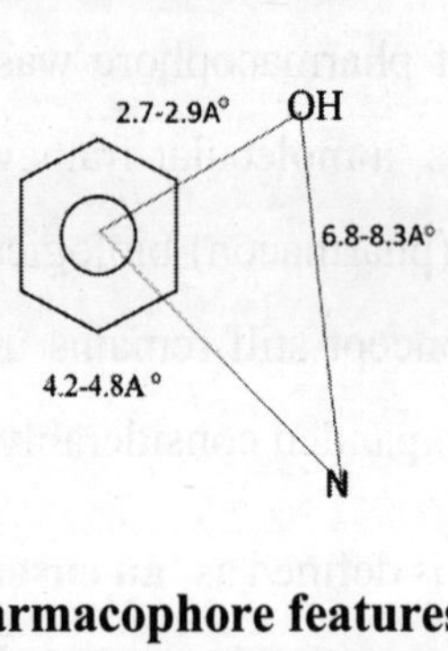


**Fig.11. 2 Pharmacophore features for Dopamine Receptor**

Different molecules can be compared at the pharmacophore level; this usage is often described as "pharmacophore fingerprints." When only a few pharmacophore features are considered in a 3D model the pharmacophore is sometimes described as a "query." A pharmacophore model can be established either in a ligand-based manner, by superposing a set of active molecules and extracting common chemical features that are essential for their bioactivity, or in a structure-based manner, by probing possible interaction points between the macromolecular target and ligands. The software used for Pharmacophore mapping is Disco, Apex, HipHop, Gasp, Accelrys, Aladdin, Apollo and Rapid.

## 4.3 Process of Pharmacophore Model

The process for developing a pharmacophore model generally involves the following steps:

- **(i) Ligand Selection:** Molecule under pharmacophore study was chosen. Structurally diverse set of molecules under study was selected. A selected molecule must include both active and inactive compound.
- **(ii) Conformational Analysis:** The compound with low energy conformations was generated.
- **(iii) Molecular Superimposition:** The low energy conformations of the molecules are superimposed in all combination to generate pharmacophoric site considering pharmacophoric features like hydrogen bond acceptor, hydrogen bond acceptor, hydrogen bond donor electron withdrawing, hydrophobic, cationic and anionic site. Generation of site for all the atom or group of molecules are ranked on the basis of descriptors value. For example, superimposed phenyl rings might be referred to more conceptually as an 'aromatic ring' pharmacophore element. Likewise, hydroxy groups could be designated as a 'hydrogen-bond donor/acceptor' pharmacophore element.

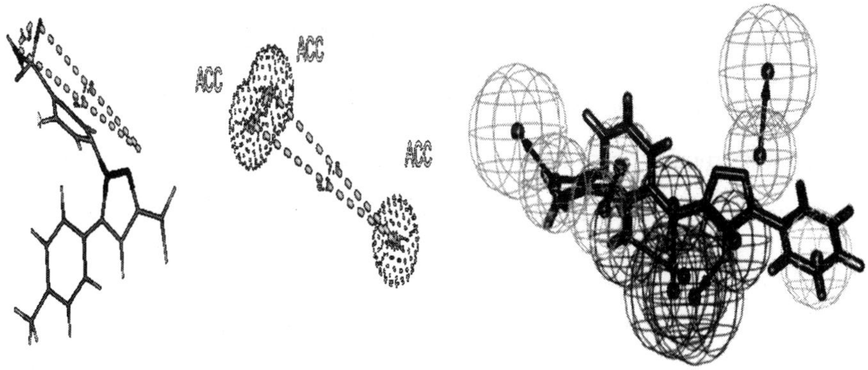

**Fig. 11.3 Model of Pharmacophore Mapping**

(iv) **Validation of Pharmacophore:** The validation parameters determine the statistical significance and predictive reliability of the selected models. The model is a *hypothesis* accounting for the observed biological activities of a set of molecules that bind to a common biological target. The model is only valid insofar as it is able to account for differences in biological activity of a range of molecules.

## 4.4 Applications of Pharmacophore Modelling

Pharmacophore modelling is extensively applied for virtual screening, lead optimization, target identification, toxicity prediction and *de novo* lead design and has a huge application in fragment-based drug design and lead design targeting protein-protein interaction interfaces and target-based classification of chemical space. Pharmacophores are often combined with molecular docking simulations to improve virtual screening. By combining docking based virtual screening with pharmacophore-based virtual screening the database of ligands can be pre-filtered using a pharmacophore query, prior to evaluation using docking simulations.

The docking simulations can be post-filtered using a pharmacophore query to remove any compounds that fail to bind according to the pharmacophore query. The method can also discard compounds that would have scored well in a pure pharmacophore search, but that fail to bind according to some hypothesis taking more information into account, such as incompatibility of the overall ligand structure with the receptor site.

Pharmacophore modelling approaches are often used for ADME-Tox prediction. The pharmacophore models can be used to identify possible interactions of drugs with drug metabolizing enzymes by matching the equivalent chemical groups of test molecules to those of drug molecules with a well-known ADME-Tox profile.

# COMBINATORIAL CHEMISTRY

Chapter 12

## 1. INTRODUCTION

Combinatorial chemistry has its earliest origin in solid phase peptide in 1960 by Bruce Merrifield. In 1980's, researchers like H. Hario Grysen developed this technique further, creating libraries of different peptide on separate supports. From 1990 onwards, there was an upsurge in combinatorial synthesis and small molecules were also synthesized as multi component mixture. Since then combinatorial chemistry has expanded from peptide to organic, organometallic, inorganic and polymer chemistry. Drug discovery is a lengthy and expensive process, within which the synthesis of exploratory compounds has been the slowest step. But in combinatorial synthesis a large number of chemical compounds can be synthesized quickly.

Combinatorial chemistry can be viewed as a tool which allows large number of compounds to be synthesized simultaneously in a time taken to prepare only handful of compounds by traditional synthetic methods.

The number of compounds produced, far exceeds the number of chemical steps required to make them. A chosen set of building blocks are reacted together to make every available product and collection of these product is referred as "library" or an "array". This collection of compounds can be synthesized as a mixture or individuals using a variety of techniques.

Combinatorial synthesis is a simultaneous synthesis of a large number of possible compounds that could be formed from a number of building blocks. The product of such process is called "**Combinatorial Library**".

For example, in orthodox synthesis, compound A would react with compound B to give product AB, which would be isolated after working up and purification. In contrast to this approach, combinatorial chemistry offers the potential to make every combination of compound $A_1$ to $A_n$ with compound $B_1$ to Bn. (Fig. 12.1).

**Fig. 12.1 Traditional Synthesis Combinatorial Synthesis**

The compounds are present as a mixture and not as individual characterized structures. The structure of compound in a mixture is not known with certainty and the compounds are not separated or purified instead, each mixture is tested for biological activity as a whole. If there is no activity, then there is no need to study the mixture any more. If the activity is observed, then the active component in the mixture is identified and separated.

This process is:

a) Faster, more efficient, cheaper and give rise to million of compounds in the same time, as it takes to make one compound.

b) If we want to find a lead compound quickly and efficiently, combinatorial chemistry provides a mean for producing this quantity of compounds.

Combinational Chemistry can be applied to:

a) Solution phase synthesis

b) Solid phase synthesis.

In solution phase synthesis, the library members are typically synthesized as individual compounds, so called parallel synthesis. On solid support, the split and mix techniques as well as parallel synthesis can be applied.

## 2. SOLID PHASE SYNTHESIS

In this method, the reaction is carried out on a solid support such as resin beads. The bead is treated with different starting materials, which bound together. Then it is mixed with another reagent to get the product. Since the products are bound to solid support, excess reagent or by-product can be easily removed by washing with appropriate solvent. Large excess of reagent solvent can be used to drive the reaction sequence are bound to the bead and need not be purified Individual beads can be separated at the end of the experiment to get individual products. The polymeric support can be regenerated and reused if appropriate cleavage conduction and suitable anchor / linker groups are chosen.

Solid phase synthesis was pioneered by Merrifield for the synthesis of peptides. As a result most early work carried out on combinational synthesis was performed on peptides. But large amount of research has been carried out in solid phase synthetic method to synthesize small non-peptide molecules.

The essential requirement for solid phase synthesis is:

- a cross linked insoluble polymeric support which is inert to synthetic condition. eg. Resin.
- an anchor or linker co-valently linked to the resin.
- a bond linking the substrate to the linker, which will be stable to the reaction condition.
- chemical protecting groups for protecting the functional group not involved in the synthesis.

i) The Solid Support

The choice of solid support depends on the type of reaction. In addition, resin is the stable and commonly used solid support. Some examples are

- Polystyrene.

The polystyrene support is normally cross linked by the addition of 1% Divinyl benzene (DVB) to the polymerization mixture. This degree of cross linking offers the best compromise between mechanical stability and swelling performance. Highly cross linked polystyrene have a higher mechanical and thermal stability, but their swelling performance and loading capacity are clearly reduced.

- Tentagel is polystyrene-polyoxa ethylene graft co-polymer.
- Pepsin is a polyamide support especially developed for peptide synthesis.
- PEGA [Poly (acrylic amide-ethylene glycol) copolymers].

Due to its amphiphilic properties, these supports are mainly used for SPOS of polar compounds.

ii) Linkers

The linker is the molecule that sits between our compound and the solid support. The linkers move the point of substrate attachment away from the surface of the bead. This has the effect of reducing steric hindrance, thereby making the reaction easier and allows the final product to cleave off in high yield.

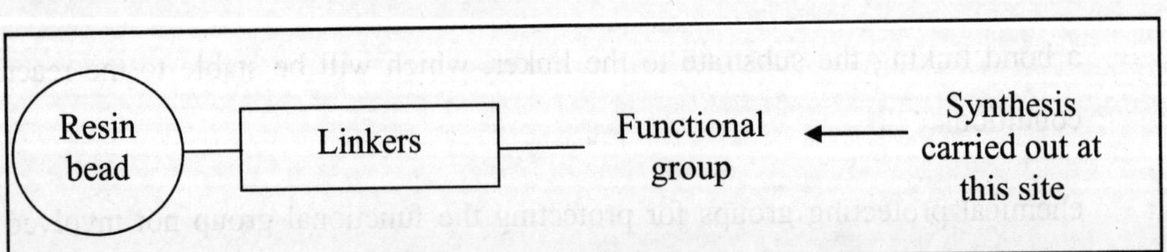


**Fig. 12.2 A Schematic Representation of the Resin Bead Used in Combinatorial Synthesis**

Different linkers are used depending on the functional group which will be present on the substrate and the functional group which is desired on the functional product once it is released. Resin having different linkers has different names.

For example

a) The Wang resin: It has linkers which is suitable for the attachment and release of carboxylic acids.

b) The Rink resin: Suitable for the attachment of carboxylic acid and the release of Carboxamide.

c) The Dihydropyran derivative resin: Suitable for the attachment of alcohol.

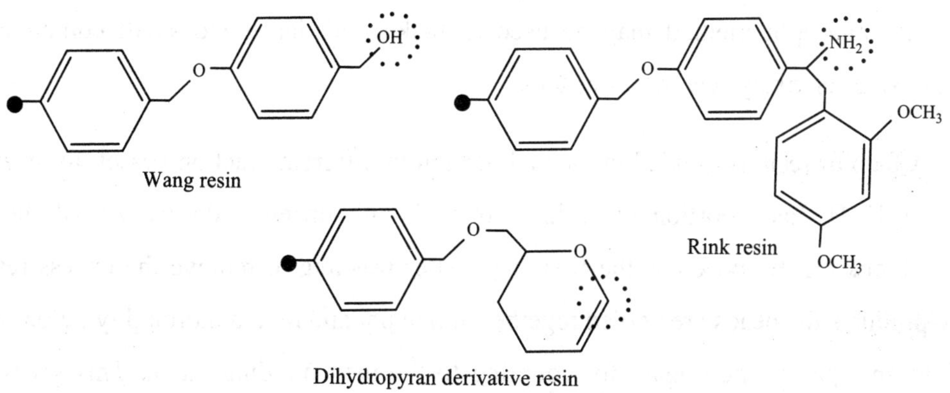


**Fig. 12.3 Various Types of Resins Circle Portion is Linkage Point**

iii) Protecting groups

Protecting groups are important for blocking and regenerating certain functional group in a reaction sequence. Some examples of protecting groups are FMOC (Fluoro methoxy carbonyl benzyl ester) and TBOC (Tertiary butyloxycarbonyl)

Combinational synthesis on solid support is usually carried out by using either parallel synthesis or Furka split and mix procedures.

## 2.1 Parallel Synthesis

In this method, the compounds are prepared in separate vessel but at the same time that is in parallel. The array of reaction vessel are taken either in a grid well in a plastic plate (if the synthesis in carried out in a bead) or pins (grid of plastic rods) called crowns. The building blocks are attached to these beads or crowns. The structure of product formed is usually identified by the grid code. Finally, the products are liberated from the resin by appropriate linked cleavage reaction and the product is isolated. The structure of these products are usually determined by following the history of the synthesis using the grid references of the wells and confirmed by instrumental methods.

## 2.2 Mix and Split Technique

Mix and split method may be used to make both large and small combinatorial libraries using relatively few reaction steps.

A bath of resin is divided into equal portion in different reaction vessel, for example three (Fig.12.4). Each portion of resin is treated with different derivatives of the first building block (A, B and C) as the first step. After washing to remove the excess reagent and by-products the beads are pooled together in one pot and mixed thoroughly before being split into an equal portion again for coupling to the next building block. This gives nine different compounds in statistically equal amount. Thus, the beads are split into portion, mixed together and re-split depending upon the number of different building blocks be used. This process is continued until the required library is synthesized.

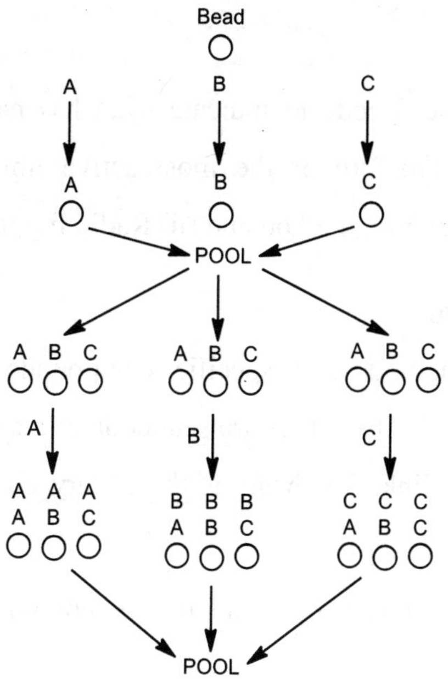

Fig. 12.4 Split and Mix Synthesis

If same building block is used at each step the maximum possible numbers of compounds that can be synthesized for the given number of different building blocks (b) are given by

$$\text{Number of compounds} = b^x..$$

Unlike in parallel synthesis, the history of the bead cannot be traced from the grid reference; it is traced by using suitable encoding method or deconvolution.

### 2.2.1 Deconvolution

Assuming that a compound mixture proves to be biologically active, the tricky job of identifying the active component now needs to be carried out. Isolation and identification of the most active compound in mixture is known as deconvoluting the mixture there are several methods of doing this. eg. Micromanipulation, Sequential release.

### 2.2.2 Encoding Methods

Encoding methods use a code to indicate what has happened at each step in the synthesis and identify the structure of the most active library member. Two popular techniques are (i) Chemical tagging method and (ii) Radio frequency tagging.

#### i) Chemical Tagging Method

Chemical tagging method uses specific compounds (tags) as a code for the individual step in the synthesis. These tags are sequentially attached in the form of polymer - like molecule to the same linker or bead as the library compound at each step in the synthesis.

At the end of the synthesis both the library compound and tag compound are liberated from the bead.

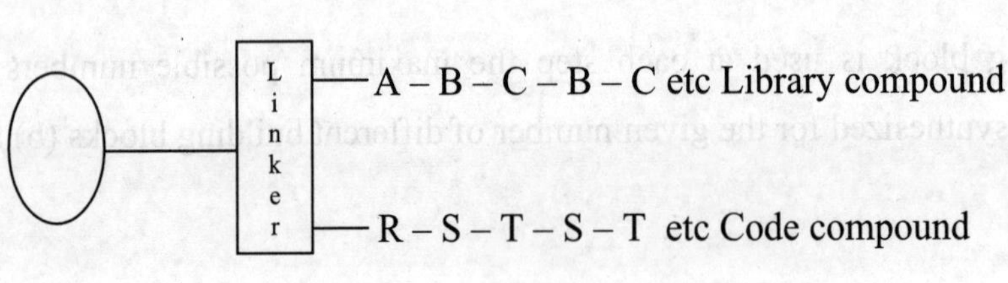


**Fig. 12.5 Chemical Encoding of Resin Bead**

Branched linkers, with one side for attaching the library compound and another for attaching the tag are often used for encoding.

#### ii) Radio Frequency (RF) Tagging

It employs a microchip tag like a bar code to label each library member. Tags are robust, encapsulated in glass casing, stable to chemical and synthetic conditions. Each individual tag code is associated with the identity of its library member - a set of building blocks used - in a data base computer and accompanied a particular portion of resin throughout its synthetic journey in a porous 'tea bag' vessel.

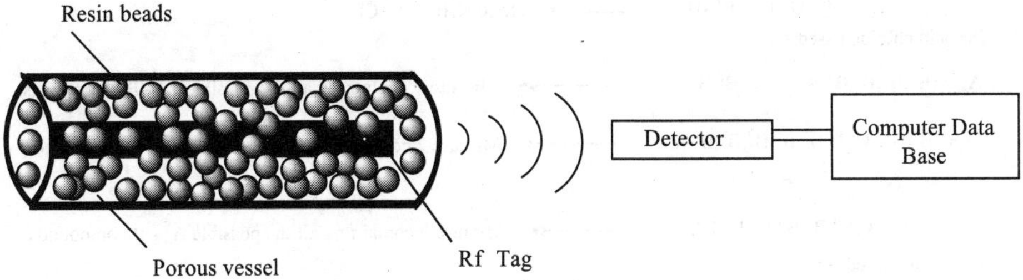


**Fig. 12.6 Schematic Representation of RF Tagging**

## 3. SOLUTION PHASE SYNTHESIS

The main problem with preparing libraries using solution chemistry is the difficulty of removing unwanted impurities at each step in the synthesis. Consequently, many of the strategies used for the preparation of libraries using solution chemistry are directed to the purification of the products of each steps of the synthesis. This and other practical problem has usually restricted the use of solution combinatorial chemistry to synthetic pathways consisting of two or three steps.

Combinatorial synthesis in solution can be used to produce libraries that consist of single compounds or mixtures using traditional organic chemistry. Single compound libraries are prepared using the parallel synthesis technique (Fig. 12.7). Libraries of mixtures are formed by separately reacting each of the members of a set of similar compounds with the same mixture of all the member of the second set of compounds. Consider, for example, a combinatorial library of amides formed by reacting a set of five acid chlorides ($A^1$ - $A^5$) with ten amines ($B^1$ - $B^{10}$). Each of the five acid chlorides is reacted separately with an equimolar mixture of all ten amine and each of the amine is reacted with an equimolar mixture of all the acid chlorides (Fig. 12.7). This produces a library consisting of a set of five mixtures based on individual acid halides and 10 mixtures based on individual amines. This means that each compound in the library is prepared twice, once from the acid chloride set and once from the amine set. Consequently, determining the most biologically active of the mixtures from the acid halide set will define the acyl part of the most active amide and similarly identifying the most biologically active of the amine-based set of mixtures will identify the amine residue of that amide. Libraries used in this manner are often referred as indexed libraries.

$RCOCl + R'NH_2 \longrightarrow RCONHR' + Cl$

The acid chloide based set

$A^1 + (B^1, B^2, B^3, B^4.B^5.B^6.B^7, B^8.B^9.N^{10} \longrightarrow$ Mixture 1 containing all the possible $A^1$ - B compounds

$A^2 + (B^1, B^2, B^3, B^4.B^5.B^6.B^7, B^8.B^9.N^{10} \longrightarrow$ Mixture 2 containing all the possible $A^2$ - B compounds

: Etc. · Etc.

$A^5 + (B^1, B^2, B^3, B^4.B^5.B^6.B^7, B^8.B^9.N^{10} \longrightarrow$ Mixture 5 containing all the possible $A^5$ - B compounds

The amine based set

$B^1 + (A^1, A^2, A^3, A^4.A^5.) \longrightarrow$ Mixture 6 containing all the possible $B^1$ - A compounds

· Etc. · Etc.

$B^{10} + (A^1, A^2, A^3, A^4.A^5.) \longrightarrow$ Mixture 15 containing all the possible $B^1$ - A compounds

**Fig. 12.7 A Schematic Representation of the Index Approach to Identifying Active Compounds in Libraries Formed in Solution**

## 4. SCREENING

The success of library depends not only on it containing the right compounds but also on the efficacy of screening procedure. Since combinatorial synthesis produces a large quantity of structure in a very short time period, biological testing should be carried out quickly and automatically. The technique used by this system is known as High throughout screening (HTS). Traditionally, compounds are automatically tested and analyzed on a plate containing 96 small wells with the capacity of 0.1 ml. But it HTS, 1536 well with capacity of 1-10 μl only used. Moreover, methods such as fluorescence and chemiluminescence's are being developed, which will allow the simultaneous identification of active compound.

## 5. APPLICATIONS

From the prospective of the pharmaceutical industry, the ultimate test for combinatorial chemistry is its application to the discovery of commercially successful drugs. The overall aim is to identify a chemical lead with *in vitro* activity in a particular screening assay that is amenable to further chemical and biological optimization.

The synthesis analogues of existing lead structure, elucidate the structure activity relationships and to improve biological activity *in vitro* (eg. affinity, efficacy, selectivity) and *in vivo* (eg. behavioral pharmacology, metabolism, kinetics).

In short, this technique is applied to both lead identification and lead optimization. The integration of these two has established combinatorial chemistry as a useful tool for drug discovery.

# Index


**A**

Acyclovir, 78,79,83,84,**130**,131,132
Albendazole, 167,168,170,**172**
Amantadine hydrochloride, 129,**134**
Amodiaquine, 91,92,95,**97**
Amoxicillin, 16,19,**24**
Amphotericin-B, 148,**149**
Ampicillin, 12,16,19,**23,**24,29,41,42,68,70,78
Arsphenamine, 64
Artemether, 92,**103**,104
Artesunate, 92,103,**104**
Aspirin, 75
Atovaquone, 101,102,**105**,161,**165**
Azithromycin, 30,57,58,**60**
Aztreonam, **42**,43

**B**

Bacampicillin**,** 12,68,78
Benzathine penicillin, **25**
Benzocaine, 80
Benzyl penicillin, 9,15,16,18,**21**,26
Butoconazole, 155,**156**

**C**

Capreomycin sulphate, 107,**111**
Carbapenam, 5
Carbenicillin, 1,12,19,**24**
Carumonam, 42,**44**
Cefaclor, 32
Cefadroxil, 30,31,**36**
Cefalexin, 30,**36**
Cefalotin, 32,**36**
Cefamandole, 32
Cefazolin, 32,**37**
Cefepime, **39**
Cefixime, 33,**38**
Cefoperazone, 34
Cefotaxime, 33,**37**
Cefotetan, 33
Cefoxitin, 33
Cefpirome, **38**
Cefpodoxime, 33,**38**
Cefprozil, 32
Cefradine, 32,
Ceftaroline, **39**
Ceftazidime, 34
Ceftizoxime, 33
Ceftobiprole, **39**
Ceftriaxone, 34
Cefuroxime, 32,**37**
Cephalothin, 2,26,29,32,**36**
Cephem, 5
Chloramphenicol, **62**,69
Chloroquine, 91,92,**95**,194
Chlorpropamide, 88
Chlortetracycline, 49,52,**54**
Ciprofloxacin, 115,116,117,**119**
Clarithromycin, 57,**59**
Clavulanic acid, 30,**40**
Clindamycin, **61,**75,76
Clotrimazole, 154,**155**
Cloxacillin, 16,19,**22**
Cotrimoxazole, **192**
Cycloguanil pamoate, 86,92,**101**
Cycloserine, 107,**113**

**D**

Dapsone, 185,**191**
Delavirdine, 129,136,**141**
Demeclocycline, **52**
Diazepam, 87
Dicloxacillin, **19**
Didanosine, 129,**138**
Diethylcarbamazine citrate, 167,**168**
Diloxanide, 161,**164**
Dopamine, 87
Doxycycline, 52,**55**

**E**

Econazole, 155,**156**
Eflornithine, 161,**166**

Enalapril, 79
Enoxacin, 115,**119**
Erythromycin, 57,75,**58**
Ethambutol, 107,**109**
Ethionamide, 107,**110**
Etoposide, 79

**F**

Fluconazole, 155,**158**
Fluocinolone, 80
Fluphenazine, 85
Furazolidone, 115,**124**

**G**

Ganciclovir, 129,**132**
Gatifloxacin, 115,**122**
Griseofulvin, 148,**152**

**I**

Idoxuridine, 129,**132**
Indinavir, 129,136,**143**
Iodoquinol, 161,**164**
Isoniazid, **107**
Itraconazole, 155,**159**
Ivermectin, 167,168,**174**

**K**

Kanamycin, 45,**48**
Ketoconazole, 155,**158**

**L**

Lamivudine, 129,136,**140**
Lincomycins, 61
Lomefloxacin, 115,**121**
Loviride, 129, 136,**142**

**M**

Mafenide acetate, 184,185,**190**
Mebendazole, 167,168,**170**
Meclocycline, 52
Mefloquine, 92,**105**
Mepacrine hydrochloride, **100**
Methacycline, 52
Methenamine, 115,**125**
Methicillin, 16,**22**
Metronidazole, 75,**161**
Mezlocillin, 7
Miconazole, 155,**157**
Minocycline, 52,**56**
Monobactams, 42
Moxifloxacin, 115,**123**

**N**

Naftifine hydrochloride, 148,**153**
Nalidixic acid, 115,**118**
Natamycin, 148,**151**
Neomycin, **47**
n-Heptyl penicillin, 18
Niclosamide, 167, 168,**174**
Nicotinic acid, 75
Nitrofurantoin, 115,**124**
Nocardicin A, 42,**43**
Nordazepam, 87
Norfloxacin, 115,**118**
Nystatin, 148,**150**

**O**

Ofloxacin, 115,**120**
Ornidazole, 161,**163**
Oxacillin, 18
Oxamniquine, 167,**173**
Oxiconazole, 155,**156**
Oxophenazine, 64
Oxytetracycline, 52,**55**

**P**

Pamaquine, 92,**98**
Para amino salicylic acid, 107,**109**
Paracetamol, 65
Penam, 5,8
Penicillanic acid, 8
Penicillin - F, 18
Penicillin - G, 18
Penicillin – K, 18
Penicillin- X, 18
Penicillin-V, 18
Pentamidine isethionate, 161,**165**

Phenacetin, 65
Phenoxymethylpenicillin, 15,**21**
p-Hydroxy benzyl penicillin, 15
Piperacillin, 7,13,19,**25**,41
Pivampicillin, 12,68,78
Praziquantel, 167,168,**173**
Prednisolone, 78
Primaquine phosphate, 92,**100**
Procaine penicillin, **26**
Proguanil, 92,**101**
Prontosil, 65
Pyrazinamide, 107,**108**
Pyrimethamine, 92,**102**

**Q**

Quinacrine hydrochloride, 92,**100**
Quinine sulphate, 92,**93**,

**R**

Ribavirin, 129,**135**
Rifabutin, 107,**113**
Rifampicin, 107,**112**
Rimantadine hydrochloride, 129,**134**
Ritonavir, 129,136,**143**

**S**

Salicylic acid, 75
Saquinavir, 129,136,**142**
Sparfloxacin, 115,**122**
Streptomycin, 45,**46**
Succinyl sulfathiazole, 86
Sulbactam, **41**
Sulfacetamide, 182,**189**
Sulfadiazine, **183,186**
Sulfadimidine, **187**
Sulfafurazole, **188**
Sulfamethazine, 183,**187**
Sulfamethizole, 183,**188**
Sulfamethoxazole, 183,**187**
Sulfapyridine, 70,182,**186**
Sulfasalazine, 70,**189**
Sulfathiazole, **183**
Sulfisoxazole, 75,183,**188**

**T**

Tabtoxin, 42,**44**
Tazobactam, 30,40,**41**
Terconazole, 154,155,**159**
Tetracycline, 49,52,**54**
Thiabendazole, 167,170,**172**
Ticarcillin, 11,**19**
Tigemonam, 42,**43**
Tinidazole, 161,**163**
Tioconazole, 155,**157**
Tolbutamide, 88
Tolmetin sodium, 86
Tolnaftate, 148,**153**
Trifluridine, 129,**133**
Trimethoprim, 165,176,179, 181,191,**192**

**V**

Valacyclovir, 79

**Z**

Zalcitabine, 129,**139**
Zidovudine, 129,136,**139**

Phenacetin, 65
Phenoxymethylpenicillin, 15,**21**
p-Hydroxybenzyl penicillin, 15
Piperacillin, 7,13,19,25,**41**
Pivampicillin, 12,68,73
Praziquantel, 167,168,**173**
Prednisolone, 78
Primaquine phosphate, 92,**100**
Procaine penicillin, **26**
Proguanil, 92,**101**
Prontosil, 65
Pyrazinamide, 107,**108**
Pyrimethamine, 92,**102**

**Q**

Quinacrine hydrochloride, 92,**100**
Quinine sulphate, 92,93

**R**

Ribavirin, 129,**135**
Rifabutin, 107,**112**
Rifampicin, 107,**112**
Rimantadine hydrochloride, 129,**134**
Ritonavir, 129,136,**143**

**S**

Salicylic acid, 75
Saquinavir, 129,136,**142**
Sparfloxacin, 115,**122**
Streptomycin, 45,46
Succinyl sulfathiazole, 86
Sulbactam, **41**
Sulfacetamide, 182,**185**
Sulfadiazine, 183,**186**
Sulfadimidine, **187**
Sulfafurazole, **188**
Sulfamethazine, 183,**187**
Sulfamethizole, 183,**188**
Sulfamethoxazole, 183,**187**
Sulfapyridine, 70,182,**186**
Sulfasalazine, 70,**189**
Sulfathiazole, **183**
Sulfisoxazole, 75,183,**188**

**T**

Tabtoxin, 42,**44**
Tazobactam, 30,40,**41**
Terconazole, 154,155,**159**
Tetracycline, 49,52,**54**
Thiabendazole, 167,170,**172**
Ticarcillin, 11,**19**
Tigemonam, 42,**43**
Tinidazole, 161,**163**
Tioconazole, 155,**157**
Tolbutamide, 88
Tolmetin sodium, 86
Tolnaftate, 148,**153**
Trifluridine, 129,**133**
Trimethoprim, 165,176,179, 181,191,**192**

**V**

Valacyclovir, 79

**Z**

Zalcitabine, 129,**139**
Zidovudine, 129,136,**139**